HEALTHWATCH
Personal Medical Record & Disease Prevention Guide

KIM HENDRICKSON LEFFLER

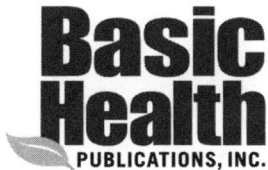

The information contained in this book is based upon the research and personal and professional experiences of the author. It is not intended as a substitute for consulting with your physician or other healthcare provider. Any attempt to diagnose and treat an illness should be done under the direction of a healthcare professional.

The publisher does not advocate the use of any particular healthcare protocol but believes the information in this book should be available to the public. The publisher and author are not responsible for any adverse effects or consequences resulting from the use of the suggestions, preparations, or procedures discussed in this book. Should the reader have any questions concerning the appropriateness of any procedures or preparation mentioned, the author and the publisher strongly suggest consulting a professional healthcare advisor.

Basic Health Publications, Inc.
8200 Boulevard East
North Bergen, NJ 07047
1-201-868-8336

Library of Congress Cataloging-in-Publication Data

Leffler, Kim Hendrickson.
　　HealthWatch : personal medical record and disease prevention guide / Kim Hendrickson Leffler.
　　　　p. cm.
　　Includes bibliographical references and index.
　　ISBN 1-59120-123-3
　1. Medical records. 2. Medicine, Preventive. I. Title.
　　R864.L446　　2004
　　613—dc22

2004007262

Copyright © 2004 by Kim Hendrickson Leffler

All rights reserved. No part of this publication may be reproduced, stored in a retrieval system, or transmitted, in any form or by any means, electronic, mechanical, photocopying, recording, or otherwise, without the prior written consent of the copyright owner.

Editors: Carol Rosenberg and Karen Anspach
Typesetting/Book design: Gary A. Rosenberg
Cover design: Mike Stromberg

Printed in the United States of America

10　9　8　7　6　5　4　3　2　1

This Personal Medical Record Belongs to

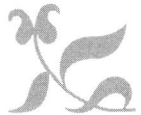 

_____

My Health History at a Glance
(Chronic or Serious Medical Conditions—Diagnosed and/or Treated)

_____
_____
_____
_____
_____
_____
_____
_____
_____
_____
_____
_____
_____
_____
_____
_____
_____
_____
_____
_____
_____
_____

For Ray, Andrew, and Christina,
Always

Contents

Acknowledgments, vii

Introduction, 1

How to Use This Book, 2

Risk Factors, 3

General Guidelines for a Healthy Lifestyle, 5

PART ONE • MEDICAL HISTORY

Personal Medical History, 12

Infections and/or Illnesses Requiring Medical Treatment, 14

Prescription Record, 15

Over-the-Counter Medications, Herbs, and Other Products, 19

Allergies, 20

Pregnancy and Childbirth History, 21

Contraceptive History, 23

Hereditary Conditions, 25

Medical Conditions That Tend to Run in Families, 29

Family Medical History, 34

PART TWO • WHAT TO DO AND WHEN TO DO IT

Recommended Tests for Children and Adults, 41

Immunizations, 62

Bone Density Screenings, 77

Cholesterol Screenings, 79

Colon Cancer Screenings, 83

Dental Records and Checkups, 87

Diabetes Screenings, 96

Eye Medical Records, 98

Tests for Men, 100

Tests for Women, 103

Menstrual Record, 109

PART THREE • HEALTHCARE PROVIDERS

Physicians, 125

Dentists, 129

Eye-Care Specialists, 132

Other Practitioners, 135

Insurance Companies, 138

Medicare/Medicaid Information, 140

Definitions of Medical Practices and Practitioners, 141

PART FOUR • THE IMPORTANCE OF NUTRIENTS

Vitamins, Minerals, and Trace Elements, 143

Vitamin and Mineral Intake, 144

Vitamins

Vitamin A, 146

Vitamin B_1 (Thiamine), 149

Vitamin B_2 (Riboflavin), 150

Vitamin B_3 (Niacin), 151

Vitamin B_6 (Pyridoxine), 152

Vitamin B_{12} (Cobalamin), 153

Vitamin C (Ascorbic Acid), 155

Vitamin D (Calciferol), 156

Vitamin E (Tocopherol), 158

Vitamin K, 160

Biotin, 161

Choline, 162

Folic Acid (Folate), 163

Pantothenic Acid, 165

Minerals

Calcium, 166

Magnesium, 167

Phosphorus, 169

Potassium, 170

Sodium, 171

Trace Elements

Chromium, 173

Copper, 174

Fluoride, 175

Iodine, 176

Iron, 177

Manganese, 180

Molybdenum, 181

Selenium, 182

Zinc, 183

PART FIVE • DISEASE PREVENTION GUIDE

The Bladder, 187

The Blood Supply, 190

The Bones, 197

The Brain, 202

The Breasts, 207

The Cervix, 210

The Circulatory System, 212

The Ears, 217

The Esophagus, 220

The Eyes, 222

The Gallbladder, 228

The Hands, 229

The Heart, 231

The Hormones, 235

The Immune System, 238

The Intestines, 243

The Joints, 248

The Kidneys, 251

The Liver, 254

The Lungs, 259

The Lymphatic System, 263

The Mouth, 265

The Muscles, 267

The Nervous System, 269

The Nose, 272

The Ovaries, 274

The Pancreas, 277

The Penis, 280

The Prostate, 282

The Rectum, 284

The Skin, 287

The Spine, 290

The Stomach, 293

The Teeth, 296

The Testicles, 299

The Throat, 301

The Thyroid, 303

The Urinary Tract, 305

The Uterus, 308

The Vagina, 310

References, 313

Index, 315

About the Author, 327

Acknowledgments

This book would not have been possible without the help of several important and invaluable individuals who generously reviewed the manuscript. Any errors are mine.

    Thomas Hubbard, M.D., Family Practitioner

    James Ratliff, M.D., Urology

    Louise Korpics, D.D.S., Dentistry

    Peter Goldmann, M.D., Ophthalmology

    Todd Billett, M.D., Obstetrics-Gynecology

    Peter D'Adamo, N.D., Naturopath

    Joseph Longacher, M.D., Gastroenterology

    Katherine Harris, Dental Hygienist

I also am eternally grateful to my parents, Jack and Audra Hendrickson, my brothers and sisters-in-law Reyn and Vivianne Hendrickson, Peter and Doreen Hendrickson, Rob and Rhonda Hendrickson, and my stepdaughters and stepsons-in-law Katie and Scott Edwards, and Cheryl and Michael Wyer, who proofed, advised, and supported me through the entire process, my children, Andrew and Christina, whose births stimulated an engrossing interest in health maintenance, and especially my husband, Ray, who worked with me all the way in composing and formatting the book.

Introduction

When you buy an automobile, you get an owner's manual with instructions on maintenance and recommended service intervals, tire pressure, and fluids. Everything you need to know to keep your car or truck in top running condition is found within that manual. Even vacuum cleaners and food processors come with instructions.

But humans don't come with owner's manuals. The most complicated, ingenious mechanical system in the world doesn't come with instructions! The human body has more than 200 bones, 800 muscles, yards of intestines, thousands of miles of veins and arteries, a brain more powerful than the most advanced computer, an immune system capable of defeating millions of enemy invaders, a sophisticated breathing apparatus that functions automatically, a circulatory system that efficiently delivers oxygen, transports wastes, and removes carbon dioxide—thousands of moving parts that work together, twenty-four hours a day, seven days a week.

Theoretically, we don't need an owner's manual. Theoretically, the human system can function quite well without much help from us.

In reality, however, things can and do go wrong. Although it may be no fault of our own, we are exposed to hazards, such as infectious diseases, environmental pollutants, and foodborne contaminants. We may even be born with genetic characteristics that put us at risk for certain illnesses.

For thousands of years people have been searching for ways to identify health risks and prevent or minimize them. Significant progress has been made, especially in the last hundred years: vaccines have been developed to protect against infectious diseases that once killed or crippled millions; diagnostic equipment and techniques have been designed to screen for early signs of cancer and heart disease; statistics have been accumulated to help identify both risk factors and the populations most at risk. All of this research and development is ultimately good, but the negative result is an almost overwhelming amount of information.

The average bewildered man or woman is left wondering, "What immunizations am I supposed to have, and when should I get them?" "How many annual checkups and screenings should I get, and for what?" "What kind of vitamins do I need?" "How do I know if I am at risk for a certain type of cancer?"

There are hundreds of medical books and other resources that help identify symptoms and treatments for every medical condition under the sun. This is not one of those books. This book *can* act as an instruction manual for your body, taking into account your personal risk factors.

How to Use This Book

The *HealthWatch Personal Medical Record and Disease Prevention Guide* is designed to help you stay healthy from the moment of your birth. Use Part One, Medical History, to store your personal medical record and to keep track of your personal and family medical histories. Part Two provides a list of recommended schedules for health screening tests, immunizations, and checkups, with descriptions of these tests. Here you can record the results of mammograms, prostate exams, colonoscopies, cholesterol screenings, bone density exams, blood glucose tests, eye exams, and dental checkups.

Use Part Three to keep track of your doctors, dentists, ophthalmologists, and other healthcare providers and insurance companies, including dates of service. It contains a glossary of definitions of medical practices and practitioners. Part Four explains the importance of nutrients and provides comprehensive information about vitamins and minerals so you can determine the supplements you need.

Part Five, the Disease Prevention Guide, is devoted to the various organs and other body parts. Each section includes an illustration of the specific part, its key components, its location in the body, and the following sections, where applicable:

Function

Keeping [the body part] Healthy

Beneficial Foods and Nutrients

Other Tips

What Can Go Wrong

Medical Conditions That Can Affect [the body part]

Risky Behavior and Possible Consequences

It is important to note that the Disease Prevention Guide is not meant to be a diagnostic tool. You will not find descriptions of symptoms or suggested treatments for specific conditions. Instead, the focus is on learning what the average person needs to do to keep that part of the body healthy. When specific diseases or conditions are mentioned, it is for the purpose of identifying factors that may put you at risk of developing that disease. Some of the factors are immutable—in other words, unchangeable—because you were born with certain characteristics. Some factors are lifestyle choices and *can* be changed to minimize the risk. It is up to you.

The *HealthWatch Personal Medical Record and Disease Prevention Guide* was written in the belief that the more people know about their own health, their personal history, their family history, and their risk factors for certain diseases, the more control they can take over their lives, lifestyle, and well-being.

Ongoing Online Support

Medical news is made daily, as researchers discover more about causes and cures for various health conditions. Sometimes this information makes the headlines, but more often than not it is buried amid the clutter of other news topics. Your life is busy enough without having to be a medical detective as well, so *HealthWatch* makes the job easier by providing an online resource for owners of this book. Everything that you need to stay informed about new immunizations, health tips, and risk factors is available—at no charge—at www.healthwatchguide.com. Visit the site at your convenience for updates. At the end of each calendar year, the updates will be assembled into a printed supplement, which will be available for purchase. Health care is a lifelong concern, and *HealthWatch* is committed to providing a comprehensive, trustworthy lifelong resource for you and your family and friends.

Risk Factors

Risk factors are characteristics that can increase our vulnerability to certain medical conditions. These characteristics have been shown to be common and consistent and are used as guideposts to help individuals and their doctors take a proactive position on health care.

Sometimes the risk factors can be linked directly to the condition; for instance, menopause signals a drastic decline in the production of estrogen, a female hormone vital to bone health. Thus, menopause is a risk factor for osteoporosis. Other risk factors are not as clear-cut. In many cases doctors don't know why some people become ill and others do not. Why does testicular cancer strike men between the ages of fifteen and forty? Why do whites have a greater risk for this disease than Hispanics, Asians, Native Americans, and blacks? Currently no one knows. Medical knowledge is advancing rapidly, though, and perhaps someday we will learn the answers. Meanwhile, physicians have learned that, almost without exception, testicular cancer occurs within this twenty-five-year window. Knowing this, men can be particularly vigilant about checking themselves for lumps during these years and, if necessary, promptly seeking medical help.

It is important to remember that the presence of risk factors does not guarantee that you will develop a particular condition. Instead, risk factors are valuable tools that you can use to stay healthy for life.

There are two types of risk factors, those over which we have no control and those we choose to accept or reject.

Uncontrollable Risk Factors

Each of us has certain characteristics over which we have no control. These include:

- Age (obviously this changes the longer you live, but you can't stop getting older)
- Gender
- Ethnicity/ancestry
- Blood type
- Family history
- Personal history

Sometimes these characteristics increase our risk for various diseases. For instance, fair-skinned people are at greater risk for skin cancer than those who have darker complexions. Does this mean that fair-skinned people are doomed to develop melanomas? Not at all. It just means that they need to learn about the *risk factors over which they have control.* If you know that exposure to ultraviolet radiation increases your chances of developing skin cancer, then you can take steps to minimize the risk, such as wearing sunblock and/or avoiding the sun between 10:00 A.M. and 3:00 P.M.

Controllable Risk Factors

Most controllable risk factors are lifestyle choices. If you make certain choices, you take certain chances. Going boating without wearing a life jacket is your choice, but you increase your chances of drowning if the boat sinks. From a health standpoint, there are many controllable risk factors, but the big five are:

- Obesity
- Smoking
- Poor nutrition
- Lack of physical exercise
- Unprotected sexual intercourse

Most of the diseases that plague humans, especially Americans in the twenty-first century, can be traced, in part, to one or more of these top-five risky behaviors. The Disease Prevention Guide lists hundreds of risky behaviors and their possible consequences. Making lifestyle choices that minimize your controllable risks is one of the most important steps you can take toward a more healthful life.

Regular Screenings to Counter Risks

Although you cannot eliminate your uncontrollable risk factors, you can help to offset them by tracking your personal health to find out about problems at an early stage. Simple tests can detect early forms of cancer, including breast, cervix, colon, prostate, and rectum cancers, and can also identify high blood pressure, elevated cholesterol levels, and dangerous diabetic precursors. Use of these tests can save millions of lives. This book identifies the tests recommended for everyone, plus those specifically for men and women, and includes charts where you can keep track of test results.

General Guidelines for a Healthy Lifestyle

Each of us is a unique individual with our own genetic makeup and heritage—no one else is *exactly* like you. However, as human beings we share some universal traits with regard to health maintenance. Wisdom accumulated over thousands of years has identified several elements essential to the good health of almost everyone on the planet. Much of this wisdom is based on the time-tested truth of the axiom "moderation in all things." For instance, we all need daily exposure to the sun, but *too much* sunlight is harmful. We all need to eat, but *too much* food, or *too much* of the *wrong foods,* can be dangerous to your health. Other health advice is based on scientific evidence. For instance, good hygiene is essential to reduce the spread of germs. Most of the universal health guidelines are simple and obvious, but adhering to them can help you to stay healthy.

1. Get fifteen to twenty minutes of sunlight per day without sunblock. This amount of sunshine is necessary to produce vitamin D for strong bones and melatonin for healthful sleep cycles.

2. Guard against skin cancer. Use sunblock and wear a hat the rest of the time you are outdoors.

3. Don't smoke. Almost every form of cancer and heart disease, and many other serious health issues, are related to smoking. Risks include bladder cancer, leukemia, stroke, transient ischemic attacks, cervical cancer, atherosclerosis, high blood pressure, ear infections (from secondhand smoke), GERD, esophageal cancer, Dupuytren's contracture (affects the hands), heart disease, weakened immune system, colon polyps, liver cancer, bronchial cancer, lung cancer, chronic bronchitis, emphysema, sudden infant death syndrome (SIDS), cancers of the lip, tongue, gums, cheeks, and salivary glands, cancers of the nose and sinuses, type II diabetes, pancreatic cancer, stomach cancer, ulcers, cancer of the larynx, low-birth-weight babies, early menopause, and asthma in children exposed to secondhand smoke.

4. Exercise daily. At the very least, walk a mile a day. This way you'll get exercise and exposure to sunlight (if you walk during daytime hours).

5. Eat dark green and/or deep orange/red fruits and vegetables. These fruits and vegetables contain the most vitamins and beta-carotene.

6. Wash your hands often and thoroughly. Lather up and count to twenty while washing. This is the best way to avoid catching and spreading germs. Minimize your use of antibiotic cleansers.

7. Know your blood type. There is a significant connection between blood type and the digestive and immune systems. Dr. Karl Landsteiner first identified the four blood types, A, B, AB, and O, in 1900. Since then, thousands of studies have documented the association between blood type and disease. Research in this field is still fairly new, but enough evidence has accumulated to show that one's blood type, in conjunction with other factors, may contribute to a greater risk of developing specific diseases. For instance, blood type A has the highest levels of clotting factors, leading to a greater risk of heart disease and stroke (cerebral thrombosis). In other diseases, blood type is important because of the immune system's response to foods and microbes containing antigens that resemble "foreign" blood types.

8. Know your family history. Being aware of inherited health risks gives you a definite advantage in protecting yourself.

9. Maintain a healthful weight. Your body uses the food you eat as fuel, just as your car burns gasoline. Like any good machine, your body works best with the right amount and kind of fuel. Your body can't function efficiently if you don't eat enough food and are underweight. In order to survive, the body may have to shut down some of its systems. For instance, girls and women who are severely underweight will stop menstruating. An underweight body will begin to consume its own muscle tissue.

Being overweight is equally unhealthful. For one thing, every extra pound you carry stresses the heart. For another, estrogen is stored in fat cells, putting overweight women at an increased risk of breast and uterine cancer. Obesity is a growing problem in the United States. The following list highlights some of the hazards of obesity in children and adults.

- Obesity contributes to insulin resistance, which leads to a risk of diabetes.
- Obesity is a risk factor for hypothyroidism, which is caused by an underactive thyroid.
- Obesity suppresses the production of growth hormone, a particular concern for obese children.
- Obesity restricts the production of androgen, one of the male hormones.
- Obesity contributes to the overproduction of cortisol, a stress hormone.
- Obesity in young girls contributes to early puberty, which increases their lifetime production of estrogen and thereby increases their risk of breast and uterine cancer.
- Obesity increases the risk of developing most cancers.

> Children's stomachs are about the size of their closed fist—not very big. So they don't need to eat very much in order to feel full. If they are hungry between meals, offer fruit and vegetables as snacks instead of crackers, chips, and cookies.

10. Practice safe sex. This is incredibly important! Sexually transmitted diseases (STDs) are rampant, and can also be spread through the shared use of infected needles, or even from mother to baby through the placenta. If you have a baby while you are infected with herpes, HIV, syphilis, gonorrhea, or chlamydia, your baby has an enormous risk of being born blind, or with brain damage or any of a number of other irreversible conditions.

The safest sex is no sex. Abstinence until you are ready to commit your life to someone else is by far the best way to avoid STDs. But if you aren't willing to abstain, then protect yourself. Remember that your partner may have been infected by someone else and may have a disease with minimal symptoms.

Before you have sex with anyone, educate yourself concerning the signs of these diseases. Learn to recognize genital warts, colors and odors of various discharges, and other symptoms. Ask your prospective sexual partner about his or her sexual history. And think about it—if you don't feel that you know this person well enough to ask such personal questions, do you really know them well enough to have intercourse?

Remember, some STDs can *never* be cured. You certainly don't want to spend the rest of your life treating herpes or worrying about your risk of cancer because you slept with the wrong person. Be careful not to spread infection yourself—don't have sex if you are suffering a herpes outbreak or a urinary tract infection. Remember that oral contraceptives do not protect you from STDs. Only barrier products like condoms can do that, and even they are not 100 percent effective.

If you are homosexual, be aware that anal intercourse is an extremely high-risk activity that contributes to anal cancer, bladder infections, and parasitic infections, in addition to STDs.

If you *do* become infected with an STD, be prepared to give your physician the names of anyone you may have infected, so that they can be contacted for treatment.

Calculating Your Body Mass Index (BMI)

Are you at a healthful weight? One way to find out is by calculating your body mass index (BMI), which is a measurement of the ratio between your height and weight. Multiply your weight in pounds by 705. Divide the answer by your height in inches. Divide that answer by your height in inches (again). The final answer is your BMI.

For example, if you weigh 140 pounds, and are 5'5" tall, you would multiply 140 by 705. The answer is 98,700. Divide 98,700 by 65 (your height in inches). The answer is 1,518. Now divide that (again) by 65. The answer is 23, your body mass index. A healthful range is between 19 and 25; a range between 25 and 30 indicates overweight, and over 30 is considered obese.

General Guidelines for a Healthy Lifestyle

11. Get regular checkups. It only makes sense that something caught early is easier to correct. Americans have gotten in the habit of waiting until we are unwell before we go to the doctor. We need to change this approach and perform regular maintenance on ourselves instead, just as we do on our cars. One easy way to remember to do this is by giving yourself a birthday present—have all your necessary screenings done in the month of your birth. Get an annual physical, visit the dentist for a six-month checkup, see the eye doctor, go to the chiropractor, have a colonoscopy. If you are a woman, have a mammogram, see your ob/gyn (obstetrician/gynecologist), and get a Pap smear. Men should have a prostate exam and get a PSA reading. Obviously, everyone's screening requirements will be different depending on health conditions and age, but setting aside one time of the year to do it all helps ensure that these important screenings aren't overlooked.

12. Get the necessary immunizations and vaccinations. No one need face illness and possible death from communicable diseases like measles, mumps, rubella, polio, diphtheria, influenza, tetanus, and whooping cough.

If you plan to become pregnant, be sure to get the vaccination against rubella (German measles). Contracting this disease while pregnant increases the risk that your baby will be born with birth defects, mental retardation, or may be stillborn.

Guidelines for Managing Your Health

It would be really nice to think that your family doctor regarded you as his or her only or, at least, most important patient. That when you called, he or she would know you, your family history, personal history, prescription records, and drug allergies without having to look up this information. Better yet, your doctor would make a house call if you were really sick. Maybe doctors were like this once upon a time, but not now, and maybe never again. The sad reality is that you are in charge of your own health, and perhaps that of your young children. The good news is that this is something you can manage.

When You Go to the Doctor, Dentist, or Ophthalmologist

1. Write down any symptoms that you have been experiencing.
2. Write down any questions you have about your illness, injury, or general condition.

A Special Note for Parents of Infants and Toddlers

Please remember that everything in which you walk comes into the house on your shoes or boots. This could include fertilizer, pesticides, animal droppings, chemicals from the workplace, oil from the driveway, and so on. Your small children who are crawling or putting things in their mouths will wind up ingesting these substances, and even tiny amounts can make them very sick. The odds are you would not even know what they encountered, which would make it hard to treat them properly. Get in the habit of changing into inside shoes when you come indoors. Leave the (potentially) contaminated footwear outside.

---

3. *Take this book with you*. It will have your medical history stored in it.
4. Ask the doctor or nurse to tell you your temperature, pulse, and blood pressure readings.

If the Doctor Prescribes Medications

1. Ask for the name of the drug, and why it is being prescribed. Ask for the spelling and write it down.
2. If you are taking the medication to correct a condition, such as high cholesterol, find out what your numbers are now, and what you are shooting for. Keep track of the numbers for your own information.
3. Ask if the doctor is prescribing the generic version of the medication. If not, why not?
4. Get precise instructions—how many days should the drug be taken, how many times a day, and in what quantity? If the instructions say you are to take the drug three times a day, does that mean during waking hours or over a twenty-four-hour period?
5. Tell the doctor what other medicines you are taking, including vitamins, herbs, and over-the-counter products, such as cough medicine or sleeping tablets, and particularly about any antacids containing aluminum.
6. Make sure your doctor is aware of all your medical conditions, especially those being treated by another physician or specialist.

7. Ask if you should avoid taking alcohol while on the medication, and remember that many common over-the-counter cough and cold remedies have alcohol in their formulation.
8. Ask if the doctor will need to take periodic blood tests while you take the medication.
9. Ask if the medication has any side effects.
10. Ask what you should do in case of an allergic reaction to the medication. Should you keep antihistamines on hand, just in case?
11. Ask if you should avoid certain foods or beverages while taking the medication.
12. Ask how many refills you will need. Will you need authorization for refills?
13. Ask if the doctor will need to re-examine you periodically before refills are authorized.
14. Ask how to store the medication. Some require refrigeration.
15. Ask if your ethnicity affects the drug's potency.
16. Ask if your age or weight affects the amount of medication you will be taking.
17. Ask if you can or should take pain medication while on prescription antibiotics if, for instance, you are running a fever.

When You Go to the Pharmacy

1. Confirm that the prescription label has the right drug name on it.
2. Ask the pharmacist to tell you what medication they have provided to you.
3. If the prescription is a refill, make sure the pills, capsules, or tablets look familiar.
4. Ask if you should take the medication with food or on an empty stomach. If on an empty stomach, how long before or after eating?

Lastly, remember to follow the prescription procedures to the letter and take all of the medicine unless your doctor specifically says it is all right to stop—for example, stopping a pain medication after pain subsides. It is especially important to take the full prescription of medicines such as antibiotics. People who feel better after a couple of days and stop taking the antibiotic often suffer a serious relapse. This is because the antibiotic first killed off the majority of the weaker germs, but the survivors soon regroup and multiply, and now form the stronger, antibiotic-resistant majority. The doctor then needs to prescribe stronger antibiotics to combat them; meanwhile, the patient has been infecting other people with the stronger germs, so they become really sick as soon as they are infected.

Also, remember that antibiotics are effective against *bacteria*, not viruses. Your doctor won't prescribe antibiotics if you are suffering from a viral infection, like a cold or the flu.

Life is full of health risks, beginning with the moment of conception when your genetic code is established. Some risks are inherited; others are encountered during the course of your daily activities. Many risks simply cannot be avoided, but every one can be mitigated. *Knowing your risk factors puts you in control.* This book has been written to help you determine what you need to know to stay healthy for your whole life. I wish you all the best.

General Guidelines for Pregnant Women

*Source: **The Centers for Disease Control and Prevention***

A Avoid exposure to toxic substances and chemicals such as cleaning solvents, lead, and mercury, some insecticides, and paint. Pregnant women should avoid exposure to paint fumes.

B Be sure to see your doctor, and get prenatal care as soon as you think you're pregnant. It's important to see your doctor regularly throughout your pregnancy, so be sure to keep all your prenatal-care appointments. And . . .

Breastfeeding is the healthiest choice for both you and your baby. Talk to your doctor, your family and friends, and your employer about how you choose to feed your baby and how they can support you in your decision.

C Cigarette smoking during pregnancy can result in low-birth-weight babies. It has been associated with infertility, miscarriage, tubal pregnancies, infant mortality, and childhood morbidity. Additionally, cigarette smoking may also cause long-term learning disabilities. If you smoke, you should try to quit. Secondhand smoke may also harm a mother and her developing baby. It is a good idea to ask people to stop smoking around you during your pregnancy and after the baby is born.

D Drink extra fluids (water is best) throughout your pregnancy to help your body keep up with the increases in your blood volume. Drink at least six to eight glasses of water, fruit juice, or milk each day. A good way to know if you're drinking enough fluid is when your urine looks like almost-clear water or is a very light yellow.

E Eat healthfully to get the nutrients you and your unborn baby need. Your meals should include the five basic food groups. Each day you should get the following: six to eleven servings of grain products, three to five servings of vegetables, two to four servings of fruit, four to six servings of milk and milk products, three to four servings of meat and protein foods. Foods low in fat and high in fiber are important to a healthy diet.

F Take 400 micrograms of folic acid **daily both before pregnancy and during the first few months of pregnancy** to reduce the risk of birth defects of the brain and spine. All women who could possibly become pregnant should take a vitamin pill with folic acid, every day. It is also important to eat a healthful diet with fortified foods (enriched grain products, including cereals, rice, breads, and pastas) and foods with natural sources of folate (orange juice, leafy green vegetables, beans, peanuts, broccoli, asparagus, peas, and lentils).

G Genetic testing should be done as appropriate. It's important to know your family history. Have there been problems with pregnancies or birth defects in your family? If so, report these to your doctor. Also, genetic counselors can provide you with the information you might need in making decisions about having a family. You can call a major medical center in your area for help in finding a board-certified genetic counselor.

H Hand-washing is important throughout the day, especially after handling raw meat or using the bathroom. This can help prevent the spread of many bacteria and viruses that cause infection.

I Take 30 milligrams of iron during your pregnancy as prescribed by your doctor to reduce the risk of anemia later in pregnancy. All women of childbearing age should eat a diet rich in iron.

J Join a support group for moms-to-be, or join a class on parenting or childbirth.

K Know your limits. Let your physician know if you experience any of the following: pain of any kind, strong cramps, uterine contractions at twenty-minute intervals, vaginal bleeding, leaking of amniotic fluid, dizziness, fainting, shortness of breath, palpitations, tachycardia (rapid beating of the heart), constant nausea and vomiting, trouble walking, edema (swelling of joints), or if your baby has decreased activity.

L Legal drugs such as alcohol and caffeine are important issues for pregnant women. There is no safe amount of alcohol a woman can drink while pregnant. Fetal alcohol syndrome, a disorder characterized by growth retardation, facial abnormalities, and central nervous system dysfunction, is caused by a woman's use of alcohol during pregnancy. Be sure to read labels when trying to cut down on caffeine during pregnancy. More than 200 foods, beverages, and over-the-counter medications contain caffeine!

M Medical conditions such as diabetes, epilepsy, and high blood pressure should be treated and kept under control. Ask your doctor about any medications that may need to be changed or adjusted during pregnancy. If you are currently taking any medications, ask your doctor if it is safe to take them while you're pregnant. Also, be sure to discuss any herbs or vitamins you are taking. They are medicines, too! Discuss with your doctor all medications, prescribed and over-the-counter, that you are taking.

N Never hesitate to ask your doctor or healthcare provider any questions about your health. It is better to take all precautions and discuss any questions or concerns you may have.

O Over-the-counter cough and cold remedies may contain alcohol or other ingredients that should be avoided during pregnancy. Ask your healthcare provider about prescription or over-the-counter drugs that you are taking or may consider taking while pregnant.

P Physical activity during pregnancy can benefit both you and your baby by lessening discomfort and fatigue, providing a sense of well-being, and increasing the likelihood of early recovery after delivery. Light to moderate exercise during pregnancy strengthens the abdominal and back muscles, which help to improve posture. Practicing yoga, walking, swimming, and cycling on a stationary bicycle are usually safe exercises for pregnant women. But always check with your doctor before beginning any kind of exercise, especially during pregnancy.

Q Queasiness, stomach upset, and morning sickness are common during pregnancy. Foods that you normally love may make you feel sick to your stomach. You may need to substitute other nutritious foods. Eating five or six small meals a day instead of three large ones may make you feel better.

R Read about and make plans to baby proof your home. This is important for making your home a safe environment for your baby.

S Saunas, hot tubs, and steam rooms should be avoided while you are pregnant. Excessive high heat may be harmful during your pregnancy.

T Toxoplasmosis is an infection caused by a parasite that can seriously harm an unborn baby. Avoid eating undercooked meat and handling cat litter, and be sure to wear gloves when gardening.

U Uterus size increases during the first trimester, which, along with more efficient functioning of your kidneys, may cause you to feel the need to urinate more often. You may also leak urine when sneezing, coughing, or laughing. This is due to the growing uterus pressing against your bladder, which lies directly in front of and slightly under the uterus during the first few months of pregnancy. Be sure to tell your doctor if you experience burning along with frequency of urination.

V Vaccinations are an important concern for pregnant women. Get needed vaccines before pregnancy. The Centers for Disease Control has clear guidelines for the use of vaccines during pregnancy. Review the list and be sure to discuss it with your doctor.

W Being overweight or underweight during pregnancy may cause problems. Try to get within fifteen pounds of your ideal weight before pregnancy. Remember, pregnancy is not a time to be dieting! Don't stop eating or start skipping meals as your weight increases. Both you and your baby need the calories and nutrition you receive from a healthy diet. Be sure to consult with your doctor about your diet.

X Avoid x-rays. If you must have dental work or diagnostic tests, tell your dentist or physician that you are pregnant so that extra care can be taken.

Y Your baby loves you, and you should show your baby that you love her, too. Give your baby a healthy environment to live in while you are pregnant. Infants and children require constant care and guidance. Their health and safety should be carefully watched at all times.

Z Get your ZZZZZZZZZZZs. . . . Be sure to get plenty of rest. . . . Resting on your side as often as possible, especially on your left side, is advised, as it provides the best circulation to your baby and helps reduce swelling.

Disclaimer: Please consult your doctor on any and all issues regarding your pregnancy. Although these may be good general pregnancy tips, every pregnancy is different, and each deserves the attention of a doctor or healthcare provider.

And (a final note from *HealthWatch*)—it is important to take care of your teeth during pregnancy. Periodontitis is a bacterial infection of the gums that can be treated if found in the early stages. If left untreated in pregnant women, it can lead to serious health risks for your baby, including premature delivery and low birth weight. Oral bacteria also can pass through the placenta and infect the unborn baby with cavity-causing germs. Be sure to visit your dentist for regular checkups and cleanings during this time, and don't forget to brush and floss at least twice a day.

PART ONE
MEDICAL HISTORY

The following pages provide space for you to record your personal and family medical histories. This is important because everything that happens to one part of your body may affect other organs and systems. You may also have inherited genetic or familial conditions from your parents or grandparents. This is why physicians ask for your personal and family medical histories. Your physician may also ask about medications your mother took while pregnant with you because some *may* lead to cancers in your adult years. And remember that medications prescribed by one physician may interact with medications for other conditions. This part of the book is a convenient and portable place to store this vital information to take with you when you visit doctors.

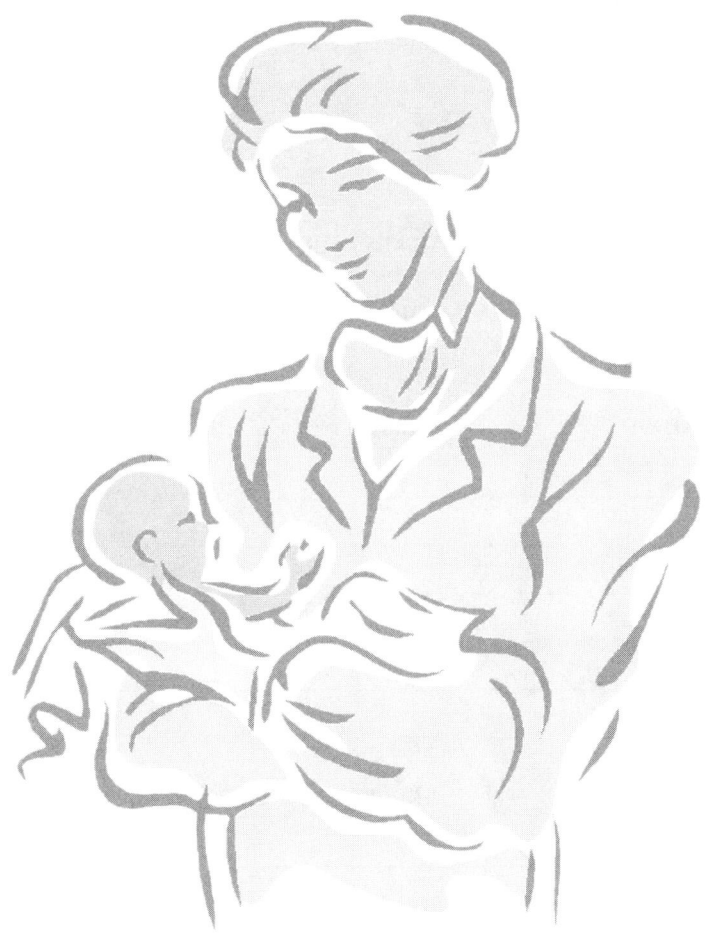

Personal Medical History

Name_____ Birth Date_____ Time of Birth_____ A.M./P.M. Blood Type_____

Birth Weight_____ Birth Length_____ Distinguishing Marks_____

Mother's Name_____ Father's Name_____

Physician or Midwife_____ Hospital_____

City and/or County_____ State_____ Country_____

Mother's medications during pregnancy_____

Mother's medications during delivery_____

Complications, if any_____

Type of Delivery: Vaginal / Caesarean

Breastfed: Yes / No   If yes, how long_____

Formula: Yes / No   If yes, how long_____ Type_____

For women: Age at first period_____ Date menopause began_____ Natural / Surgical

For men: Circumcised Yes / No Age:_____ Complications, if any_____

Surgical History

WHAT	DATE	HOSPITAL	SURGEON	COMMENTS

Broken Bones

WHAT	DATE	HOSPITAL/CLINIC	OFFICE/PHYSICIAN

Other Important Personal Data

Infections and/or Illnesses Requiring Medical Treatment

INFECTION/ILLNESS	DATE	HOSPITAL/CLINIC/OFFICE	PHYSICIAN(S)	TREATMENT

Prescription Record

(If necessary, make photocopies and attach additional pages.)

Date_____ Physician_____ Illness/Condition_____

Medication_____ Pharmacy_____ Dosage_____ # Refills_____

Date_____ Physician_____ Illness/Condition_____

Medication_____ Pharmacy_____ Dosage_____ # Refills_____

Date_____ Physician_____ Illness/Condition_____

Medication_____ Pharmacy_____ Dosage_____ # Refills_____

Date_____ Physician_____ Illness/Condition_____

Medication_____ Pharmacy_____ Dosage_____ # Refills_____

Date_____ Physician_____ Illness/Condition_____

Medication_____ Pharmacy_____ Dosage_____ # Refills_____

Date_____ Physician_____ Illness/Condition_____

Medication_____ Pharmacy_____ Dosage_____ # Refills_____

Date_____ Physician_____ Illness/Condition_____

Medication_____ Pharmacy_____ Dosage_____ # Refills_____

Date_____ Physician_____ Illness/Condition_____

Medication_____ Pharmacy_____ Dosage_____ # Refills_____

Date_____ Physician_____ Illness/Condition_____

Medication_____ Pharmacy_____ Dosage_____ # Refills_____

Date_____ Physician_____ Illness/Condition_____

Medication_____ Pharmacy_____ Dosage_____ # Refills_____

Date_____ Physician_____ Illness/Condition_____

Medication_____ Pharmacy_____ Dosage_____ # Refills_____

Date_____ Physician_____ Illness/Condition_____

Medication_____ Pharmacy_____ Dosage_____ # Refills_____

Date_____ Physician_____ Illness/Condition_____

Medication_____ Pharmacy_____ Dosage_____ # Refills_____

Date_____ Physician_____ Illness/Condition_____

Medication_____ Pharmacy_____ Dosage_____ # Refills_____

Date_____ Physician_____ Illness/Condition_____

Medication_____ Pharmacy_____ Dosage_____ # Refills_____

Date_____ Physician_____ Illness/Condition_____

Medication_____ Pharmacy_____ Dosage_____ # Refills_____

Date_____ Physician_____ Illness/Condition_____

Medication_____ Pharmacy_____ Dosage_____ # Refills_____

Date_____ Physician_____ Illness/Condition_____

Medication_____ Pharmacy_____ Dosage_____ # Refills_____

Date_____ Physician_____ Illness/Condition_____

Medication_____ Pharmacy_____ Dosage_____ # Refills_____

Date_____ Physician_____ Illness/Condition_____

Medication_____ Pharmacy_____ Dosage_____ # Refills_____

Date_____ Physician_____ Illness/Condition_____

Medication_____ Pharmacy_____ Dosage_____ # Refills_____

Date_____ Physician_____ Illness/Condition_____

Medication_____ Pharmacy_____ Dosage_____ # Refills_____

Date_____ Physician_____ Illness/Condition_____

Medication_____ Pharmacy_____ Dosage_____ # Refills_____

Date_____ Physician_____ Illness/Condition_____

Medication_____ Pharmacy_____ Dosage_____ # Refills_____

Date_____ Physician_____ Illness/Condition_____

Medication_____ Pharmacy_____ Dosage_____ # Refills_____

Date_____ Physician_____ Illness/Condition_____

Medication_____ Pharmacy_____ Dosage_____ # Refills_____

Date_____ Physician_____ Illness/Condition_____

Medication_____ Pharmacy_____ Dosage_____ # Refills_____

Date_____ Physician_____ Illness/Condition_____

Medication_____ Pharmacy_____ Dosage_____ # Refills_____

Date_____ Physician_____ Illness/Condition_____

Medication_____ Pharmacy_____ Dosage_____ # Refills_____

Date_____ Physician_____ Illness/Condition_____

Medication_____ Pharmacy_____ Dosage_____ # Refills_____

Date_____ Physician_____ Illness/Condition_____

Medication_____ Pharmacy_____ Dosage_____ # Refills_____

Date_____ Physician_____ Illness/Condition_____

Medication_____ Pharmacy_____ Dosage_____ # Refills_____

Date_____ Physician_____ Illness/Condition_____

Medication_____ Pharmacy_____ Dosage_____ # Refills_____

Date_____ Physician_____ Illness/Condition_____

Medication_____ Pharmacy_____ Dosage_____ # Refills_____

Date_____ Physician_____ Illness/Condition_____

Medication_____ Pharmacy_____ Dosage_____ # Refills_____

Date_____ Physician_____ Illness/Condition_____

Medication_____ Pharmacy_____ Dosage_____ # Refills_____

Date_____ Physician_____ Illness/Condition_____

Medication_____ Pharmacy_____ Dosage_____ # Refills_____

Date_____ Physician_____ Illness/Condition_____

Medication_____ Pharmacy_____ Dosage_____ # Refills_____

Date_____ Physician_____ Illness/Condition_____

Medication_____ Pharmacy_____ Dosage_____ # Refills_____

Date_____ Physician_____ Illness/Condition_____

Medication_____ Pharmacy_____ Dosage_____ # Refills_____

Date_____ Physician_____ Illness/Condition_____

Medication_____ Pharmacy_____ Dosage_____ # Refills_____

Date_____ Physician_____ Illness/Condition_____

Medication_____ Pharmacy_____ Dosage_____ # Refills_____

Date_____ Physician_____ Illness/Condition_____

Medication_____ Pharmacy_____ Dosage_____ # Refills_____

Over-the-Counter Medications, Herbs, and Other Products

PRODUCT	DOSAGE	DATE

Allergies

ALLERGIC TO	DATE OF INITIAL DIAGNOSIS	TREATMENT, IF ANY	COMMENTS

NOTES

Pregnancy and Childbirth History

Number of Pregnancies_____   Number of Live Births_____

CHILDREN			
	CHILD ONE	**CHILD TWO**	**CHILD THREE**
Name			
Date of birth			
Sex			
Birth weight			
Vaginal or caesarean			
Medication (epidural, other)			
Ob/gyn name			
Hospital			
Breastfed duration			
Formula fed duration, type			
	CHILD FOUR	**CHILD FIVE**	**CHILD SIX**
Name			
Date of birth			
Sex			
Birth weight			
Vaginal or caesarean			
Medication (epidural, other)			
Ob/gyn name			
Hospital			
Breastfed duration			
Formula fed duration, type			

Miscarriages

DATE	COMPLICATIONS, IF ANY

Abortions

DATE	COMPLICATIONS, IF ANY

NOTES

Contraceptive History

ORAL			
Brand	Dates of use	Prescribed by	Became pregnant while using Y/N

IUD			
Brand	Dates of use	Prescribed by	Became pregnant while using Y/N

DIAPHRAGM			
Brand	Dates of use	Prescribed by	Became pregnant while using Y/N

CONDOM		
Brand	Dates of use	Became pregnant while using Y/N

RHYTHM		
Dates of use	Prescribed by	Became pregnant while using Y/N

SPONGE		
Brand	Dates of use	Became pregnant while using Y/N

INJECTION

Brand	Dates of use	Prescribed by	Became pregnant while using Y/N

VAGINAL PATCH

Brand	Dates of use	Prescribed by	Became pregnant while using Y/N

VAGINAL RING

Brand	Dates of use	Prescribed by	Became pregnant while using Y/N

OTHER

Brand	Dates of use	Prescribed by	Became pregnant while using Y/N

NOTES

Hereditary Conditions

Medical science has identified many diseases or conditions that are inherited from parents. Other conditions are called "congenital defects," meaning that something unpredictable happened to the baby during pregnancy. These spontaneous occurrences are unfortunate but are usually not indicative of similar risk to future children.

However, many conditions that occur as a result of genetic defects are identifiable and predictable, and are passed to offspring by anyone who has the condition or is a carrier of the malformed gene. The list of genetically inherited birth defects is growing rapidly as scientists map the genetic code, and this knowledge gives prospective parents a better understanding of the risks their future children may face.

Genetically Inherited Defects— Background Information

An egg (from the mother) *always* contains an X (female) chromosome and twenty-two other chromosomes loaded with genes containing information regarding hair color, height, blood type, and so forth. A sperm (from the father) contains *either* an X (female chromosome) *or* a Y (male chromosome) and twenty-two other chromosomes that, like those of the egg, contain information about various characteristics. The sex chromosomes of the parents combine in the new baby. The mother always contributes an X sex chromosome. The sex chromosome carried by the father determines the sex of the baby: If the sperm has an X, the new baby will have the sex chromosomes XX, and will be a girl. If the sperm has a Y, the baby will be XY, and will be a boy.

The other twenty-two chromosomes contributed by each parent combine for a total of forty-four chromosomes that determine the physical characteristics of the new baby. Each of these characteristics is controlled by whichever parent's gene is dominant for that trait. Either parent can contribute dominant and recessive genes.

In many inherited diseases (*autosomal dominant*), the abnormal gene is dominant over the normal gene. A child will develop the condition if the abnormal gene is on a chromosome passed on by either parent.

In other inherited diseases (*autosomal recessive*), a child must receive abnormal genes from both parents in order to develop the condition. If the child receives only one abnormal gene, the normal gene they receive from the other parent will dominate. The child may exhibit only mild symptoms of the condition, or no symptoms at all. However, the child will still be capable of passing the recessive gene on to their offspring. If a parent has one abnormal and one normal gene for a characteristic and passes on the normal gene, their child will not inherit the condition, and in turn cannot pass it on to their offspring.

In *X-linked* inherited conditions, the disease is *always* carried on the X chromosome. If the disease is *X-recessive*, and the mother carries the abnormal X, but the father does not have the disease, girls will not be affected because their other (normal) X chromosome (provided by the father) will be dominant. However, these girls will have one normal and one abnormal X chromosome, so they will still be able to pass the abnormal gene on to their offspring.

However, sons have a fifty-fifty chance of developing the condition because they will always get a normal Y from the father, but they could get either a normal X or an abnormal X from the mother. Without a normal X to counter the abnormal X, the XY son will have the condition and will always pass it on to his female children.

If the father carries the abnormal X, and the mother two normal Xs, all of their daughters will be normal but carriers, and all of their sons will be normal. This is because the father's abnormal X will pass only to daughters, and the mother's normal X will be dominant in the girls.

If the mother has a normal X and an abnormal X, and the father has an abnormal X, then each of their daughters has a fifty-fifty chance of having the condition and/or being a carrier, and each son has a fifty-fifty chance of having the disease or being normal.

For a disease to be considered *X-dominant*, other circumstances apply. For instance, if the father carries the abnormal X chromosome, all of his daughters will have the condition and be carriers, but all of the sons will be normal (because they inherit only a Y from the father).

If the mother has the disease and the father does not, each of their children, male or female, has a fifty-fifty chance of having the disease. The girls could inherit a normal X from the mother and a normal X from the father, or an abnormal X from the mother and a normal X from the father. The boys could each inherit a normal Y from the father and either a normal or an abnormal X from the mother. For boys and girls, the abnormal X would dominate the normal gene.

Partial List of Hereditary Conditions

The following lists are by no means complete. The conditions identified are examples of autosomal recessive, autosomal dominant, X-linked recessive, and X-linked dominant conditions. *Some conditions can be inherited in several forms. Some conditions are mild; some are devastating. Keep track of any inherited conditions that run in your family. You may want to meet with a genetic counselor regarding your plans to have children if any such conditions are present.*

AUTOSOMAL RECESSIVE CONDITIONS (TWO GENES NEEDED, ONE FROM EACH PARENT)			
CONDITION	INCIDENCE IF KNOWN	AREA AFFECTED	ETHNICITY/ANCESTRY FACTORS
Albinism		eyes, skin, hair	
Canavan disease		brain	Ashkenazi Jews
Charcot-Marie-Tooth disease		nervous system	
Clinical thalassemia		blood supply	
Crigler-Najjar syndrome		brain, liver	
Cystic fibrosis		lungs, stomach, intestines	
Ellis-van Creveld syndrome		multiorgan, skin	Amish
Familial dysbetalipo-proteinemia	1/10,000	circulatory system, heart	
Galactosemia	1/60,000	liver, brain, eyes, kidneys	
Gaucher's disease—type 1	1/500–1,000	spleen, bones, liver	Ashkenazi Jews
Hemochromatosis	1/250	liver, blood, heart	British, Celtic, N. European
Krabbe's disease	1/150,000	nervous system	Scandinavian
Pernicious anemia		blood supply	
Phenylketonuria (PKU)		brain	
Porphyria		blood supply	
Riley-Day syndrome		nervous system	Ashkenazi Jews
Sanfilippo syndrome		brain, muscles, speech	
Scheie syndrome		joints, eyes	
Selective IgA deficiency	1/700	immune system	Europeans
Sickle-cell anemia	1/12	blood supply	African American
Spinal muscular atrophy	4/100,000	muscles	
Tay-Sachs disease	1/2,500	brain, nervous system	Ashkenazi Jews

PART ONE • MEDICAL HISTORY

AUTOSOMAL DOMINANT CONDITIONS (ONE GENE NEEDED, FROM EITHER PARENT)

CONDITION	INCIDENCE IF KNOWN	AREA AFFECTED	ETHNICITY/ANCESTRY FACTORS
Albinism		eyes, skin, hair	
Alzheimer's disease (early onset)	1/625	brain	
Charcot-Marie-Tooth disease		nervous system	
Congenital cataracts		eyes	
Facioscapulohumeral muscular dystrophy		muscles	
Familial hypercholesterolemia	7/1,000	circulatory system, heart	
Familial hypertriglyceridemia	1/300	circulatory system, heart, pancreas	
Familial tremor		nervous system	
Hereditary amyloidosis		multiorgan	
Hereditary elliptocytosis	1/4,000	blood supply	
Huntington's disease		nervous system, brain	
Marfan syndrome	2/10,000	bones, heart, eyes, skin	
Medullary cystic disease		kidneys	
Neurofibromatosis-1		nervous system	
Noonan syndrome	1/2,500	bones, heart, brain	
Osler-Weber-Rendu syndrome		blood supply	
Osteogenesis imperfecta		bones	
Peutz-Jeghers syndrome		intestines	
Polycystic kidney disease	1/1,000	kidneys	
Selective IgA deficiency	1/700	immune system	European
Tourette's syndrome	2% total population	nervous system	

X-LINKED RECESSIVE CONDITIONS (CARRIED BY EITHER PARENT, PRIMARILY AFFECTS MALES, ALTHOUGH SOME FEMALES MAY SHOW SLIGHT SYMPTOMS)

CONDITION	INCIDENCE IF KNOWN	AREA AFFECTED	ETHNICITY/ANCESTRY FACTORS
Becker's muscular dystrophy		muscles	
Charcot-Marie-Tooth disease		nervous system	
Color blindness		eyes	
Duchenne muscular dystrophy		muscles	
G-6-PD deficiency	10–14%	blood supply	African American
Hemophilia A	1/5,000	blood supply	
Medullary cystic disease		kidneys	
Reifenstein syndrome		testicles	

X-LINKED DOMINANT CONDITIONS (CARRIED BY EITHER PARENT, CAN AFFECT BOTH MALES AND FEMALES)

CONDITION	INCIDENCE IF KNOWN	AREA AFFECTED	ETHNICITY/ANCESTRY FACTORS
Incontentia pigmenti (Bloch-Sulzberger syndrome)	mostly girls, may be lethal in boys	skin	
Rett syndrome		brain	

X-LINKED (DOMINANCE FACTORS NOT ESTABLISHED)

CONDITION	INCIDENCE IF KNOWN	AREA AFFECTED	ETHNICITY/ANCESTRY FACTORS
Fragile X syndrome	1/2,000 boys 1/4,000 girls	brain	

CHROMOSOMAL DEFECTS (CAUSED BY PROBLEMS ON SPECIFIC CHROMOSOMES OTHER THAN X OR Y)

CONDITION	INCIDENCE IF KNOWN	AREA AFFECTED	ETHNICITY/ANCESTRY FACTORS
Chronic myelogenous leukemia		blood supply	
Cri du chat syndrome (missing chromosome)		brain	
Klinefelter syndrome (extra X chromosome)	men only	testicles	
Prader-Willi syndrome (chromosome 15)		brain, muscles, testicles	
Turner syndrome	1/3,000 girls	bones, eyes, heart, sexual organs	

AUTOSOMAL OR CHROMOSOMAL CONDITIONS THAT HAVE BEEN IDENTIFIED IN MY FAMILY

CONDITION	FAMILY MEMBERS	RELATIONSHIP

Medical Conditions That Tend to Run in Families

These are conditions for which there is no known chromosomal or genetic link *at this time*. Science in this area is advancing rapidly, however, so some of these may eventually be added to the list of definite hereditary disorders. Meanwhile, if you know that your family has a predisposition for any of the following conditions, you can take any necessary precautions to minimize the impact on your life. *Note: Some conditions are not normally considered serious, such as male-pattern baldness, but if they are known to run in families, they have been included in the list.*

CONDITION	AREA AFFECTED	FAMILY MEMBERS AND RELATIONSHIP
Achalasia	esophagus	
Acute glaucoma	eyes	
Acute otitis media (ear infection)	ears	
Allergies	lungs, nose, skin	
Alopecia areata	hair	
Alzheimer's disease (late onset)	brain	
Amblyopia	eyes	
Anemia of vitamin B_{12} deficiency	blood supply	
Ankylosing spondylitis	spine	
Anorchism	testicles (missing)	
Arthritis	joints (inflammation)	
Asthma	lungs	
Atrial myxoma	heart (tumors)	
Attention deficit disorder	brain	
Autism	brain	
Benign hypermobility joint syndrome	joints	
Berger's disease (IgA nephropathy)	kidney	
Bipolar affective disorder	brain	
Bladder cancer	bladder	
Bleeding disorders	blood supply	
Breast cancer	breasts	
Cataracts	eyes	
Celiac disease (sprue)	intestines	

CONDITION	AREA AFFECTED	FAMILY MEMBERS AND RELATIONSHIP
Cholelithiasis (gallstones)	gallbladder	
Chronic fatigue syndrome	immune system	
Chronic glaucoma	eyes	
Chronic lymphocyte leukemia	blood supply	
Chronic thyroiditis (Hashimoto's)	thyroid	
Chylomicronemia syndrome	blood supply	
Cleft lip or palate	mouth	
Clubfoot	feet	
Colorectal cancer	intestines	
Colorectal polyps	intestines	
Congenital platelet function defects*	blood supply	
Congenital protein C or S deficiency*	blood supply	
Congenital spherocytic anemia*	blood supply	
Coronary artery disease	heart	
Crohn's disease	intestines	
Dementia	brain	
Diaphragmatic hernia	diaphragm	
Down syndrome	chromosome abnormality	
Duodenal ulcers	duodenum	
Eczema	skin	
Ehlers-Danlos syndrome (many forms)	connective tissue	
Endometriosis	uterus	
Enuresis (bed-wetting)	bladder, nervous system	
Epilepsy	brain	
Essential tremor	nervous system	
Exstrophy of the bladder	bladder	
Familial Mediterranean fever	abdomen, lungs	
Farsightedness (hyperopia)	eyes	

*Although the condition includes the word "congenital," implying that it is a random, unanticipated event, in this case the condition is one that does tend to run in families.

CONDITION	AREA AFFECTED	FAMILY MEMBERS AND RELATIONSHIP
Febrile seizures	brain, nervous system	
Fibrocystic breast disease	breasts	
Fibromyalgia	muscles, nerves	
Giant cell arteritis	circulatory system	
Glaucoma	eyes	
Goiter	thyroid	
Goodpasture's syndrome	kidneys	
Gout	joints	
Headache (migraine)	brain	
Heart attacks (early)	heart	
Heart disease	heart	
Hereditary angioedema	immune system	
Hirsutism	excess hair, especially facial	
Hypertension (high blood pressure)	circulatory system	
Hypogonadism	testicles	
Hypospadias	penis	
Ichthyosis vulgaris	skin	
Juvenile rheumatoid arthritis	joints	
Lactose intolerance	stomach	
Lamellar ichthyosis	skin	
Limb-girdle muscular dystrophies	muscles	
Lupus nephritis	kidneys	
Macular degeneration	eyes	
Male-pattern baldness	hair	
Manic-depressive disorder	brain	
Maple syrup urine disease	brain	
Melanoma skin cancer	skin	
Mitral valve prolapse	heart	
Multiple endocrine neoplasia (MEN) I	pancreas	

CONDITION	AREA AFFECTED	FAMILY MEMBERS AND RELATIONSHIP
Multiple endocrine neoplasia (MEN) II	thyroid	
Multiple myeloma	blood supply	
Multiple sclerosis	nervous system	
Narcolepsy	brain	
Nearsightedness	eyes	
Nephrolithiasis (kidney stones)	kidneys	
Neurosarcoidosis	nervous system	
Olivopontocerebellar atrophy	brain	
Osteitis fibrosa	bones	
Osteoarthritis	bones, joints	
Osteoporosis	bones (brittle)	
Osteosarcoma (bone cancer)	bones	
Otosclerosis	ears (hearing loss)	
Ovarian cancer	ovaries	
Pancreatic cancer	pancreas	
Parkinson's disease (early onset)	brain	
Pernicious anemia	blood	
Peyronie's disease	penis	
Pick's disease	brain	
Plummer-Vinson syndrome	esophagus	
Prognathism	jawbones, teeth	
Prostate cancer	prostate	
Psoriasis	skin	
Psoriatic arthritis	joints	
Recurrent cystitis	urinary tract	
Rheumatoid arthritis	joints	
Russell-Silver syndrome	bones	
Sarcoidosis	lymph glands, lungs, skin, liver, eyes	

PART ONE • MEDICAL HISTORY

CONDITION	AREA AFFECTED	FAMILY MEMBERS AND RELATIONSHIP
Schizophrenia	brain	
Scoliosis	spine	
Seborrheic dermatitis	skin	
Selective mutism	brain	
Sjögren's syndrome	immune system	
Sleepwalking	brain	
Spina bifida	spine	
Stein-Leventhal syndrome	ovaries	
Stomach (gastric) cancer	stomach	
Strabismus	eyes	
Stroke	brain	
Stuttering	nervous system	
Sudden infant death syndrome (SIDS)	n/a	
Systemic lupus erythematosus	immune system	
Testicular cancer	testicles	
Thyroid cancer	thyroid	
Transient ischemic attack (TIA)	brain	
Type I diabetes (juvenile)	pancreas	
Type II diabetes (mellitus)	pancreas	
Ulcerative colitis	intestines, rectum	
Varicose veins	circulatory system	
Vitiligo	skin	
Von Willebrand's disease	blood supply	
Wilms' tumor	kidney	

NOTES

Family Medical History

FEMALE RELATIVES

Great-Grandmothers

Name _____ Born _____

Died _____ Cause of Death _____

Known Medical Conditions _____

Name _____ Born _____

Died _____ Cause of Death _____

Known Medical Conditions _____

Name _____ Born _____

Died _____ Cause of Death _____

Known Medical Conditions _____

Name _____ Born _____

Died _____ Cause of Death _____

Known Medical Conditions _____

Grandmothers

Name _____ Born _____

Died _____ Cause of Death _____

Known Medical Conditions _____

Name _____ Born _____

Died _____ Cause of Death _____

Known Medical Conditions _____

Part One • Medical History

Mother

Name _____ Born _____

Died _____ Cause of Death _____

Known Medical Conditions _____

Aunts

Name _____ Born _____

Died _____ Cause of Death _____

Known Medical Conditions _____

Name _____ Born _____

Died _____ Cause of Death _____

Known Medical Conditions _____

Name _____ Born _____

Died _____ Cause of Death _____

Known Medical Conditions _____

Name _____ Born _____

Died _____ Cause of Death _____

Known Medical Conditions _____

Name _____ Born _____

Died _____ Cause of Death _____

Known Medical Conditions _____

Name _____ Born _____

Died _____ Cause of Death _____

Known Medical Conditions _____

Sisters

Name _____ Born _____

Died _____ Cause of Death _____

Known Medical Conditions _____

Name _____ Born _____

Died _____ Cause of Death _____

Known Medical Conditions _____

Name _____ Born _____

Died _____ Cause of Death _____

Known Medical Conditions _____

Name _____ Born _____

Died _____ Cause of Death _____

Known Medical Conditions _____

Name _____ Born _____

Died _____ Cause of Death _____

Known Medical Conditions _____

Name _____ Born _____

Died _____ Cause of Death _____

Known Medical Conditions _____

NOTES

MALE RELATIVES

Great-Grandfathers

Name _____ Born _____

Died _____ Cause of Death _____

Known Medical Conditions _____

Name _____ Born _____

Died _____ Cause of Death _____

Known Medical Conditions _____

Name _____ Born _____

Died _____ Cause of Death _____

Known Medical Conditions _____

Name _____ Born _____

Died _____ Cause of Death _____

Known Medical Conditions _____

Grandfathers

Name _____ Born _____

Died _____ Cause of Death _____

Known Medical Conditions _____

Name _____ Born _____

Died _____ Cause of Death _____

Known Medical Conditions _____

Father

Name _____ Born _____

Died _____ Cause of Death _____

Known Medical Conditions _____

Uncles

Name _____ Born _____

Died _____ Cause of Death _____

Known Medical Conditions _____

Name _____ Born _____

Died _____ Cause of Death _____

Known Medical Conditions _____

Name _____ Born _____

Died _____ Cause of Death _____

Known Medical Conditions _____

Name _____ Born _____

Died _____ Cause of Death _____

Known Medical Conditions _____

Name _____ Born _____

Died _____ Cause of Death _____

Known Medical Conditions _____

Name _____ Born _____

Died _____ Cause of Death _____

Known Medical Conditions _____

Brothers

Name _____ Born _____

Died _____ Cause of Death _____

Known Medical Conditions _____

PART ONE • MEDICAL HISTORY

Brothers (cont.)

Name _____ Born _____

Died _____ Cause of Death _____

Known Medical Conditions _____

Name _____ Born _____

Died _____ Cause of Death _____

Known Medical Conditions _____

Name _____ Born _____

Died _____ Cause of Death _____

Known Medical Conditions _____

Name _____ Born _____

Died _____ Cause of Death _____

Known Medical Conditions _____

Name _____ Born _____

Died _____ Cause of Death _____

Known Medical Conditions _____

NOTES

ADDITIONAL NOTES

PART TWO

WHAT TO DO AND WHEN TO DO IT

As pointed out in the introduction, every appliance you own, from toasters to trucks, comes with an owner's manual. If you own a car, the manual recommends oil weight, filters, gasoline, spark plugs, and tire pressure, and lists service intervals for tune-ups and parts replacement. Up until now, there has not been an owner's manual for humans.

This part has compiled the recommended service intervals for average adults and children. Following the guidelines and tracking the results will give you the information you need to monitor your health and stay healthy.

Recommended Tests for Children and Adults

This section provides a list of recommended schedules for health screening tests, immunizations, and checkups, and descriptions of these tests. Everyone has different health issues, and you may need additional, or more frequent, screenings for existing medical conditions. In that case, follow your doctor's recommendations. For most people, the tests, examinations, and immunizations that follow are the standard tools used to *prevent* health problems and to promptly identify any that occur. The guidelines and recommendations are those issued by the American Academy of Pediatrics and the American Academy of Family Physicians.

Tests for Children

Your child's pediatrician performs many tests at each regular checkup. These tests help to monitor your child's growth and development. Some tests will be performed periodically, not annually, and not every test is required for every child. Most tests are simple and painless. Record the results on the "Recommended Tests for Children" charts (pages 44–45).

Blood pressure. Annually, beginning at age three.

Body mass index. Annually, beginning from birth.

Eye exam. Eye exams are recommended on the following schedule:

- *From birth to two years*—a basic eye exam at each checkup; be sure to mention any family history of vision problems

- *Age two to five*—a more comprehensive exam at age three or as recommended for specific conditions
- *Age six to seventeen*—once every three years; every eighteen months if corrective lenses are used

Head size. At every checkup, through age two.

Hearing. At birth and periodically at checkups, especially if problems are suspected. A thorough exam should be done once between the ages of four and ten, and every three years thereafter until age seventeen.

Height. Every checkup through age one, annually thereafter.

Hematocrit or Hemoglobin. A test for anemia should be done between nine and twelve months, and annually from then on for children at risk. Girls who are menstruating should have an annual hematocrit.

Teeth. The first visit to the dentist between nine months and two years, every six months thereafter.

Testicular self-exam. Boys should perform a monthly testicular self-exam beginning at about age thirteen.

Urinalysis. The pediatrician should test the child's urine at age five.

Weight. Measured at every checkup through age one, annually thereafter.

Other Childhood Tests That May Be Needed

In addition to the standard examinations listed above, your doctor may recommend tests based on your child's particular health issues. For instance, sexually active teens should be screened regularly for sexually transmitted diseases.

Cholesterol. Annually, beginning at age two for children at risk.

Genetic screenings. In the first month after birth, where required by state law.

Lead. At each checkup between nine and twelve months, and again at age two for children at risk.

Pelvic exam. Annually, for sexually active girls.

STD screening. Annually, for boys and girls at risk (sexually active, or victims of sexual abuse).

Tuberculosis. Test at twelve, fifteen, and eighteen months, and annually thereafter if the child is at high risk.

Urinalysis. Annually for sexually active girls.

Tests for Adults

Many adult tests and examinations are recommended on an annual basis. They usually are performed at your yearly physical. Dental checkups should take place every six months, and other exams are recommended every two, three, or ten years.

Blood pressure. A baseline arm-cuff test at age twenty. If the readings are in the normal range, test every two years. Test every year if the pressure is slightly elevated, test every other month or per your physician's advice if the readings are high (120/80 or higher).

Bone density screening. Recommended for the following:
- All women over the age of sixty-five
- All postmenopausal women under age sixty-five who have one or more risk factors for osteoporosis (see the section "The Bones" in the Disease Prevention Guide)
- All postmenopausal women who have ever had a bone fracture
- All women who have taken hormone replacement therapy (HRT) for an extended period of time
- Men with low levels of testosterone

Breast exam. Women should perform a breast self-exam every month, and should have a clinical breast exam at their doctor's office every one to two years from age eighteen through age forty, and annually after age forty.

Cholesterol. Simple blood test for LDL, HDL, total cholesterol, and triglycerides:

- *From age twenty through age forty*—every five years
- *From age forty-one through age fifty*—every two years
- *After age fifty*—every year, or per your physician's advice

Colon cancer. Most gastroenterologists screen average-risk patients with a colonoscopy every eight to ten years. Some doctors recommend an air-contrast barium enema with flexible sigmoidoscopy every five years with an annual fecal occult blood test (*occult* means "hidden"—this is a test for blood in your stool). Fecal occult blood tests are seldom done if a colonoscopy is performed every ten years. Discuss your specific needs with your physician. *If colon cancer has affected a parent or sibling, you should consider having a colonoscopy every five years, beginning at an age ten years younger than the age at which your relative was diagnosed.*

Diabetes. If your blood sugar level is normal, have a fasting plasma glucose or oral glucose-tolerance blood test every three years beginning at age forty-five. Get checked every year if the levels are high, or per your physician's advice.

Digital prostate exam. Men should have this exam annually, beginning at age forty for blacks and men with a family history of prostate cancer, and at age fifty for all other men.

Eye exam. Recommended eye exams:
- *Age eighteen to age forty*—once every three years; once every eighteen months if corrective lenses are used
- *Over age forty*—at least once every two years; every eighteen months if contact lenses or glasses are used, or as recommended for specific conditions; every two years for glaucoma, beginning at age forty for blacks, diabetics, and anyone who has sleep apnea, is very nearsighted, or has a family history of glaucoma, and beginning at age sixty-five for everyone else

Hearing. Annually after age sixty-five.

Height and weight. Check these periodically, or at your annual physical exam.

Mammogram. The American Cancer Society recommends that a woman have her first mammogram by age forty, followed by one every one to two years up to age forty-nine, and annually thereafter, unless you have a family history of breast cancer or other risk factors. *Note: Screening recommendations change with every new study on the subject. The best advice for your mammogram schedule will come from your physician.*

Pap smear. Annually, beginning at age eighteen, or earlier if sexually active.

Prostate-specific antigen. Men should have this blood test annually, beginning at age forty for blacks and men with a family history of prostate cancer, and age fifty for all other men.

Teeth. Have a dental checkup every six months, or per your dentist's advice.

Testicular self-exam. Men should perform this exam on a monthly basis.

Other Adult Tests That May Be Needed

In addition to the general tests recommended for all adults, some individuals may need other tests. For instance, people with genetic markers for cancer, sexually active men and women, or anyone with diabetes or kidney disease should follow their doctor's advice about the nature and frequency of these tests.

Cancer screenings. As recommended by your physician.

Chlamydia. Annually or more often, for sexually active women aged twenty-five and younger, and sexually active men and women of any age if there is a risk of exposure to STDs. Follow your doctor's advice.

Thyroid screening. Women over age fifty should have this test, per their physician's advice, especially if there is a personal history of high cholesterol or a family history of thyroid disease. Make sure your physician knows your personal and family medical histories.

Urinalysis. Periodically, per your physician's advice, after age fifty. This test often is performed at regular checkups to look for early signs of disease. Urinalysis also is used to evaluate conditions such as kidney disease, and so may be performed more frequently.

Temperature and Blood Pressure—What Is Normal?

Although the accepted standard for a normal temperature is 98.6°F, researchers are discovering that this is not the norm for everyone. Many people have normal temperatures of 97.6°F or 99.6°F. Take your temperature at various times of the day during a month when you are not ill in order to learn your normal temperature. This will help your doctor determine whether or not you are running a fever the next time you are sick.

Blood exerts pressure against the walls of the arteries as it is pumped through the body. Your blood pressure is a measurement of that force and provides valuable information about the amount of blood being pumped and the condition of the arteries.

Understanding Your Blood Pressure Reading

The blood pressure reading consists of two numbers, displayed one above the other. The upper number represents the maximum pressure in your arteries when the heart is pumping (pressure is greatest at this time). This is called the systolic number. The lower of the two numbers, called the diastolic number, shows pressure between heartbeats (when it is lowest). A normal blood pressure reading is considered to be anything under 120/80; however, lower readings are better for your arteries.

AGE	PULSE RATE	RESPIRATION	BLOOD PRESSURE	
			SYSTOLIC	DIASTOLIC
Newborn	125	N/A	60 +/– 10	37 +/– 8
1 year	120	20–30	96 +/– 30	66 +/–25
2–3 years	115	N/A	99 +/– 25	64 +/– 25
4–5 years	100	N/A	99 +/– 20	65 +/– 20
6–9 years	100	12–25	100 +/– 20	65 +/– 15
10–12 years	75	N/A	112 +/– 20	68 +/– 15
14 years and up	70	12–18	120 +/– 20	75 +/– 15

Source: P. C. Jordan, "Multiple Trauma," in *Emergency Medicine—Concepts and Clinical Practice*, 3rd edition, eds. P. Rosen, R. Barkin, et al. (St. Louis: Mosby, 1990), 281–282. http://www.emedicine.com.

RECOMMENDED TESTS FOR CHILDREN

Age	Body Mass Index	Head Size	Height	Weight	Blood Pressure	Hematocrit	Urinalysis
1 month							
2 months							
4 months							
6 months							
9 months							once	
12 months							
15 months							
18 months							
2							
3							
4							
5							
6							
7							
8							
9							
10							
11							
12							
13							
14							
15							
16							
17							

Check the appropriate shaded box when the test has been completed.

RECOMMENDED TESTS FOR CHILDREN

Hearing	Eye Exam					Physician or Clinic
once						

RECOMMENDED ADULT TESTS AND EXAMINATIONS FOR WOMEN

Age	Height	Weight	Blood Pressure	Fecal Occult Blood*	Urinalysis—Periodically After Age 50	Hearing—Periodically After Age 65	Vision*	Glaucoma
18								
19								
20								
21								
22								
23								
24								
25								
26								
27								
28								
29								
30								
31								
32								
33								
34								
35								
36								
37								
38								

Check the appropriate shaded box when the test has been completed.   *Record these results in the charts provided in the appropriate section.

RECOMMENDED ADULT TESTS AND EXAMINATIONS FOR WOMEN

Clinical Breast Exam	Mammo-gram*	Pap Smear*	Cholesterol*	Diabetes*			Physician or Clinic

RECOMMENDED ADULT TESTS AND EXAMINATIONS FOR WOMEN

Age	Height	Weight	Blood Pressure	Fecal Occult Blood*	Urinalysis—Periodically After Age 50	Hearing—Periodically After Age 65	Vision*	Glaucoma
39								
40								
41								
42								
43								
44								
45								
46								
47								
48								
49								
50								
51								
52								
53								
54								
55								
56								
57								
58								
59								

Check the appropriate shaded box when the test has been completed.   *Record these results in the charts provided in the appropriate section.

RECOMMENDED ADULT TESTS AND EXAMINATIONS FOR WOMEN

Clinical Breast Exam	Mammo-gram*	Pap Smear*	Cholesterol*	Diabetes*			Physician or Clinic

RECOMMENDED ADULT TESTS AND EXAMINATIONS FOR WOMEN

Age	Height	Weight	Blood Pressure	Fecal Occult Blood*	Urinalysis—Periodically After Age 50	Hearing—Periodically After Age 65	Vision*	Glaucoma
60								
61								
62								
63								
64								
65								
66								
67								
68								
69								
70								
71								
72								
73								
74								
75								
76								
77								
78								
79								
80								

Check the appropriate shaded box when the test has been completed.   *Record these results in the charts provided in the appropriate section.

RECOMMENDED ADULT TESTS AND EXAMINATIONS FOR WOMEN

Clinical Breast Exam	Mammo-gram*	Pap Smear*	Cholesterol*	Diabetes*			Physician or Clinic

RECOMMENDED ADULT TESTS AND EXAMINATIONS FOR WOMEN

Age	Height	Weight	Blood Pressure	Fecal Occult Blood*	Urinalysis— Periodically After Age 50	Hearing— Periodically After Age 65	Vision*	Glaucoma
81								
82								
83								
84								
85								
86								
87								
88								
89								
90								
91								
92								
93								
94								
95								
96								
97								
98								
99								
100								

Check the appropriate shaded box when the test has been completed.   *Record these results in the charts provided in the appropriate section.

RECOMMENDED ADULT TESTS AND EXAMINATIONS FOR WOMEN

Clinical Breast Exam	Mammo-gram*	Pap Smear*	Cholesterol*	Diabetes*			Physician or Clinic

RECOMMENDED ADULT TESTS AND EXAMINATIONS FOR MEN

Age	Height	Weight	Blood Pressure	Fecal Occult Blood*	Colono-scopy*	Urinalysis—Periodically After Age 50	Hearing—Periodically After Age 65	Vision*
18								
19								
20								
21								
22								
23								
24								
25								
26								
27								
28								
29								
30								
31								
32								
33								
34								
35								
36								
37								
38								

Check the appropriate shaded box when the test has been completed.   *Record these results in the charts provided in the appropriate section.

RECOMMENDED ADULT TESTS AND EXAMINATIONS FOR MEN

Glaucoma	Digital Prostate Exam*†	PSA (Prostate Specific Antigen)*†	Cholesterol*	Diabetes*			Physician or Clinic

†*Annually after age 50 or age 40 for high risk*

RECOMMENDED ADULT TESTS AND EXAMINATIONS FOR MEN

Age	Height	Weight	Blood Pressure	Fecal Occult Blood*	Colono-scopy*	Urinalysis—Periodically After Age 50	Hearing—Periodically After Age 65	Vision*
39								
40								
41								
42								
43								
44								
45								
46								
47								
48								
49								
50								
51								
52								
53								
54								
55								
56								
57								
58								
59								

Check the appropriate shaded box when the test has been completed.   *Record these results in the charts provided in the appropriate section.

RECOMMENDED ADULT TESTS AND EXAMINATIONS FOR MEN

Glaucoma	Digital Prostate Exam*†	PSA (Prostate Specific Antigen)*†	Cholesterol*	Diabetes*			Physician or Clinic

†Annually after age 50 or age 40 for high risk

RECOMMENDED ADULT TESTS AND EXAMINATIONS FOR MEN

Age	Height	Weight	Blood Pressure	Fecal Occult Blood*	Colono-scopy*	Urinalysis—Periodically After Age 50	Hearing—Periodically After Age 65	Vision*
60								
61								
62								
63								
64								
65								
66								
67								
68								
69								
70								
71								
72								
73								
74								
75								
76								
77								
78								
79								
80								

Check the appropriate shaded box when the test has been completed.   **Record these results in the charts provided in the appropriate section.*

RECOMMENDED ADULT TESTS AND EXAMINATIONS FOR MEN

Glaucoma	Digital Prostate Exam*†	PSA (Prostate Specific Antigen)*†	Cholesterol*	Diabetes*			Physician or Clinic

†Annually after age 50 or age 40 for high risk

RECOMMENDED ADULT TESTS AND EXAMINATIONS FOR MEN

Age	Height	Weight	Blood Pressure	Fecal Occult Blood*	Colono-scopy*	Urinalysis—Periodically After Age 50	Hearing—Periodically After Age 65	Vision*
81								
82								
83								
84								
85								
86								
87								
88								
89								
90								
91								
92								
93								
94								
95								
96								
97								
98								
99								
100								

Check the appropriate shaded box when the test has been completed.   *Record these results in the charts provided in the appropriate section.

RECOMMENDED ADULT TESTS AND EXAMINATIONS FOR MEN

Glaucoma	Digital Prostate Exam*†	PSA (Prostate Specific Antigen)*†	Cholesterol*	Diabetes*			Physician or Clinic

†Annually after age 50 or age 40 for high risk

Immunizations

Immunizations against communicable diseases are incredible medical achievements. Vaccines are now available to protect against fifteen devastating diseases, illnesses that once left children and adults blind, mentally retarded, sterile, scarred, crippled, or dead. In some cases, immunization programs have been so successful that diseases have been completely eradicated. Smallpox, for instance, is no longer a natural threat in the United States, and today children are not even vaccinated against it. The World Health Organization hopes to eradicate polio worldwide by the end of 2004. Many other diseases, however, still put people at risk. Immunizations against known health risks are important safeguards for yourself, your children, and your grandchildren.

These immunizations are recommended by the American Academy of Pediatrics and the American Academy of Family Physicians. Record the date and place of the immunizations on pages 66–75.

Childhood Immunizations

Parents often wonder if there is any need to immunize their children against diseases that seem to have disappeared. Sometimes parents worry about the safety of vaccines. The reality is that *because* of immunizations many diseases have all but disappeared, but they *haven't* been eradicated. In 1974, many parents in Japan stopped vaccinating their children against pertussis (whooping cough) because only 393 cases were reported, and no deaths occurred. By 1976, only 10 percent of Japanese children were being immunized. In 1979, a major whooping cough outbreak occurred, with 13,000 cases nationwide and 41 deaths. The disease hadn't disappeared; it had just gone underground.

With regard to the safety of vaccines, the most common side effects are sore arms and mild fevers, both of which are temporary. According to the Centers for Disease Control, the risk of death from vaccines is so low that it is hard to assess the risk statistically. On the other hand, the risk of death from measles is one in five hundred; the risk of death from diphtheria is one in twenty. Boys and men who contract mumps have a very serious risk of sterility. One last note: many parents have become alarmed at reports of a possible link between the use of the measles, mumps, rubella vaccine and autism. This possibility was first raised in an article in the British medical journal *The Lancet*, in February 1998. Since then, researchers worldwide have conducted extensive studies to validate or disprove this theory. No evidence at all was found to support the hypothesis that the MMR vaccine causes autism. In March 2004, the authors of the original paper retracted the controversial interpretation of their findings.

MMR: Measles, Mumps, Rubella (German Measles)

The MMR vaccine protects against three highly contagious viruses that can have serious and possibly fatal consequences. The vaccine is given in two series, the first between twelve and fifteen months of age, and the second between four and six years of age. If the second series is missed, it can be given when the child is eleven or twelve years old. It confers lifelong immunity from these diseases:

- Measles—complications from this disease can include ear infections, bronchitis, pneumonia, brain damage, and seizures.

- Mumps—complications from this disease can include deafness, meningitis, inflammations of the testicles or ovaries, sterility in males, and death.

- Rubella (German measles)—can lead to serious birth defects in babies of women who become infected while pregnant.

DTaP: Diphtheria, Tetanus, Pertussis (Whooping Cough)

The DTaP vaccine protects against three bacterial diseases. It is given in five series, the first at two months of age, the second at four months of age, the third at six months of age, the fourth at fifteen to eighteen months of age, and the fifth between four and six years of age. A tetanus/diphtheria (Td) booster should be given every ten years from then on. Immunity to pertussis is lifelong, but tetanus and diphtheria boosters are needed every ten years for life.

DTaP protects against:

- Diphtheria—an infectious disease with complications that can include heart failure, nerve damage, paralysis, kidney damage, and death (in 10 percent of cases).

- Tetanus—an infectious disease caused by exposure to a toxic bacillus (a type of bacteria), that enters the body through a wound, especially punctures and deep lacerations. Complications include muscle spasms and rigidity, such as lockjaw, nerve damage, heart failure, fractures, pneumonia, and death.

- Pertussis (whooping cough)—a highly contagious disease with complications that can include apnea, pneumonia, convulsions, permanent brain damage, nosebleeds, ear infections, bleeding in the brain, permanent seizure disorders, and developmental retardation. The disease can be fatal in children under six months of age.

Pneumococcal Conjugate

Streptococcus pneumoniae is a highly contagious bacterial infection. Complications can include meningitis, blood infections, ear infections, deafness, and brain damage. Children under age two have the highest risk of infection.

The pneumococcal conjugate vaccine confers long-term benefits. It is given in four series, the first at two months of age, the second at four months of age, the third at six months of age, and the fourth at twelve to fifteen months of age. Boosters can be given, per your physician's advice, from two years old on.

HIB: H. Influenza Type B

Haemophilus influenza B is a severe and possibly fatal childhood infection. Complications can include infections of the joints, the bones, and the blood, as well as meningitis and pneumonia.

The vaccine confers long-term protection. It is given in four series, the first at two months of age, the second at four months of age, the third at six months of age, and the fourth at twelve to fifteen months of age.

Hepatitis B

Hepatitis B is a serious infection spread through contact with blood and body fluids of infected people. Mothers can infect their babies during delivery. Complications can include cirrhosis of the liver, liver cancer, chronic liver disease, and death due to chronic infection.

The vaccine confers long-term protection. It is given in three series, the first shortly after birth, the second between two to four months of age, and the third between six and eighteen months of age.

VZV: Varicella (Chicken Pox)

Chicken pox is a highly contagious viral disease. Complications can include birth defects for babies born to infected mothers, encephalitis, Reye's syndrome, pneumonia, heart muscle inflammation, temporary arthritis, and a lifelong risk of shingles.

The vaccine confers long-term immunity. *It is usually given between twelve to eighteen months of age, but can be given any time after that. Individuals over the age of thirteen will need two doses.*

IPV or OPV (Polio)

Poliomyelitis is caused by a contagious viral infection. Complications can include permanent paralysis, fluid in the lungs, pneumonia, high blood pressure, intestinal paralysis, lung paralysis, heart muscle inflammation, and death. Children under age five are most at risk.

Polio vaccine confers lifetime immunity, although boosters may be advised for travel to countries where polio is still found. It is given in four series, the first at two months of age, the second at four months of age, the third between six and eighteen months of age, and the fourth between four and six years of age.

Other Childhood Immunizations That May Be Required

Occasionally, specific immunizations are recommended if a serious health risk exists for a certain segment of the population. For instance, children aged six months to twenty-three months often are at high risk for complications from severe strains of influenza, and may be advised to get the "flu shot" during this time.

Hepatitis A

Hepatitis A is an inflammation of the liver caused by exposure to the virus, usually from contaminated water or food, or by contact with an infected person.

Immunization is recommended where advised by the public health authorities. *Check with your physician as to its need.* It is given in three doses and confers lifetime protection.

Influenza

Influenza is a highly contagious, viral respiratory infection. Complications can include other bacterial infections, pneumonia, and inflammation of the brain.

Immunizations may be recommended for children with medical conditions that increase their risk of complications from the flu. The vaccination confers short-term protection.

Adulthood Immunizations

Many vaccinations we receive as children confer lifetime immunity to diseases, but others wear off over time and need to be supplemented. Other immunizations are required if we missed the vaccination as children, or never contracted the disease. The influenza immunization is needed every year, as the disease itself mutates, mandating a new form of vaccine. The following is a list of immunizations most commonly required by adults.

Rubella (German Measles)

Rubella is a highly contagious viral infection that can lead to serious birth defects in babies of women who become infected while pregnant. *Caution: this vaccination should not be done during pregnancy.*

The vaccine is given once during a woman's childbearing years, if she didn't have an immunization or infection as a child. It confers lifetime protection.

Tetanus-Diphtheria Booster

This booster is needed every ten years to supplement the vaccines given during childhood. It protects against:

- Diphtheria—an infectious bacterial disease. Complications can include heart failure, nerve damage, paralysis, kidney damage, and death (in 10 percent of cases).
- Tetanus—an infectious disease caused by exposure to a toxic bacillus (a type of bacteria) that enters the body through a wound, especially punctures and deep lacerations. Complications include muscle spasms and rigidity, such as lockjaw, nerve damage, heart failure, fractures, pneumonia, and death.

Pneumococcal Polysaccharide

Pneumonia (inflammation of the lungs) can be caused by a fungal, viral, or bacterial infection. There are many kinds of pneumonia, but the one most common in adults is *Streptococcal pneumoniae*. Complications can include meningitis and respiratory failure.

The vaccine is recommended for at risk groups over the age of two, and for all adults over the age of sixty-five. One dose is usually sufficient and confers long-term protection. Discuss your specific needs with your physician.

Meningitis

Meningococcal meningitis is a bacterial infection. Complications can include brain damage, heart muscle inflammation, deafness, paralysis, mental retardation, seizures, strokes, and can be fatal in up to 15 percent of cases.

The vaccine is given once, usually at eighteen years of age, if not earlier, and confers lifelong immunity. Many colleges require incoming freshmen to be vaccinated against meningitis.

Influenza

Influenza is a highly contagious, viral respiratory infection. Complications can include other bacterial infections, pneumonia, and inflammation of the brain.

The vaccination confers short-term protection. Because the most common form of influenza mutates often, rendering the new strains immune to previous vaccines, a new vaccination is required annually, especially for high-risk individuals of any age, and everyone over the age of fifty.

Other Adult Immunizations That May Be Required

Children today routinely are vaccinated against hepatitis B, chicken pox, measles, mumps, and rubella, but if you didn't receive these immunizations and never contracted the disease as a child, you are at high risk for serious complications if you develop the disease as an adult. Adults who contract "childhood" diseases generally become very ill and have a long recovery period. Discuss your immunization requirements with your doctor.

Hepatitis B

Hepatitis B is a serious infection spread through contact with blood and body fluids of infected people. Mothers can infect their babies during delivery. Complications can include cirrhosis of the liver, liver cancer, chronic liver disease, and death due to chronic infection.

The vaccine confers long-term protection and is given in three doses. *It may be recommended up until age twenty-four if the person was not immunized as a child. If you are at risk, your doctor may recommend the immunization after age twenty-five as well.*

VZV: Varicella (Chicken Pox)

Chicken pox is a highly contagious viral disease. Complications can include birth defects for babies born to infected mothers, encephalitis, Reye's syndrome, pneumonia, heart muscle inflammation, temporary arthritis, and a lifelong risk of shingles.

This vaccine may be an option if you weren't immunized and never contracted chicken pox. It confers long-term immunity. Anyone over age thirteen will need two doses.

Lyme Disease

Vaccination against this tick-borne disease may be an option if you live in a high-risk area.

MMR: Measles, Mumps, Rubella (German Measles)

Vaccinations may be recommended if you have no history of infection or immunization. Check with your physician.

CHILDHOOD IMMUNIZATIONS

Age	MMR (Measles, Mumps, Rubella)	DTaP (Diphtheria, Tetanus, Pertussis)	Pneumococcal Conjugate	HIB (H. Influenza Type B)	Hepatitis B	VZV: Varicella (Chicken pox)	IVP or OPV (Polio)
Birth					1st		
1 month							
2 months		1st	1st	1st	2nd		1st
4 months		2nd	2nd	2nd			2nd
6 months		3rd	3rd	3rd	3rd		3rd
9 months							
12 months	1st		4th	4th			
15 months		4th					
18 months							
2			if required				
3							
4	2nd	5th					4th
5							
6							
8							
10							
11, 12	if 2nd series missed	tetanus booster				if not vaccinated or infected	
14							
16							
17							

Shaded areas indicate the recommended time frame for vaccinations.

CHILDHOOD IMMUNIZATIONS

Hepatitis A*	Influenza*					Physician or Clinic

* Where advised by public health authority

ADULT IMMUNIZATIONS

Age	Rubella*	Tetanus-Diphtheria Booster	Pneumococcal Polysaccharide	Meningitis	Influenza— Annually
18	Once				
19				physician/clinic	
20					
21					
22		physician/clinic			
23					
24					
25					
26					
27					
28					
29					
30					
31					
32		physician/clinic			
33					
34					
35					
36					
37					
38					

Shaded areas indicate the recommended time frame for vaccinations.   ** For women of childbearing age, if not already immunized*

ADULT IMMUNIZATIONS

				Physician or Clinic

ADULT IMMUNIZATIONS

Age	Rubella*	Tetanus-Diphtheria Booster	Pneumococcal Polysaccharide	Meningitis	Influenza—Annually
39					
40					
41					
42		physician/clinic			
43					
44					
45					
46					
47					
48					
49					
50					
51					
52		physician/clinic			
53					
54					
55					
56					
57					
58					
59					

Shaded areas indicate the recommended time frame for vaccinations.   ** For women of childbearing age, if not already immunized*

ADULT IMMUNIZATIONS

				Physician or Clinic

ADULT IMMUNIZATIONS

Age	Rubella*	Tetanus-Diphtheria Booster	Pneumococcal Polysaccharide	Meningitis	Influenza— Annually
60					
61		*			
62		physician/clinic			
63					
64					
65			once		
66					
67					
68					
69					
70					
71					
72		physician/clinic			
73					
74					
75					
76					
77					
78					
79					
80					

Shaded areas indicate the recommended time frame for vaccinations.   ** For women of childbearing age, if not already immunized*

ADULT IMMUNIZATIONS

				Physician or Clinic

ADULT IMMUNIZATIONS

Age	Rubella*	Tetanus-Diphtheria Booster	Pneumococcal Polysaccharide	Meningitis	Influenza—Annually
81					
82		physician/clinic			
83					
84					
85					
86					
87					
88					
89					
90					
91					
92		physician/clinic			
93					
94					
95					
96					
97					
98					
99					
100					

Shaded areas indicate the recommended time frame for vaccinations.   * *For women of childbearing age, if not already immunized*

ADULT IMMUNIZATIONS

				Physician or Clinic

NOTES ON TESTS AND IMMUNIZATIONS

Bone Density Screenings

Bone mineral density (BMD) screenings are performed to detect and manage the demineralization of bones, or osteoporosis. Osteoporosis is a serious health risk for postmenopausal women because estrogen, a hormone vital to bone production, is significantly reduced after menopause. Men with certain medical conditions also are at risk. BMD screenings usually are performed with low-dose x-ray machines and are painless. Your doctor will monitor your BMD score and may advise future screenings and/or medications.

Your first bone density scan will be taken as a baseline screening. These measurements will be compared to established standards for bone density based on the age of the person taking the test. Future tests are compared to this baseline screening, to determine the rate of bone loss (if any) and whether the loss is within acceptable standards.

Bone density scans are recommended for the following individuals:

- All women over the age of sixty-five
- All postmenopausal women under age sixty-five who have one or more risk factors for osteoporosis (see "The Bones" in Part Five)
- All postmenopausal women who have ever had a bone fracture
- All women who have taken hormone replacement therapy (HRT) for an extended period of time
- Men with low levels of testosterone

Recommended frequency. Per the advice of your physician.

What your reading means. Screening results are reported as "T scores" and "Z scores." The T score compares your bone density to that of a typical thirty-year-old, while the Z score provides a comparison between your score and that of other people your age, race, and gender. A score of 0 is normal. A score of –1.0 means that your bone mass is 10 percent below normal. A reading of –2.0 means that the bone mass is 20 percent below normal and indicates early stages of osteoporosis. See the section "The Bones" in the Disease Prevention Guide for more information on osteoporosis.

\multicolumn{5}{c}{BONE DENSITY SCREENINGS}
AGE	DATE	PHYSICIAN OR CLINIC	DENSITY READING	COMMENTS

BONE DENSITY SCREENINGS (cont.)

AGE	DATE	PHYSICIAN OR CLINIC	DENSITY READING	COMMENTS

NOTES

Cholesterol Screenings

A cholesterol screening is one way to evaluate your risk of heart disease. Cholesterol is manufactured in the liver and actually is a vital component that the body uses to build cell membranes and synthesize hormones, acids, and vitamin D, but sometimes too much cholesterol accumulates in the arteries. Often this excess cholesterol results from a diet high in saturated fats. (Cholesterol is found in foods of animal origin only, never in fruits, vegetables, or grains.) Excess cholesterol (plaque) lines the walls of your arteries in much the same way that grease coats your kitchen-sink pipes. The more narrow the arteries, the more easily a blood clot or piece of plaque can get stuck, resulting in heart attack or stroke.

A cholesterol screening measures three components:

- LDL (low-density lipoprotein)—the kind of cholesterol that clogs your arteries
- HDL (high-density lipoprotein)—the good factor that takes excess cholesterol to the liver for excretion
- Triglycerides—compounds that move fatty acids through the body; high levels signal danger

The test is performed on a small sample of your blood. The results usually are provided to you by component—LDL, HDL, triglycerides, and total cholesterol. Knowing your numbers and keeping track of them can help you to make any necessary changes to your diet and exercise program. Cholesterol screenings are available at many locations, including your doctor's office, public health departments, and pharmacies.

Recommended frequency. Once every five years until age forty, every two years until age fifty, annually from then on, or per your physician's advice.

	TOTAL CHOLESTEROL		LDL		TRIGLYCERIDES
	Adults (over age 19)	Children (age 2–19)	Adults (over age 19)	Children (age 2–19)	Adults (over age 19)
Desirable	Less than 200 mg/dL*	Less than 170	Less than 130 mg/dL	Less than 110	Less than 150 mg/dL
Borderline high risk	200–239 mg/dL	170–199	130–159 mg/dL	110–129	150–199 mg/dL
High risk	240 mg/dL and over	200 and over	160 mg/dL or higher	130 and over	200–499 mg/dL
Very high risk	240 mg/dL and over	200 and over	160 mg/dL or higher	130 and over	500 mg/dl and over

*mg/dL—milligrams per deciliter

HDL Levels

The higher the HDL number, the better.

Men: Below 40 mg/dL increases your risk of heart disease. Above 60 mg/dL decreases your risk. (Some studies have shown that high doses of therapeutic testosterone, progesterone, and some steroids lower HDL.)

Women: Average 50–60 mg/dL. Estrogen raises HDL. Premenopausal women usually have a low risk of heart disease because of this. However, only your doctor can advise you whether you should take estrogen postmenopause.

Dangerous for men and women: Less than 40 mg/dL.

Cholesterol Ratio

When you have your cholesterol levels checked, your physician may give you a *ratio* of your cholesterol counts. The ratio provides one measurement of your readings but should not serve as a substitute for the individual HDL, LDL, triglycerides, and total cholesterol values. Be sure to ask for those numbers, too. *To calculate your cholesterol ratio, divide your total cholesterol number by the HDL number. For example, a person with a total cholesterol of 200 mg/dL and an HDL* cholesterol level of 50 mg/dL would have a ratio of 4:1. The optimum ratio is 5:1 or less.

Hints for Taking and Tracking Cholesterol Screenings

1. For the most accurate results you should fast for nine to twelve hours before the test. Drink as much water as you like during this time, but caffeinated beverages, such as coffee, tea, and soft drinks can skew the readings.

2. Certain medical conditions and medications can affect the readings. Be sure to discuss your test results with your physician.

3. Track your results in the chart provided below. If your blood is screened more than once a year, divide each age row into two, three, or four parts.

\multicolumn{8}{c	}{CHOLESTEROL SCREENINGS}
AGE	DATE	LDL	HDL	TRIGLYCERIDES	TOTAL CHOLESTEROL	RATIO	PHYSICIAN/ CLINIC
20							
25							
30							
35							
40							
42							
44							
46							
48							
50							
51							
52							
53							
54							
55							
56							
57							
58							
59							
60							

CHOLESTEROL SCREENINGS (cont.)

AGE	DATE	LDL	HDL	TRIGLYCERIDES	TOTAL CHOLESTEROL	RATIO	PHYSICIAN/ CLINIC
61							
62							
63							
64							
65							
66							
67							
68							
69							
70							
71							
72							
73							
74							
75							
76							
77							
78							
79							
80							
81							
82							
83							
84							
85							
86							
87							

CHOLESTEROL SCREENINGS (cont.)

AGE	DATE	LDL	HDL	TRIGLYCERIDES	TOTAL CHOLESTEROL	RATIO	PHYSICIAN/ CLINIC
88							
89							
90							
91							
92							
93							
94							
95							
96							
97							
98							
99							
100							

NOTES

Colon Cancer Screenings

Colon cancer is the second leading cause of cancer deaths in the United States. Some 150,000 cases are diagnosed annually. This disease is completely treatable if caught early, which is the reason colon cancer screenings are so important. There are several kinds of tests available, and your doctor will recommend the one most appropriate for you, based on your health history and risk factors.

The fecal occult blood test and the colonoscopy are standard tests used to screen for precancerous and cancerous conditions in the large intestine and colon. They are especially useful for detecting cancer in its early stages before symptoms begin to display. They are particularly important for individuals with a personal or family history of polyps or colorectal cancer, but are important tests for all adults.

For more information on risk factors, see "The Intestines" in the Disease Prevention Guide. Use the following charts to record the results of your colon cancer screenings.

Fecal Occult Blood Test

The fecal occult blood test is sometimes called a stool guaiac or hemoccult test. This test screens for blood in your stool and is performed by the patient, who collects small stool samples over a three-day period using a kit the doctor provides. The kit is then mailed to the testing laboratory. Detailed instructions on use are provided with the kit. This is a safe, noninvasive test that is quick and easy to do. There are times when the test should not be performed, including:

- If you have an anal fissure or active bleeding from hemorrhoids
- If you are experiencing blood in your urine
- *Women:* during your period or within three days after your period

There can be false positives with this test since blood present in the stool may have come from other sources along the digestive tract, such as an ulcer or because of medications or foods. Speak to your doctor about medications and supplements to avoid and dietary changes to make in the days prior to the test.

Recommended frequency. Test for fecal occult blood every year beginning at age fifty, unless your doctor recommends otherwise.

COLON CANCER SCREENINGS			
AGE	DATE	PHYSICIAN OR CLINIC	COMMENTS
20			
25			
30			
35			
40			
42			
44			
46			

COLON CANCER SCREENINGS (cont.)

AGE	DATE	PHYSICIAN OR CLINIC	COMMENTS
48			
50			
51			
52			
53			
54			
55			
56			
57			
58			
59			
60			
61			
62			
63			
64			
65			
66			
67			
68			
69			
70			
71			
72			
73			
74			

COLON CANCER SCREENINGS (cont.)

AGE	DATE	PHYSICIAN OR CLINIC	COMMENTS
75			
76			
77			
78			
79			
80			
81			
82			
83			
84			
85			
86			
87			
88			
89			
90			
91			
92			
93			
94			
95			
96			
97			
98			
99			
100			

COLONOSCOPY

The colonoscopy checks for bleeding, polyps, inflammatory bowel disease, tumors, or diverticulosis. A colonoscopy is the most efficient method of viewing the entire large intestine (colon). A physician, often a gastroenterologist, using a flexible fiber optic tube with a camera on it, performs the procedure. Preparation for the test requires the complete emptying of the bowel, usually with the help of special laxatives. Because intravenous fluids and sedatives are given during the procedure to ease discomfort, outpatients are required to have someone drive them home. The procedure usually takes less than an hour.

Your doctor will inform you of the test results and the need, if any, for additional exams. *A new "virtual" colonoscopy is available. This test does not use a fiber optic tube and eliminates the need for sedation, but it does require a completely empty bowel.*

Recommended frequency. Have a colonoscopy every ten years after the age of fifty, or per your physician's advice. Most gastroenterologists screen average-risk patients with a colonoscopy every eight to ten years.

If colon cancer has affected a parent or sibling, you should consider having a colonoscopy every five years, beginning ten years younger than the age at which your relative was diagnosed.

COLONOSCOPY

AGE	DATE	PHYSICIAN OR CLINIC	COMMENTS
50			
60			
70			
80			
90			
100			

NOTES

Dental Records and Checkups

Teeth are the hardest structures in the body and serve several important functions. We use teeth to bite and chew our food, thus starting the process of digestion, and, with the tongue, to help us form certain sounds necessary for speech.

Teeth begin to develop when the fetus is six weeks old, although baby teeth usually don't emerge until the baby is four to six months old. Adult teeth begin to emerge when a child is around six years old. Dental care should begin at birth, and regular checkups can help to ensure a lifetime of healthy teeth and gums. See the section on "The Teeth" in the Disease Prevention Guide for more dental-care advice.

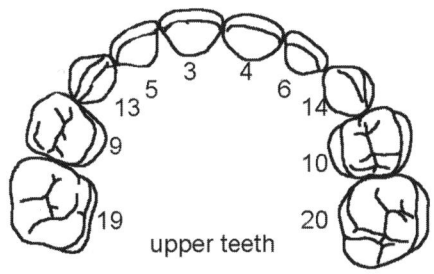
upper teeth

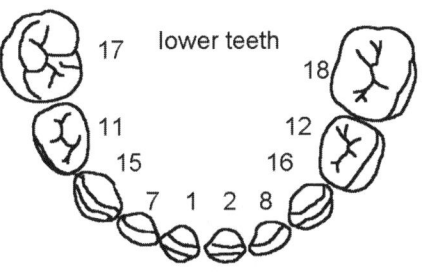
lower teeth

BABY TEETH

Baby Teeth

Use this chart to track the history of your baby teeth. Identify the dates on which each tooth emerged and fell out, as well as any treatment required.

DENTAL RECORDS—BABY TEETH			
TOOTH	EMERGED	LOST	TREATMENT, IF ANY
1			
2			
3			
4			
5			
6			
7			
8			
9			
10			
11			
12			
13			
14			
15			
16			
17			
18			
19			
20			

Permanent Teeth

Use this chart to track the history of your permanent teeth. Identify the date on which each tooth emerged, as well as any treatment required, such as filling, capping, crowning, removal, and so forth.

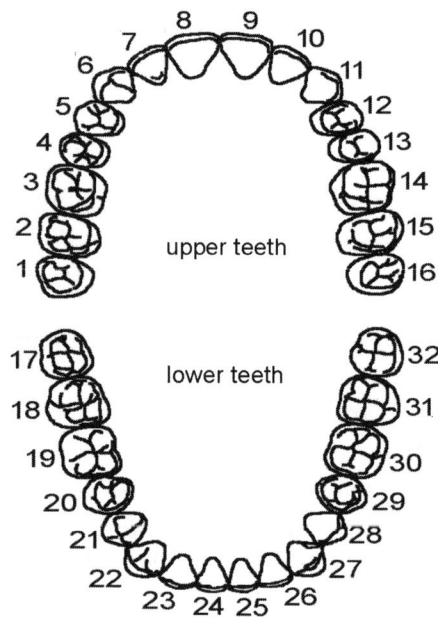

ADULT TEETH

DENTAL RECORDS—PERMANENT TEETH		
TOOTH	EMERGED	TREATMENT, IF ANY
1		
2		
3		
4		
5		
6		
7		
8		
9		
10		
11		
12		
13		
14		
15		
16		
17		
18		
19		
20		

DENTAL RECORDS—PERMANENT TEETH (cont.)

TOOTH	EMERGED	TREATMENT, IF ANY
21		
22		
23		
24		
25		
26		
27		
28		
29		
30		
31		
32		

NOTES

Dental Examinations and Treatments

Use this chart to track dental examinations, x-rays, cleanings, or other general treatments, and any orthodontic, periodontal, or other dental work.

Recommended schedule. Every six months or more frequently, per your dentist's advice.

DENTAL EXAMINATIONS AND TREATMENTS			
AGE	DATE	DENTIST OR CLINIC	COMMENTS/TREATMENT
2			
2.5			
3			
3.5			
4			
4.5			
5			
5.5			
6			
6.5			
7			
7.5			
8			
8.5			
9			
9.5			
10			
10.5			
11			
11.5			
12			
12.5			
13			
13.5			
14			
14.5			
15			
15.5			
16			
16.5			
17			

DENTAL EXAMINATIONS AND TREATMENTS (cont.)

AGE	DATE	DENTIST OR CLINIC	COMMENTS/TREATMENT
17.5			
18			
18.5			
19			
19.5			
20			
20.5			
21			
21.5			
22			
22.5			
23			
23.5			
24			
24.5			
25			
25.5			
26			
26.5			
27			
27.5			
28			
28.5			
29			
29.5			
30			
30.5			
31			
31.5			
32			
32.5			
33			
33.5			
34			
34.5			

DENTAL EXAMINATIONS AND TREATMENTS (cont.)

AGE	DATE	DENTIST OR CLINIC	COMMENTS/TREATMENT
35			
35.5			
36			
36.5			
37			
37.5			
38			
38.5			
39			
39.5			
40			
40.5			
41			
41.5			
42			
42.5			
43			
43.5			
44			
44.5			
45			
45.5			
46			
46.5			
47			
47.5			
48			
48.5			
49			
49.5			
50			
50.5			
51			
51.5			
52			

DENTAL EXAMINATIONS AND TREATMENTS (cont.)

AGE	DATE	DENTIST OR CLINIC	COMMENTS/TREATMENT
52.5			
53			
53.5			
54			
54.5			
55			
55.5			
56			
56.5			
57			
57.5			
58			
58.5			
59			
59.5			
60			
60.5			
61			
61.5			
62			
62.5			
63			
63.5			
64			
64.5			
65			
65.5			
66			
66.5			
67			
67.5			
68			
68.5			
69			
69.5			

DENTAL EXAMINATIONS AND TREATMENTS (cont.)

AGE	DATE	DENTIST OR CLINIC	COMMENTS/TREATMENT
70			
70.5			
71			
71.5			
72			
72.5			
73			
73.5			
74			
74.5			
75			
75.5			
76			
76.5			
77			
77.5			
78			
78.5			
79			
79.5			
80			
80.5			
81			
81.5			
82			
82.5			
83			
83.5			
84			
84.5			
85			
85.5			
86			
86.5			
87			

DENTAL EXAMINATIONS AND TREATMENTS (cont.)

AGE	DATE	DENTIST OR CLINIC	COMMENTS/TREATMENT
87.5			
88			
88.5			
89			
89.5			
90			
90.5			
91			
91.5			
92			
92.5			
93			
93.5			
94			
94.5			
95			
95.5			
96			
96.5			
97			
97.5			
98			
98.5			
99			
99.5			
100			

NOTES

Diabetes Screenings

Diabetes is a lifelong, irreversible condition that results from an imbalance of glucose and insulin. Glucose is a sugar used by the body as fuel. Insulin is a hormone produced by the pancreas to regulate blood sugar amounts. Diabetes can occur when the pancreas does not produce enough insulin, or because the body's cells do not respond properly to insulin. Some people are born with diabetes (type I), but more than 90 percent of diabetics have type II (also know as "adult onset") diabetes, which usually results from obesity and a lack of exercise. Seventeen million Americans are diabetic.

Diabetes screenings are performed to test the levels of glucose in the blood. A fasting glucose test is the most common form and requires the patient to refrain from eating for six hours before the test. A small amount of blood is drawn from a vein in the arm.

Normal values are 64–110 mg/dL (milligrams per deciliter). Results that are higher than this will alert your physician to your increased risk of diabetes.

Recommended frequency. People over age forty-five *who are not at high risk for diabetes* should have their blood glucose levels checked every three years. Anyone at risk for diabetes or gestational (pregnancy) diabetes should have tests more often, according to your doctor's advice. (See "The Pancreas" in the Disease Prevention Guide for risk factors.) Diabetics usually test their own blood glucose levels on a daily basis.

AGE	DATE	PHYSICIAN OR CLINIC	TYPE OF TEST	RESULTS
45				
48				
51				
54				
57				
60				
63				
66				
69				
72				
75				
78				
81				

DIABETES SCREENINGS (cont.)

AGE	DATE	PHYSICIAN OR CLINIC	TYPE OF TEST	RESULTS
84				
87				
90				
93				
96				
99				
100				

NOTES

Eye Medical Records

The eye is an organ that collects light rays and sends them to the brain in the form of electronic messages, which are then converted into pictures.

Regular eye examinations can help to identify and correct vision problems.

Recommended frequency. Eye exams are recommended on the following schedule:

- *From birth to two years*—the pediatrician should do a basic eye exam at each checkup; be sure to mention any family history of vision problems
- *Age two to five*—a more comprehensive exam at age three or as recommended for specific conditions
- *Age six to forty*—once every three years; once every eighteen months if corrective lenses are used
- *Over age forty*—at least once every two years, including a glaucoma test (glaucoma tests should be done more frequently for blacks or anyone with a family history of glaucoma); every eighteen months for contact lenses or glasses, or as recommended for specific conditions.

Eye Conditions and Treatments

Use this chart to track eye conditions. Identify dates of diagnosis or treatment, including laser surgery or other similar surgery.

EYE COLOR: _____

Note: Eye exams are tracked on the examination charts on pages 44–61.

EYE (R OR L)	CONDITION	DATE DIAGNOSED	TREATMENT, IF ANY	PHYSICIAN/ CLINIC
	amblyopia			
	astigmatism			
	cataracts			
	glaucoma			
	hyperopia			
	macular degeneration			
	myopia			
	presbyopia			
	retinitis pigmentosa			
	sarcoidosis			
	strabismus			

Eye Prescriptions

Use this chart to track eye prescriptions for glasses and contact lenses. Identify the date of the prescription, vision, a description of the glasses (progressive lenses, other lens treatments), and brand name of the contact lenses.

EYE PRESCRIPTIONS				
DATE	VISION R	L	GLASSES (REGULAR, BIFOCAL, TRIFOCAL, OR OTHER)	CONTACT LENSES

NOTES

Tests for Men

In addition to the tests recommended for all individuals, men are advised to have regular examinations for testicular and prostate cancer. The good news is that both conditions can be successfully treated if caught early. Tests for both diseases are easy to perform.

Testicular Self-Exam

A monthly testicular self-exam (TSE) is the best way to identify testicular cancer in its earliest stages. This is a risk-free, painless exam that can be life saving and can save fertility. This test is particularly important for men with a history of an undescended testicle. If you had a childhood hernia that was fixed, you will want to check to find out if this was the cause.

How to perform a TSE: Right after a warm shower, when the skin of the scrotum is relaxed, gently roll the testicle between your thumb and fingers, feeling for a small, firm, painless lump or swelling. If you find one, call your doctor right away. Chances are that it is nothing more than a harmless cyst or enlarged blood vessel, but if it is cancer, early treatment is highly successful.

Prostate Exams

Prostate tests are recommended for all men. Prostate cancer is the most common cancer in men (other than skin cancer) and the second leading cause of cancer death in men, after lung cancer. Close to 200,000 new cases are diagnosed each year in the United States. Fortunately, this is a very-slow-growing cancer with an excellent prognosis if caught in time. Physicians routinely perform digital rectal exams at annual physicals because it is easy to feel the outline of an enlarged prostate. Another test, the prostate-specific antigen (PSA) test, has become a standard examination tool, as well. The PSA test has triggered some concerns because it sometimes fails to detect cancers, so it usually is used in conjunction with a digital rectal exam. A new screening test, AMACR, now under study, detects the presence of a specific protein that appears only in cancer cells and has been effective in finding 90 percent of prostate cancers in research subjects.

Treatment of prostate cancers is variable and depends on the stage of the tumor.

Recommended frequency. Annually beginning at age forty for black men and men who have a family history of prostate cancer, and at age fifty for all others.

Annual Prostate-Specific Antigen (PSA) Blood Test

Prostate-specific antigen is a substance found in the blood of all men, but levels are increased in most men with prostate cancer. Although not foolproof, the PSA test can alert your physician to early stages of cancer. The PSA test is performed using a small amount of blood drawn from a vein in the arm. Normal values are less than 4 ng/ml (nanograms per milliliter).

What to look for: Any reading under 4 is generally considered to be good, however, any significant increase from the reading the year before is a warning sign. A reading between 4 and 10 is a sign that all is not right, and a reading over 10 reveals a high risk of cancer. The good news is that prostate cancer grows very slowly and, if caught early, has an excellent prognosis for recovery. *Note: Avoid ejaculation for forty-eight hours before the PSA blood test—it may boost the readings.*

Digital Rectal Exam

A digital rectal exam is the time-tested method of evaluating the condition of the prostate gland. With a gloved finger, your doctor can easily feel the outline of the prostate through the inside wall of your rectum and can tell if it is hardening and/or changing shape, either one of which could indicate cancer. The exam itself takes only seconds. Although mildly uncomfortable, it could save your life.

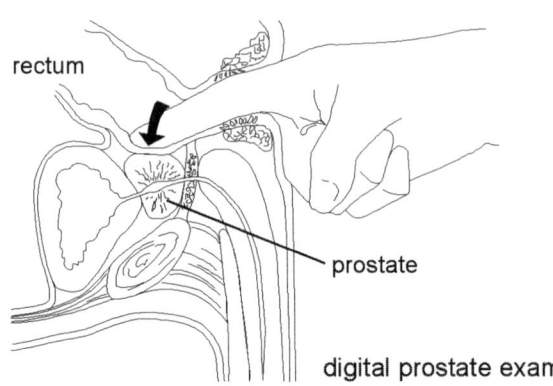

digital prostate exam

PROSTATE EXAMS

AGE	DATE	PHYSICIAN	COMMENTS/PSA READING
40			
41			
42			
43			
44			
45			
46			
47			
48			
49			
50			
51			
52			
53			
54			
55			
56			
57			
58			
59			
60			
61			
62			
63			
64			
65			
66			
67			
68			
69			
70			
71			
72			
73			
74			

PROSTATE EXAMS (cont.)

AGE	DATE	PHYSICIAN	COMMENTS/PSA READING
75			
76			
77			
78			
79			
80			
81			
82			
83			
84			
85			
86			
87			
88			
89			
90			
91			
92			
93			
94			
95			
96			
97			
98			
99			
100			

NOTES

Tests for Women

In addition to the regular tests recommended for everyone, women are advised to have examinations to detect uterine, cervical, and breast cancer at their earliest stages. Some of these tests are self-performed; others require a visit to the doctor or the radiographer. These cancers can be deadly if not caught in time, so be sure to make the examinations priorities. The following pages provide recommended schedules and charts to track your results.

Pap Smears

The *Pap test* is named for its developer, George Papanicolaou. The test evaluates cells scraped from the wall of your cervix, the entrance to the uterus. Pap smears are taken at your doctor's office. The doctor inserts an instrument called a "speculum" (Latin for "observer") into your vagina and uses a small wooden scraper to gently remove some cells from your cervical tissues. A laboratory then performs a microscopic analysis of the cells, looking for abnormalities. A negative result means that no abnormalities were found. If abnormalities are found, your doctor will advise you have another Pap smear, as false positives are not uncommon.

The test is only mildly uncomfortable. With early detection, treatment of problems can begin right away.

Unless you have had a hysterectomy, you should have regular Pap tests and pelvic exams to catch any problems early. If you had a hysterectomy because of cervical cancer, you still need to have Pap smears taken. There is no age limit for Pap smears—you are never too old, even after menopause. The older you get, the greater the risk of developing cervical cancer, especially if you have a history of early age of first intercourse, multiple sexual partners, or infection from HPV.

Note: Have this test when you are not menstruating—ten to twenty days after the first day of your period is best. Avoid douching or using any creams, lotions, foams, and so on (including spermicidal) except as prescribed by your physician, for two days before the Pap smear.

Recommended frequency. Annually beginning at age eighteen, or earlier if sexually active.

PAP SMEARS			
AGE	DATE	PHYSICIAN OR CLINIC	RESULTS/COMMENTS
18			
19			
20			
21			
22			
23			
24			
25			
26			
27			
28			
29			
30			
31			

PAP SMEARS (cont.)

AGE	DATE	PHYSICIAN OR CLINIC	RESULTS/COMMENTS
32			
33			
34			
35			
36			
37			
38			
39			
40			
41			
42			
43			
44			
45			
46			
47			
48			
49			
50			
51			
52			
53			
54			
55			
56			
57			
58			
59			
60			
61			
62			
63			
64			
65			
66			
67			
68			
69			

PAP SMEARS (cont.)

AGE	DATE	PHYSICIAN OR CLINIC	RESULTS/COMMENTS
70			
71			
72			
73			
74			
75			
76			
77			
78			
79			
80			
81			
82			
83			
84			
85			
86			
87			
88			
89			
90			
91			
92			
93			
94			
95			
96			
97			
98			
99			
100			

NOTES

Breast Exams

No one knows your body as you do, and it is absolutely true that a breast lump is clearly distinguishable from the ordinary lumpiness of an average breast. Early detection means early treatment.

Breast Self-Exams

Self-exams find 90 percent of breast lumps, so this easy test can be critical in catching breast cancer early. All women *over age twenty* should perform this test. It is best done in the shower, every month after your period (so the breasts are not swollen or painful).

Mammograms

Mammograms are not the most fun you will have, but they are extremely effective at finding breast cancers in the early stages. Ninety to 95 percent of breast cancers too small to be felt are found through mammography. Mammograms are performed using x-ray equipment. Each breast is compressed onto an x-ray plate and several pictures are taken. The radiographer will notify you and your doctor of the results.

The American Cancer Society recommends that a woman get her first mammogram by age forty, followed by one every one to two years up to age forty-nine, and yearly thereafter, unless you have a family history of breast cancer or other risk factors. Try to go to the same facility each time for better tracking of your history, and make sure that a report is sent to your ob/gyn. Scheduling your annual mammogram about a month before your ob/gyn visit will give your physician the latest information. Many women schedule their annual mammogram on or near their birthday as a healthful present to themselves.

Recommended frequency. Screening recommendations change with every new study on the subject. The best advice on your mammogram schedule will come from your ob/gyn.

AGE	DATE	LOCATION	TECHNICIAN	COMMENTS
40				
41				
42				
43				
44				
45				
46				
47				
48				
49				
50				
51				
52				
53				
54				
55				
56				
57				

BREAST EXAMS (cont.)

AGE	DATE	LOCATION	TECHNICIAN	COMMENTS
58				
59				
60				
61				
62				
63				
64				
65				
66				
67				
68				
69				
70				
71				
72				
73				
74				
75				
76				
77				
78				
79				
80				
81				
82				
83				
84				
85				
86				
87				
88				
89				
90				

BREAST EXAMS (cont.)

AGE	DATE	LOCATION	TECHNICIAN	COMMENTS
91				
92				
93				
94				
95				
96				
97				
98				
99				
100				

Names and Addresses of Mammographers

1. _____

_____

2. _____

_____

3. _____

_____

4. _____

_____

NOTES

Menstrual Record

Menstruation is a perfectly normal event in the lives of most women. Because a certain amount of body fat is necessary to sustain a healthy pregnancy, menstruation begins when a girl weighs about 100 pounds, usually around age twelve or thirteen, although some girls begin to menstruate much earlier or later. (Because early menstruation is a risk factor for breast and uterine cancer, these women should be extra vigilant about Pap smears and mammograms.)

Menstruation usually occurs every twenty-eight to thirty days, although in the early years periods are apt to be erratic. A period typically lasts three to seven days, often starting off light, gradually getting heavier on the second and third days, and then tapering off. Some women experience cramping, clotting, flooding, water gain, breast tenderness, headaches, mood swings, acne, and bursts of energy before and during their periods. Menstruation stops during pregnancy and menopause. Other reasons why you might miss periods include extreme weight loss, high-intensity exercise programs, obesity, stress, and endocrine disorders (such as thyroid disease). Changes in your cycle are important indicators of your overall health, and your doctor will usually want to know the date of your last period at medical checkups.

Use this chart to comment on unusually heavy or light flow, clotting, cramping or pain, other symptoms, medications, or treatments used, if any.

MENSTRUAL RECORD		
DATE PERIOD STARTED	DATE PERIOD ENDED	COMMENTS

MENSTRUAL RECORD

DATE PERIOD STARTED	DATE PERIOD ENDED	COMMENTS

MENSTRUAL RECORD

DATE PERIOD STARTED	DATE PERIOD ENDED	COMMENTS

MENSTRUAL RECORD

DATE PERIOD STARTED	DATE PERIOD ENDED	COMMENTS

MENSTRUAL RECORD		
DATE PERIOD STARTED	DATE PERIOD ENDED	COMMENTS

MENSTRUAL RECORD

DATE PERIOD STARTED	DATE PERIOD ENDED	COMMENTS

MENSTRUAL RECORD		
DATE PERIOD STARTED	**DATE PERIOD ENDED**	**COMMENTS**

MENSTRUAL RECORD

DATE PERIOD STARTED	DATE PERIOD ENDED	COMMENTS

MENSTRUAL RECORD		
DATE PERIOD STARTED	DATE PERIOD ENDED	COMMENTS

MENSTRUAL RECORD

DATE PERIOD STARTED	DATE PERIOD ENDED	COMMENTS

MENSTRUAL RECORD

DATE PERIOD STARTED	DATE PERIOD ENDED	COMMENTS

MENSTRUAL RECORD

DATE PERIOD STARTED	DATE PERIOD ENDED	COMMENTS

MENSTRUAL RECORD		
DATE PERIOD STARTED	DATE PERIOD ENDED	COMMENTS

MENSTRUAL RECORD

DATE PERIOD STARTED	DATE PERIOD ENDED	COMMENTS

MENSTRUATION NOTES

ADDITIONAL NOTES

PART THREE

HEALTHCARE PROVIDERS

Today's society is increasingly mobile. People are constantly relocating, changing insurance companies, adding and replacing physicians, and consulting specialists. Use this section for recording the names, addresses, and dates of service for doctors, dentists, ophthalmologists, and other healthcare providers and insurance companies.

Physicians

Family Practice, Obstetrics and Gynecology, and Specialists

Name_____

Address_____

Clinic or Hospital_____

Telephone_____ Fax_____

Dates of Service *from* _____ *to* _____

Type of Practice_____

Name_____

Address_____

Clinic or Hospital_____

Telephone_____ Fax_____

Dates of Service *from* _____ *to* _____

Type of Practice_____

Family Practice, Obstetrics and Gynecology, and Specialists (cont.)

Name _____

Address _____

Clinic or Hospital _____

Telephone _____ Fax _____

Dates of Service *from* _____ *to* _____

Type of Practice _____

Name _____

Address _____

Clinic or Hospital _____

Telephone _____ Fax _____

Dates of Service *from* _____ *to* _____

Type of Practice _____

Name _____

Address _____

Clinic or Hospital _____

Telephone _____ Fax _____

Dates of Service *from* _____ *to* _____

Type of Practice _____

Name _____

Address _____

Clinic or Hospital _____

Telephone _____ Fax _____

Dates of Service *from* _____ *to* _____

Type of Practice _____

Family Practice, Obstetrics and Gynecology, and Specialists (cont.)

Name _____

Address _____

Clinic or Hospital _____

Telephone _____ Fax _____

Dates of Service *from* _____ *to* _____

Type of Practice _____

Name _____

Address _____

Clinic or Hospital _____

Telephone _____ Fax _____

Dates of Service *from* _____ *to* _____

Type of Practice _____

Name _____

Address _____

Clinic or Hospital _____

Telephone _____ Fax _____

Dates of Service *from* _____ *to* _____

Type of Practice _____

Name _____

Address _____

Clinic or Hospital _____

Telephone _____ Fax _____

Dates of Service *from* _____ *to* _____

Type of Practice _____

Family Practice, Obstetrics and Gynecology, and Specialists (cont.)

Name _____

Address _____

Clinic or Hospital _____

Telephone _____ Fax _____

Dates of Service *from* _____ *to* _____

Type of Practice _____

Name _____

Address _____

Clinic or Hospital _____

Telephone _____ Fax _____

Dates of Service *from* _____ *to* _____

Type of Practice _____

Name _____

Address _____

Clinic or Hospital _____

Telephone _____ Fax _____

Dates of Service *from* _____ *to* _____

Type of Practice _____

Name _____

Address _____

Clinic or Hospital _____

Telephone _____ Fax _____

Dates of Service *from* _____ *to* _____

Type of Practice _____

Dentists

Dentists, Orthodontists, Endodontists, and Periodontists

Name _____

Address _____

Clinic or Hospital _____

Telephone _____ Fax _____

Dates of Service from _____ to _____

Type of Practice _____

Name _____

Address _____

Clinic or Hospital _____

Telephone _____ Fax _____

Dates of Service from _____ to _____

Type of Practice _____

Name _____

Address _____

Clinic or Hospital _____

Telephone _____ Fax _____

Dates of Service from _____ to _____

Type of Practice _____

Dentists, Orthodontists, Endodontists, and Periodontists (cont.)

Name _____

Address _____

Clinic or Hospital _____

Telephone _____ Fax _____

Dates of Service *from* _____ *to* _____

Type of Practice _____

Name _____

Address _____

Clinic or Hospital _____

Telephone _____ Fax _____

Dates of Service *from* _____ *to* _____

Type of Practice _____

Name _____

Address _____

Clinic or Hospital _____

Telephone _____ Fax _____

Dates of Service *from* _____ *to* _____

Type of Practice _____

Name _____

Address _____

Clinic or Hospital _____

Telephone _____ Fax _____

Dates of Service *from* _____ *to* _____

Type of Practice _____

Dentists, Orthodontists, Endodontists, and Periodontists (cont.)

Name _____

Address _____

Clinic or Hospital _____

Telephone _____ Fax _____

Dates of Service *from* _____ *to* _____

Type of Practice _____

Name _____

Address _____

Clinic or Hospital _____

Telephone _____ Fax _____

Dates of Service *from* _____ *to* _____

Type of Practice _____

Name _____

Address _____

Clinic or Hospital _____

Telephone _____ Fax _____

Dates of Service *from* _____ *to* _____

Type of Practice _____

Name _____

Address _____

Clinic or Hospital _____

Telephone _____ Fax _____

Dates of Service *from* _____ *to* _____

Type of Practice _____

Eye-Care Specialists

Ophthalmologists, Optometrists, and Opticians

Name _____

Address _____

Clinic or Hospital _____

Telephone _____ Fax _____

Dates of Service *from* _____ *to* _____

Type of Practice _____

Name _____

Address _____

Clinic or Hospital _____

Telephone _____ Fax _____

Dates of Service *from* _____ *to* _____

Type of Practice _____

Name _____

Address _____

Clinic or Hospital _____

Telephone _____ Fax _____

Dates of Service *from* _____ *to* _____

Type of Practice _____

Ophthalmologists, Optometrists, and Opticians (cont.)

Name _____

Address _____

Clinic or Hospital _____

Telephone _____ Fax _____

Dates of Service *from* _____ *to* _____

Type of Practice _____

Name _____

Address _____

Clinic or Hospital _____

Telephone _____ Fax _____

Dates of Service *from* _____ *to* _____

Type of Practice _____

Name _____

Address _____

Clinic or Hospital _____

Telephone _____ Fax _____

Dates of Service *from* _____ *to* _____

Type of Practice _____

Name _____

Address _____

Clinic or Hospital _____

Telephone _____ Fax _____

Dates of Service *from* _____ *to* _____

Type of Practice _____

Ophthalmologists, Optometrists, and Opticians (cont.)

Name _____

Address _____

Clinic or Hospital _____

Telephone _____ Fax _____

Dates of Service from _____ to _____

Type of Practice _____

Name _____

Address _____

Clinic or Hospital _____

Telephone _____ Fax _____

Dates of Service from _____ to _____

Type of Practice _____

Name _____

Address _____

Clinic or Hospital _____

Telephone _____ Fax _____

Dates of Service from _____ to _____

Type of Practice _____

Name _____

Address _____

Clinic or Hospital _____

Telephone _____ Fax _____

Dates of Service from _____ to _____

Type of Practice _____

Other Practitioners

Chiropractors, Physical Therapists, and Other Practitioners

Name _____

Address _____

Clinic or Hospital _____

Telephone _____ Fax _____

Dates of Service *from* _____ *to* _____

Type of Practice _____

Name _____

Address _____

Clinic or Hospital _____

Telephone _____ Fax _____

Dates of Service *from* _____ *to* _____

Type of Practice _____

Name _____

Address _____

Clinic or Hospital _____

Telephone _____ Fax _____

Dates of Service *from* _____ *to* _____

Type of Practice _____

Chiropractors, Physical Therapists, and Other Practitioners (cont.)

Name _____

Address _____

Clinic or Hospital _____

Telephone _____ Fax _____

Dates of Service *from* _____ *to* _____

Type of Practice _____

Name _____

Address _____

Clinic or Hospital _____

Telephone _____ Fax _____

Dates of Service *from* _____ *to* _____

Type of Practice _____

Name _____

Address _____

Clinic or Hospital _____

Telephone _____ Fax _____

Dates of Service *from* _____ *to* _____

Type of Practice _____

Name _____

Address _____

Clinic or Hospital _____

Telephone _____ Fax _____

Dates of Service *from* _____ *to* _____

Type of Practice _____

Chiropractors, Physical Therapists, and Other Practitioners (cont.)

Name _____

Address _____

Clinic or Hospital _____

Telephone _____ Fax _____

Dates of Service *from* _____ *to* _____

Type of Practice _____

Name _____

Address _____

Clinic or Hospital _____

Telephone _____ Fax _____

Dates of Service *from* _____ *to* _____

Type of Practice _____

Name _____

Address _____

Clinic or Hospital _____

Telephone _____ Fax _____

Dates of Service *from* _____ *to* _____

Type of Practice _____

Name _____

Address _____

Clinic or Hospital _____

Telephone _____ Fax _____

Dates of Service *from* _____ *to* _____

Type of Practice _____

Insurance Companies

Name of Company _____

Policy # _____ Group # _____

Address _____

Telephone _____ Fax _____

Dates of Coverage _____ Services Covered: _____ Medical _____ Dental _____ Eye care

Employer _____ If COBRA, dates of coverage _____

Name of Company _____

Policy # _____ Group # _____

Address _____

Telephone _____ Fax _____

Dates of Coverage _____ Services Covered: _____ Medical _____ Dental _____ Eye care

Employer _____ If COBRA, dates of coverage _____

Name of Company _____

Policy # _____ Group # _____

Address _____

Telephone _____ Fax _____

Dates of Coverage _____ Services Covered: _____ Medical _____ Dental _____ Eye care

Employer _____ If COBRA, dates of coverage _____

Name of Company _____

Policy # _____ Group # _____

Address _____

Telephone _____ Fax _____

Dates of Coverage _____ Services Covered: _____ Medical _____ Dental _____ Eye care

Employer _____ If COBRA, dates of coverage _____

Insurance Companies (cont.)

Name of Company _____

Policy # _____ Group # _____

Address _____

Telephone _____ Fax _____

Dates of Coverage _____ Services Covered: _____ Medical _____ Dental _____ Eye care

Employer _____ If COBRA, dates of coverage _____

Name of Company _____

Policy # _____ Group # _____

Address _____

Telephone _____ Fax _____

Dates of Coverage _____ Services Covered: _____ Medical _____ Dental _____ Eye care

Employer _____ If COBRA, dates of coverage _____

Name of Company _____

Policy # _____ Group # _____

Address _____

Telephone _____ Fax _____

Dates of Coverage _____ Services Covered: _____ Medical _____ Dental _____ Eye care

Employer _____ If COBRA, dates of coverage _____

Name of Company _____

Policy # _____ Group # _____

Address _____

Telephone _____ Fax _____

Dates of Coverage _____ Services Covered: _____ Medical _____ Dental _____ Eye care

Employer _____ If COBRA, dates of coverage _____

Medicare/Medicaid Information

Name of Beneficiary _____

Medicare Claim Number _____ Sex: _____ M _____ F

Entitlements _____

Effective Date _____

Hospital (Part A) _____

Medical (Part B) _____

N O T E S

Definitions of Medical Practices and Practitioners

Advanced Practice Nurse (A.P.N.)—A nurse who has advanced education or experience in special areas.

Anesthesiologist—A doctor trained to deliver anesthesia for pain control or for surgery. General anesthesia puts the patient to sleep, while spinal block numbs part of the body but leaves the patient conscious. Local anesthesia is a painkiller used at the treatment site. The patient remains awake and alert during the procedure.

Cardiologist—A doctor specializing in treating disorders of the heart and circulatory system.

Certified Nurse Midwife (C.N.M.)—A registered nurse with advanced training in areas of women's health, including prenatal, labor and delivery, and postpartum care.

Certified Registered Nurse Anesthetist (C.R.N.A.)—A registered nurse with special training in anesthesiology.

Chiropractor—A therapist specializing in treatment of skeletal and muscular disorders by manipulating the spine, joints, and muscles back into proper alignment.

Clinical Nurse Specialist (C.N.S.)—A registered nurse with special training in clinical areas such as community health, cardiology, or psychiatry.

Dentist—A licensed practitioner who prevents, diagnoses, and treats diseases and injuries to the teeth, jaws, and mouth.

Dermatologist—A doctor specializing in treating disorders of the skin.

Endocrinologist—A doctor specializing in treating disorders of the hormones and the metabolic endocrine system.

Family Practitioner—A doctor specializing in general family care for patients of all ages.

Gastroenterologist—A doctor specializing in treating disorders of the digestive system, including the esophagus, stomach, and intestines.

Generalist—A doctor of medicine (M.D.) or a doctor of osteopathic medicine (D.O.) who specializes in internal medicine or family practice.

Gynecologist—A doctor specializing in treating the female reproductive tract; usually also practices obstetrics, in which case the doctor is called an obstetrician–gynecologist (ob/gyn).

Homeopath—A practitioner who treats diseases by stimulating the body's defense system. This is done by prescribing small amounts of substances that normally cause the symptoms being experienced by the patient, in order to build the body's resistance.

Immunologist—A doctor specializing in treatment of allergies and disorders of the immune system.

Intern—A physician who has graduated from medical school and is working under supervision in a hospital to gain required practical experience.

Internist—A doctor who specializes in internal medicine but does not perform surgery.

Licensed Practical Nurse (L.P.N.)—A caregiver for the sick who has been trained and licensed by the state.

Medical Doctor (M.D.)—A doctor who has graduated from medical school and is licensed to practice medicine.

Naturopath—A practitioner who prefers to treat conditions with natural agents and without drugs or surgery.

Nephrologist—A doctor specializing in diseases affecting the kidneys.

Neurologist—A doctor specializing in treating disorders of the nervous system.

Nurse Practitioner (N.P.)—A registered nurse with special training in primary care; for example, Geriatric Nurse Practitioner (G.N.P.), Adult Nurse Practitioner (A.N.P.), Pediatric Nurse Practitioner (P.N.P.), and Family Nurse Practitioner (F.N.P.). Some states allow nurse practitioners to write prescriptions.

Obstetrician—A doctor who treats women during pregnancy and delivers babies; usually also practices gynecology, in which case the doctor is called an obstetrician–gynecologist (ob/gyn).

Oncologist—A doctor specializing in the treatment of cancer.

Ophthalmologist—A doctor specializing in the treatment of eye disorders, including surgery.

Orthodontist—A dentist specializing in preventing or correcting irregularities of the teeth.

Orthopedist—A doctor specializing in treating disorders of bones and connective tissues.

Osteopath (D.O.)—A doctor of osteopathic medicine incorporates joint and spinal manipulations into a standard medical practice for a holistic approach to healing.

Otorhinolaryngologist—A doctor specializing in treatments of ENT (ear, nose, and throat) disorders.

Pediatrician—A doctor specializing in the treatment of young children.

Periodontist—A dentist specializing in treating disorders of the gums.

Physical Therapist—A specialist in techniques designed to restore normal function to injured muscles, joints, and bones.

Physician Assistant (P.A.)—A specially trained and certified individual who is allowed to provide basic medical services under the supervision of a licensed doctor.

Psychiatrist—A doctor specializing in the treatment of mental or emotional disorders.

Psychologist—A provider of clinical psychology services, such as counseling or guidance. A psychologist does not have a license to prescribe medications.

Radiologist—A doctor with specialized training in using radiology for diagnosis or treatment of various conditions.

Registered Nurse (R.N.)—A board-certified and state-licensed graduate of a nursing program.

Rehabilitative Therapist—A specialist in techniques designed to restore normal function to areas affected by injury, stroke, or illness.

Rheumatologist—A doctor specializing in the treatment of disorders of the joints and muscles.

Surgeon—A doctor with special training in performing surgical operations to treat or repair specific conditions.

Urologist—A doctor specializing in the treatment of disorders of the male and female urinary tracts, and the male reproductive tract.

PART FOUR

THE IMPORTANCE OF NUTRIENTS

Food is a basic necessity of life because it contains all of the components our bodies need to sustain life. These components, called "nutrients," are proteins, carbohydrates, fats, vitamins, and minerals. The body uses these nutrients to perform an amazing series of multifaceted and interactive chemical processes. As with any piece of intricate machinery—*and the body is one of the most complex*—the fuel mixture needs to be rather precise. Lack of specific nutrients, or too much of one or more, can upset this delicate balance. This section provides specific information on the vitamins and minerals you need to stay healthy for life.

Vitamins, Minerals, and Trace Elements

Vitamins and minerals are called "coenzymes" because they assist the body's own enzymes in performing thousands of functions. For instance, iron and vitamin A assist the body in the production of red blood cells. A deficiency of iron or vitamin A won't halt the production of red blood cells entirely, but the quantity will decline, possibly leading to anemia.

For the most part, a balanced diet will provide all the necessary vitamins and minerals, including trace elements, which are minerals the body requires in very small amounts. Occasionally, eating a balanced diet is not possible for one reason or another. Diseases, fad diets, stress, and poverty are major causes of malnutrition. For these and other reasons, nutritional supplements may be necessary.

The information that follows this introduction is divided into three sections: Vitamins, Minerals, and Trace Elements. Each contains descriptions of specific nutrients, their contribution to the body's functions, recommended dietary allowances (RDAs), food sources, deficiency risks, overdosing risks, and special concerns for people with specific health conditions.

Vitamins

Cells need vitamins to help them perform necessary metabolic work. Some vitamins may help prevent such diseases as cancer, cataracts, arthritis, and heart disease. The body does not produce vitamins, which must be obtained from food or supplements or, in the case of vitamin D, converted from sunshine.

While vitamin supplements are useful, fresh foods contain the most vitamins. The longer food sits at the store, in the truck, or in your refrigerator, the more its vitamin content degrades. When out-of-season food shows up in your grocery store, remember that it has had to travel a long way, so the frozen variety is probably a better choice because it was frozen shortly after being picked. Since boiling water destroys or releases vitamins, remember to use the smallest amount of water possible when cooking, and cook for the least amount of time necessary. Steaming vegetables is a great option. If you must boil food, consider saving the water in a freezer-safe jar to use at another time in soups or stews.

Minerals

Minerals are chemical elements required by our bodies for numerous biological and physiological processes that are necessary for the maintenance of health.

—*USFDA Center for Food Safety and Applied Nutrition, March, 1999*

Minerals commonly considered to be vital to our health include calcium, magnesium, phosphorus, sodium, potassium, sulfur, and chloride. A balanced diet will provide the recommended dietary allowance for some of these minerals. Sodium, sulfur, and chloride are usually found naturally in foods by way of the soil in which they are grown or the water supply. Additional salt (sodium chloride) often is added during food processing. Calcium and magnesium can be found in water, but the amounts usually are negligible. Calcium, magnesium, phosphorus, and potassium are all found in foods, but most of us need to supplement our intake of calcium and magnesium.

Trace Elements

Trace elements are minerals for which the daily requirement is less than 100 milligrams. Trace elements that are considered to be vital to our health include copper, chromium, iodine, iron, manganese, molybdenum, selenium, and zinc. A balanced diet generally provides the recommended dietary allowance for these minerals. Malnutrition poses a serious risk for iron and iodine deficiencies, though. Supplements for all of these minerals are available, if necessary.

Who Needs Vitamins and Minerals?

Everyone needs vitamins and minerals, especially the elderly, pregnant or nursing women, individuals under stress, dieters, and anyone taking cortisone or antibiotics.

This doesn't mean that you need to take vitamin pills, however. If you are eating a healthful diet, you are probably getting enough vitamins and minerals from your food. Each section on vitamins contains a list of food sources, for your information.

If you are in one of the above-mentioned categories, though, you may have medical conditions that mandate consumption of supplements. Some medical conditions affect the way vitamins in foods and supplements are absorbed and/or used by the body. It's also important to note that certain medications have serious interactions with vitamins and minerals.

Be sure to discuss your nutritional requirements with your doctor(s), and monitor your own body's responses and reactions. Follow your doctor's advice!

Note: Where specific benefits and dangers have been established, they are listed with each vitamin, mineral, or element. Many studies about potential benefits of supplementation for other health conditions are ongoing. Until the benefits are accepted by the medical and scientific communities they have not been included here. Please visit www.healthwatchguide.com for updates.

Using Vitamins and Minerals

Most of us take a multivitamin with a meal, usually breakfast. This may or may not be a good idea. Refer to the sections on specific vitamins and minerals for precise guidelines, but here are some general tips:

- Some B-vitamin supplements must be taken with food in order to be properly absorbed.
- Vitamin B_1 may be inactivated if taken with coffee and tea (including decaffeinated varieties).
- Too much corn in the diet can cause a vitamin B_3 deficiency.
- Large doses of folic acid may hide a vitamin B_{12} deficiency.
- Vitamin C and calcium are best absorbed when taken in several doses throughout the day.
- Vitamin E is best absorbed when taken with food.
- Fluoride-supplement absorption is decreased when taken with calcium supplements and certain antacids.
- Iron absorption is enhanced when taken with vitamin C.
- Light-colored juices enhance iron absorption. Tea and dark-colored juices inhibit iron absorption, prune juice being the exception to the rule.

Vitamin and Mineral Intake

Just how much of a specific nutrient your body needs to perform at its best is a very interesting question. The answer depends on any number of variables: your sex, weight, age, exercise regimen, fluid intake, and health. Most of us seem to get along fairly well by following commonsense advice regarding our daily diets, but having some idea of the necessary quantities of specific nutrients can be very useful. The Food and Nutrition Board of the National Academy of Sciences has developed a set of guidelines for daily vitamin and mineral intake. These guidelines are designed for the average individual, and your specific requirements may vary, so be sure to discuss your nutritional needs with your doctor.

Recommended Dietary Allowance (RDA)

Dietary reference intakes (DRIs) are reference values used for planning and assessing diets for healthy people. The recommended dietary allowance (RDA), one of the DRIs, recommends the average daily dietary intake level that is sufficient to meet the nutrient requirements of nearly all healthy individuals (97 to 98 percent) in each age and gender group. In *most* cases, nursing infants are assumed to be getting specific amounts of recommended nutrients from breast milk.

Adequate Intake (AI)

Adequate intakes are values assigned where enough research has been done on a nutrient to understand that it plays an important role in life functions, but where more information is needed for specificity.

For instance, many indicated amounts for infants are shown as adequate intakes, assuming that the baby is getting most, if not all, of its nourishment from the mother's breast milk. Formulas and processed baby foods *usually* contain vitamins and minerals to meet the AI levels.

Each section on vitamins and minerals has a chart identifying the RDA or AI for various groups of people. Values shown are from the Food and Nutrition Board of the National Academy of Sciences. For more information visit www.nap.edu.

Food Sources

Many foods naturally contain the vitamins and minerals we need. Each section on vitamins and minerals contains a list of foods containing these nutrients. Food values vary by food type and quantity. For more information on specific foods, check food package labels or go to http://dietary-supplements.info.nih.gov

Vitamin Deficiency

What if you don't get enough of a particular vitamin? This can happen for a number of reasons, such as poor nutrition or illness. Although symptoms of vitamin deficiency vary, three common symptoms are fatigue, irritability, and anxiety. Since these can also be symptoms of many other conditions, it is a good idea to talk to your doctor before self-medicating with vitamin supplements. Vitamin deficiency can result from:

- Excessive coffee drinking.
- Alcohol use and birth control pills. Talk to your doctor about your vitamin requirements.
- Vegetarian diets. Vegetarians, especially vegans, may not get enough of vitamins A, B_{12}, and D, or minerals such as phosphorus, iodine, iron, and zinc, even with an otherwise healthful diet.
- Malabsorption syndrome. This is a condition that results from diseases that inhibit the body's ability to absorb nutrients in the digestive tract. Cystic fibrosis is the leading cause of malabsorption in the United States. Other causes include abetalipoproteinenemia, acrodermatitis enteropathica, biliary atresia, bovine lactalbumin intolerance, celiac disease, lactose intolerance, parasites such as *Giardia*, threadworm, and hookworm, Schwachman-Diamond syndrome, soy milk protein intolerance, sprue, and Whipple disease. Symptoms of malabsorption syndrome include diarrhea, frequent bulky stools, a distended abdomen, and failure to thrive.

Vitamin Overdosing

Consumption of too many vitamins carries serious risks. Some vitamins can be toxic if overconsumed.

Don't exceed the recommended RDA except under a doctor's supervision. Remember that you are consuming vitamins and minerals in the food you eat, in addition to any supplements you take. The Food and Nutrition Board has established the upper limits shown on each chart. No adverse effects have been found when consumption of the supplement remains at that level or below. In some cases, no upper limits have been established, in which case no upper limit is shown on the chart.

Who Should Take Special Note of Their Intake?

Medical conditions and/or the medications used for treatment can affect the way the body is able to absorb vitamins and minerals. If you are taking any medicine, especially prescriptions, for an extended period, be sure to discuss your nutritional needs with your doctor.

Definitions of Terms

Fat-soluble vitamins—stored in the body for use as needed. Using olive oil in cooking increases their absorption.

Water-soluble vitamins—not stored in the body, so it is important to try to get the recommended dietary allowance in food or supplement form.

IU	international units
mcg or μ	micrograms
g	grams
mg	milligrams
RE	retinol equivalents
alpha-TE	alpha-tocopherol equivalent

1,000 milligrams (mg) = 1 gram (g)
1,000,000 micrograms (mcg or μ) = 1 gram (g)
1,000 micrograms (mcg or μ) = 1 milligram (mg)

VITAMINS

Vitamin A

Vitamin A is a fat-soluble vitamin stored in the liver. The body acquires vitamin A in several ways. For instance, some plant foods have very dark pigments called provitamin A carotenoids. The body can easily convert these carotenoids to vitamin A. Beta-carotene is the carotenoid that converts the most efficiently. Beta-carotene is a natural antioxidant that helps fight cancer and heart disease. The body also acquires the vitamin from foods containing retinol, also known as preformed vitamin A. Retinol is found in foods such as whole milk, liver, and whole eggs.

Necessary For

Vitamin A is required for normal vision, healthy skin, teeth, hair, bone growth, reproduction, red blood cell development, brain development, embryonic development, regulating the immune system, and night vision. Vitamin A contributes to the health of mucous membranes, which fight off bacterial infection in the mouth, urinary tract, respiratory system, and intestinal tract.

		RECOMMENDED DIETARY ALLOWANCES			
		PER DAY		UPPER LIMITS**	
		RE or MCG	IU	RE or MCG	IU
Infants (assumes breastfeeding)	0–6 months	400*	1,330	600	2,000
	7–12 months	500*	1,665	600	2,000
Children	1–3 years	300	1,000	600	2,000
	4–8 years	400	1,333	900	3,000
	9–13 years	600	2,000	1,700	5,665
Males	14–18 years	900	3,000	2,800	9,335
	19 years and up	900	3,000	3,000	10,000
Females	14–18 years	700	2,330	2,800	9,335
	19 years and up	700	2,330	3,000	10,000
Pregnancy	Up to 18 years	750	2,500	2,800	9,335
	19 years and up	770	2,565	3,000	10,000
Nursing	Up to 18 years	1,200	4,000	2,800	9,335
	19 years and up	1,300	4,335	3,000	10,000

*Adequate intake

**No adverse effects shown below these levels

Notes: RE stands for retinol equivalent. 1 RE = 1 microgram (mcg or μ) of retinol. 1 RE of vitamin A = 3.33 units of retinol and 10 units of beta-carotene.

There usually is no reason to take separate vitamin A supplements.

Vitamin A Cautions

Too much vitamin A from supplements (more than 10,000 IU daily) can lead to vitamin A toxicity. And while vitamin A has been shown to be an effective agent in controlling acne, at very high doses medicines containing vitamin A can be toxic. They also can cause birth defects: it is very important that women of childbearing age who use acne treatments containing retinoids take effective precautions against pregnancy.

No RDA guidelines have been established for beta-carotene intake. And research does not indicate that beta-carotene supplements are effective in reducing cancer risk. However, research indicates that eating 3–6 mg (3,000–6,000 mcg) daily of beta-carotene-rich foods will maintain healthful, disease-resistant blood plasma levels. Five or more daily servings of produce, including deep yellow and orange fruits and dark green, leafy vegetables, will provide an adequate amount of beta-carotene. Beta-carotene supplements (pills, capsules, or tablets) are advised *only* when they are necessary for individuals at risk of vitamin A deficiency.

Other Vitamin A Notes

The body requires an adequate supply of protein, calories, and zinc in order to manufacture retinol binding protein, which is required to transport vitamin A from the liver to the rest of the body. Iron deficiency also can limit vitamin A production.

Food Sources

Animal sources of vitamin A are well absorbed and used efficiently by the body, but too much vitamin A from these sources, especially liver and fish oils, can be dangerous. Foods include beef liver, cheddar cheese, cheese pizza, chicken liver, cod and halibut fish oils, egg substitute (fortified), milk (fortified), Swiss cheese, whole egg, and yogurt.

Plant sources of vitamin A (beta-carotene) are not as well absorbed by the body as animal sources. You can't be harmed by eating too many of these, although your skin may temporarily turn yellow! Five or more daily servings will provide an adequate amount of beta-carotene. Foods include apricots, apricot nectar, asparagus, breakfast cereal (fortified), broccoli, butternut squash, cantaloupe, carrots, carrot juice, collard greens, dandelion greens, garden cress, Hubbard squash, kale, lamb's quarters (a plant), mango, oatmeal (instant, fortified), oranges, orange juice, papaya, parsley, peaches, pumpkin, spinach, sweet potato, sweet red pepper, tomatoes, tomato juice, vegetable soup, and violet leaves.

Vitamin A Deficiency Risks

Lack of this vitamin is a major cause of xerophthalmia (corneal damage). Hundreds of thousands of children around the world still go blind from lack of vitamin A.

Symptoms of vitamin A deficiency include night blindness, dry skin, dry hair, decreased resistance to infection (especially measles), kidney stones, and broken fingernails.

A mild level of vitamin A deficiency may also contribute to respiratory and diarrheal infections, slow growth rate, slow bone development, and put children at an increased risk of dying from serious illness.

Who May Be At Increased Risk?

- Toddlers and pre-school-age children
- Children living at or below the poverty level
- Children with inadequate health care or immunizations
- Children living in areas with known nutritional deficiencies
- Recent immigrants or refugees from developing countries with high incidence of vitamin A deficiency or measles
- Children with diseases of the pancreas, liver, intestines, or with inadequate fat digestion or absorption

Who May Need Extra Vitamin A to Prevent a Deficiency?

- Children aged six months to twenty-four months who are hospitalized with measles
- Children aged six months and older who are hospitalized for any reason

What May Increase Your Risk?

- Chronic infections
- Chronic liver disease
- Diarrhea
- Eye diseases
- Intestinal diseases, such as Crohn's disease, ulcerative colitis, and short bowel syndrome

- Pancreatic disease
- Removal of the stomach

Vitamin A Overdosing Risks

Although hypervitaminosis A can occur when very large amounts of liver are regularly consumed, most cases of vitamin A toxicity result from an excess intake of vitamin A supplements. There are three major adverse effects of hypervitaminosis A: birth defects, liver abnormalities, and reduced bone mineral density that may result in osteoporosis.

Signs of toxicity include confusion, diarrhea, bleeding from the gums, dry or sore mouth, dry, cracked, or peeling lips, nausea, vomiting, headache, dizziness, blurred vision, hair loss, and increased skull pressure.

What May Increase Your Risk?

- Prolonged, excessive alcohol consumption
- Pre-existing liver disease
- Hyperlipidemia
- Severe protein malnutrition

Who Should Take Special Note of Their Intake?

The following individuals should be particularly aware of their intake:

- ***Older women.*** Older women who take supplements such as cod-liver oil and other fish oil may be getting too much vitamin A containing retinol. As a result, the body may have trouble using vitamin D to help the bones absorb calcium. This may be responsible for an increased risk of hip fractures in older women. Foods containing beta-carotene do not cause this problem. Talk to your doctor about your needs.

- ***Smokers.*** While beta-carotene and/or vitamin A have been shown to be effective in decreasing the risk of lung cancer, additional studies have indicated that smokers who take beta-carotene supplements have a 46 percent greater risk of dying from lung cancer. Until further research is done, the National Institutes of Health do not recommend beta-carotene in supplemental form for anyone not suffering a vitamin A deficiency; instead, beta-carotene should be consumed by eating appropriate fruits and vegetables.

- ***Pregnant women.*** Pregnant women who take more than 6,000 IU of vitamin A daily have a one-in-sixty chance of delivering a baby with malformations of the face, head, heart, or nervous system, including cleft lip and palate, hydrocephalus, and major heart defects. Prenatal vitamins recommended by most doctors contain 4,000–5,000 IU of vitamin A. Women taking doctor-prescribed vitamins should be careful not to take large doses inadvertently by eating foods high in vitamin A, such as fortified cereals. Beta-carotene (found in many vitamin supplements and in vitamin-A-rich foods) appears to be completely safe.

- ***Vegetarians.*** Vegetarians who do not consume dairy products or eggs need to be especially careful to eat sufficient amounts of carotenoid foods.

- ***Alcoholics.*** Excessive consumption of alcohol depletes vitamin A, but alcohol abuse may so endanger the liver as to make vitamin A supplements hazardous. A physician's evaluation is needed for anyone who drinks heavily.

- ***Individuals taking prescription drugs should be aware of possible drug interactions.*** Many prescription medicines affect the body's ability to absorb vitamin A. If you are being treated for any medical condition, be sure to discuss your nutritional requirements with your doctor.

Vitamin B₁ (Thiamine)

Vitamin B₁ (thiamine) is a water-soluble nutrient that must be replenished daily. The body extracts the vitamin from food during the digestive process. Vitamin B₁ supplements should be taken with food for proper absorption.

Necessary For

Vitamin B₁ is necessary for the body's oxidation of carbohydrates. It benefits the nervous system, muscles, heart, digestion, and appetite, and promotes proper growth.

RECOMMENDED DIETARY ALLOWANCES

		MG PER DAY**
Infants (assumes breastfeeding)	0–6 months	0.2 mg*
	7–12 months	0.3 mg*
Children	1–3 years	0.5 mg
	4–8 years	0.6 mg
	9–13 years	0.9 mg
Males	14 years and up	1.2 mg
Females	14–18 years	1.0 mg
	19 years and up	1.1 mg
Pregnancy/Nursing	All ages	1.4 mg

*Adequate intake
**No upper limits have been established for vitamin B₁

Food Sources

Animal sources of vitamin B₁ include pork, beef, chicken, and fish. Plant sources include sunflower seeds, millet, brown rice, turnip greens, dried beans and peas, sesame seeds, soybeans, wheat germ, and enriched, fortified, or whole grains.

Vitamin B₁ Deficiency Risks

Beriberi, a muscle-wasting disease, was once a very common sign of thiamine deficiency but is extremely rare in developed countries.

Symptoms of vitamin B₁ deficiency include muscle weakness, anorexia, exhaustion, paralysis, nervous irritability, insomnia, weight loss, depression, constipation, gastric distress, enlarged heart, short-term memory problems, and pain or tingling in the arms.

What May Increase Your Risk?

- Hemodialysis or peritoneal dialysis treatments
- Malabsorption syndrome
- A diet high in carbohydrates and low in thiamine
- Strenuous, prolonged exercise
- Chronic fever
- Pregnancy and nursing
- Growth spurts, particularly during adolescence
- Infection with malaria
- Hyperactive thyroid
- Alcoholism
- Liver disease

Other Vitamin B₁ Notes

Some foods, including tea and coffee, contain antithiamine factors, which inactivate thiamine when consumed at the same time. Chewing tea leaves and betel nuts (not a common habit in the United States) has the same consequence. Also, foods and beverages containing sulfites may inactivate thiamine if taken together. If you are at risk of thiamine deficiency, you may want to modify the way you take thiamine supplements.

Vitamin B₁ Overdosing Risks

There are no significant risks associated with overconsumption of thiamine.

Who Should Take Special Note of Their Intake?

The following individuals should be particularly aware of their intake:

- *Alcoholics.* Chronic alcoholism is still associated with vitamin B₁ deficiency, probably due to poor diet.

- *Individuals taking prescription drugs should be aware of possible drug interactions.* Many prescription medicines affect the body's ability to absorb vitamin B₁. If you are being treated for any medical condition, be sure to discuss your nutritional requirements with your doctor.

Vitamin B$_2$ (Riboflavin)

Vitamin B$_2$ (riboflavin) is a water-soluble nutrient that needs to be replenished daily. Riboflavin is found in a variety of foods and is extracted by the body during digestion. An important antioxidant, it also assists the functions of vitamins B$_1$, B$_6$, E, and folate (folic acid). Vitamin B$_2$ supplements should be taken with food for proper absorption.

Necessary For

Vitamin B$_2$ is important for healthy eyesight, antibody and red blood cell production, cell respiration, and healthy skin, nails, and hair. It promotes the metabolism of lipids, tryptophan, proteins, fats, and carbohydrates.

RECOMMENDED DIETARY ALLOWANCES

		MG PER DAY**
Infants (assumes breastfeeding)	0–6 months	0.3 mg*
	7–12 months	0.4 mg*
Children	1–3 years	0.5 mg
	4–8 years	0.6 mg
	9–13 years	0.9 mg
Males	14 years and up	1.3 mg
Females	14–18 years	1.0 mg
	19 years and up	1.1 mg
Pregnancy	All ages	1.4 mg
Nursing	All ages	1.6 mg

*Adequate intake
**No upper limits have been established for vitamin B$_2$

Food Sources

Animal sources of vitamin B$_2$ include dairy and milk products, organ meats, pork, and whole eggs. Plant sources include amaranth (a grain), Brazil nuts, breads and cereals (fortified), broccoli, brown rice, cantaloupe, collards, collard greens, dried peas and beans, kale, kidney bean sprouts, lentils, millet, mushrooms, oranges, peas, pecans, spinach, sunflower seeds, and white rice.

Vitamin B$_2$ Deficiency Risks

Symptoms of vitamin B$_2$ deficiency include itching, bloodshot, light-sensitive, and burning eyes; cracks and sores of the mouth, lips, and scrotum; tongue discoloration; dermatitis; growth retardation; digestive problems; trembling; sluggishness; and dry and scaly facial skin.

What May Increase Your Risk?

- Alcoholism
- Severe burns
- Cancer
- Chronic diarrhea
- Chronic fever
- Chronic illness
- Chronic infection
- Intestinal disorders
- Liver disease
- Hyperactive thyroid
- Serious injury
- Removal of the stomach
- Chronic stress
- High levels of bilirubin (jaundice) in newborns
- Poor diet

Vitamin B$_2$ Overdosing Risks

No known risks are associated with overconsumption of riboflavin.

Who Should Take Special Note of Their Intake?

The following individuals should be particularly aware of their intake:

- *Individuals taking prescription drugs should be aware of possible drug interactions.* Many prescription medicines, including oral contraceptives, affect the body's ability to absorb vitamin B$_2$. If you are being treated for any medical condition, be sure to discuss your nutritional requirements with your doctor.

Vitamin B_3 (Niacin)

Vitamin B_3 (niacin) is a water-soluble vitamin essential for many of the body's functions. It needs to be replenished daily and is easily absorbed from foods during digestion. Vitamin B_3 supplements should be taken with food for proper absorption. Excess niacin is excreted in the urine.

Necessary For

Niacin is important for healthy skin tissue, the nervous system, the tongue, the digestive system and blood circulation, reducing blood cholesterol levels and lowering high blood pressure, preventing pellagra, and promoting the energy conversion of foods.

RECOMMENDED DIETARY ALLOWANCES			
		MG PER DAY	UPPER LIMITS**
Infants (assumes breastfeeding)	0–6 months	2 mg*	N/A
	7–12 months	4 mg*	N/A
Children	1–3 years	6 mg	10 mg
	4–8 years	8 mg	15 mg
	9–13 years	12 mg	20 mg
Males	14–18 years	16 mg	30 mg
	19 years and up	16 mg	35 mg
Females	14–18 years	14 mg	30 mg
	19 years and up	14 mg	35 mg
Pregnancy	Up to 18 years	18 mg	30 mg
	19 years and up	18 mg	35 mg
Nursing	Up to 18 years	17 mg	30 mg
	19 years and up	17 mg	35 mg

*Adequate intake

**No adverse effects shown below these levels

Note: Upper limit amounts shown above include total niacin consumption from food and supplements.

Food Sources

Animal sources of vitamin B_3 include beef, poultry, salmon, and tuna. Plant sources are barley, broccoli, brown rice, cereals (fortified), coffee, collard greens, corn, dried beans, ginkgo nuts, lentils, lima beans, mushrooms, oats, peanuts, peas, sunflower seeds, whole-grain breads and bread products (enriched), and whole wheat.

Note: Too much corn can cause a niacin deficiency. However, corn processed in a lime solution (such as used in the manufacture of some tortillas) acts to increase niacin absorption.

Vitamin B_3 Deficiency Risks

The primary consequence of niacin deficiency is pellagra. Symptoms of niacin deficiency include skin disorders, gastrointestinal disturbances, nervousness, headaches, fatigue, depression, irritability, loss of appetite, insomnia, muscle weakness, indigestion, bad breath, and canker sores.

What May Increase Your Risk?

- Hemodialysis or peritoneal dialysis treatment
- Malabsorption syndrome
- Hartnup disease
- Carcinoid syndrome
- Lengthy use of certain antituberculosis drugs
- Diabetes mellitus
- Chronic diarrhea
- Chronic or prolonged fever
- Liver disease
- Hyperactive thyroid
- Alcoholism

Vitamin B_3 Overdosing Risks

According to the Food and Nutrition Board, there is no evidence of adverse effects from the consumption of naturally occurring niacin in foods. However, too much niacin from supplements may cause skin rashes, liver damage, and peptic ulcers.

Who Should Take Special Note of Their Intake?

The following individuals should be particularly aware of their intake:

- *Individuals taking prescription drugs should be aware of possible drug interactions.* Many prescription medicines affect the body's ability to absorb vitamin B_3. If you are being treated for any medical condition, be sure to discuss your nutritional requirements with your doctor.

Vitamin B_6 (Pyridoxine)

Vitamin B_6 is a water-soluble nutrient that comes in three forms—pyridoxine, pyridoxal, and pyridoxamine. Easily absorbed from foods during digestion, it needs to be replenished daily. Supplements should be taken with food for proper absorption. Vitamin B_6 converts tryptophan to niacin and assists in the function of vitamin B_3.

Necessary For

Vitamin B_6 helps in the production of more than 100 enzymes involved in protein metabolism. It is also needed for hemoglobin synthesis, preventing anemia and skin problems such as acne, maintaining healthy teeth, fighting cancer, strengthening nerves, immune system health, tryptophan conversion to niacin, and maintaining normal blood sugar levels.

RECOMMENDED DIETARY ALLOWANCES

		MG PER DAY	UPPER LIMITS**
Infants (assumes breastfeeding)	0–6 months	0.1 mg*	N/A
	7–12 months	0.3 mg*	N/A
Children	1–3 years	0.5 mg	30 mg
	4–8 years	0.6 mg	40 mg
	9–13 years	1.0 mg	60 mg
Males	14–18 years	1.3 mg	80 mg
	19–49 years	1.3 mg	100 mg
	50 years and up	1.7 mg	100 mg
Females	14–18 years	1.2 mg	80 mg
	19–49 years	1.3 mg	100 mg
	50 years and up	1.5 mg	100 mg
Pregnancy	Up to 18 years	1.9 mg	80 mg
	19 years and up	1.9 mg	100 mg
Nursing	Up to 18 years	2.0 mg	80 mg
	19 years and up	2.0 mg	100 mg

*Adequate intake

**No adverse effects shown below these levels

Note: No one should exceed the RDA without the advice of a doctor. Most people get sufficient vitamin B_6 in their diets.

Food Sources

Animal sources of vitamin B6 include beef, chicken, organ meats, pork, rainbow trout, salmon, and tuna. Plant sources are avocado, bananas, breakfast cereals (fortified), English walnuts, garbanzo beans, hazelnuts, lima beans, oatmeal (instant, fortified), peanuts, peanut butter, Persian walnuts, soybeans, soy-based meat substitutes (fortified), spinach, sunflower seeds, and wheat bran.

Vitamin B_6 Deficiency Risks

A vitamin B_6 deficiency is not very common, because there is generally an adequate amount present in the normal diet.

Symptoms include skin inflammation, glossitis (sore tongue), depression, confusion, nausea, convulsions, some types of anemia, muscle weakness, dermatitis, arm and leg cramps, hair loss, learning difficulties, and water retention.

What May Increase Your Risk?

- Advanced age
- A diet deficient in many key nutrients
- Alcoholism. Alcoholics are at risk for vitamin B_6 deficiency because of poor dietary habits, and alcohol also contributes to the destruction of vitamin B_6 in the body
- Theophylline taken by asthmatic children. Such children may need to take a B_6 supplement (under the guidance of a physician)

Vitamin B_6 Overdosing Risks

Nerve damage to the arms and legs can result from too much vitamin B_6 (more than 100 mg/day).

Who Should Take Special Note of Their Intake?

The following individuals should be particularly aware of their intake:

- *Dieters.* When caloric intake is low your body needs vitamin B_6 to help convert stored carbohydrate or other nutrients to glucose to maintain normal blood sugar levels.

Note: While a shortage of vitamin B_6 will limit these functions, supplements of this vitamin do not enhance them in well-nourished individuals. (*Source:* National Institutes of Health)

- **Individuals taking prescription drugs should be aware of possible drug interactions.** Many prescription medicines affect the body's ability to absorb vitamin B_6. If you are being treated for any medical condition, be sure to discuss your nutritional requirements with your doctor.

Vitamin B_{12} (Cobalamin)

Vitamin B_{12} (cobalamin) is released from protein during digestion by hydrochloric acid in the stomach. Vitamin B_{12} then combines with a substance called intrinsic factor before being absorbed into the bloodstream. Several forms of cobalamin are available—cyanocobalamin, hydroxocobalamin, adenosylcobalamin, and methylcobalamin. Cyanocobalamin is the form most frequently used in supplements and for fortifying foods.

Cobalamin assists folate (also called folic acid) in the synthesis of RNA and DNA, and works with vitamin B_6 and folate to lower levels of homocysteine, an amino acid which in large amounts has been found to be a factor in heart disease. Vitamin B_{12} is water soluble, so supplements should be taken with food for proper absorption.

Necessary For

Vitamin B_{12} is required for red blood cells, healthy nerve cells, and DNA and RNA synthesis.

RECOMMENDED DIETARY ALLOWANCES		MCG PER DAY**
Infants (assumes breastfeeding)	0–6 months	0.4 mcg*
	7–12 months	0.5 mcg*
Children	1–3 years	0.9 mcg
	4–8 years	1.2 mcg
	9–13 years	1.8 mcg
Males/Females	14 years and up	2.4 mcg
Pregnancy	All ages	2.6 mcg
Nursing	All ages	2.8 mcg

*Adequate intake
**No upper limits have been established for vitamin B_{12}

Food Sources

Animal sources of vitamin B_{12} include beef, beef liver, brain, cheese (American, cheddar, and mozzarella, but note that dairy products must be made with fortified milk), chicken, clams, haddock, kidneys, milk (fortified), oysters, rainbow trout, sockeye salmon, tuna, whole egg, and yogurt (made with fortified milk). Plant sources include fortified breakfast cereals.

Note: Plants and animals cannot make this vitamin. The vitamin B_{12} found in meat is made by bacterial B_{12}.

Vitamin B_{12} Deficiency Risks

Deficiency in vitamin B_{12} can result in megaloblastic macrocytic anemia and neurological dysfunction.

Symptoms of vitamin B_{12} deficiency include fatigue, weakness, nausea, flatulence, gas, constipation, loss of appetite, weight loss, numbness and tingling in the hands and feet, depression, confusion, poor memory, soreness of the mouth or tongue, difficulty maintaining balance, age-related hearing loss, Alzheimer's disease, and hyperhomocysteinemia, a condition in which levels of the amino acid homocysteine are so high as to contribute to premature coronary artery disease, and arterial and venous thrombosis.

Note: Permanent nerve damage can occur if vitamin B_{12} deficiency is not treated.

What May Increase Your Risk?

- AIDS
- Alcoholism
- A lack of intrinsic factor can lead to pernicious anemia, and usually requires intramuscular injections of vitamin B_{12}
- A vegan diet (a vegetarian diet excluding eggs, dairy, and meat)

- Being over the age of fifty (Stomach secretions decline with age, reducing the body's ability to absorb the B_{12} in food.)
- Congenital conditions such as transcobalamin II deficiency and deficient intrinsic factor production
- Drug interaction with certain medications
- Excess bacteria in the stomach and small intestine
- Kidney disease
- Metabolic disorders, such as methylmalonic aciduria and homocystinuria
- Pancreatic inefficiency
- Parasitic infections, such as worms
- Regional enteritis (inflammation of the stomach or intestines)
- Removal of all or part of the stomach or the distal ileum
- Sprue or celiac disease
- Thyroid disease

Note: Large doses of folic acid may hide the signs of B_{12} deficiency. If you are at risk of B_{12} deficiency, you may feel better by taking a lot of folic acid, but taking more than the RDA of folic acid can be dangerous and won't replace the B_{12} you need.

Vitamin B_{12} Overdosing Risks

The Institute of Medicine states that "no adverse effects have been associated with excess vitamin B_{12} intake from food and supplements in healthy individuals."

Who Should Take Special Note of Their Intake?

The following individuals should be particularly aware of their intake:

- *People with Blood Type A.* These individuals typically have low levels of hydrochloric (stomach) acid and can lack intrinsic factor. As a result, they have difficulty digesting red meat and thus fail to absorb the vitamin. This group should consider use of methylcobalamin for proper absorption of vitamin B_{12} supplements. (Visit www.dadamo.com for more information.)
- *People with Leber's disease.* This eye condition may be made worse with supplements of cobalamin. Talk to your doctor about other vitamin B_{12} options.
- *Vegetarians.* Vegetarians, specially vegans who don't eat any animal products, including eggs and dairy, may also not be consuming fortified cereals. Deficiency symptoms can take years to show up in individuals who have become vegetarians as adults because the body would have ample stores of the vitamin. However, severe symptoms of B_{12} deficiency can show up quickly in children and breast-fed infants of women who follow a strict vegetarian diet, and most often feature poor neurological development. See your doctor about appropriate supplementation for infants and children. (*Source:* National Institutes of Health)
- *Pregnant women.* Pregnant women need adequate amounts of both vitamin B_{12} and folate to ensure that their babies avoid the risk of severe neurological damage. The best advice is to start taking these supplements before you become pregnant, since most of the irreversible brain and spine damage takes place before a woman even knows she is pregnant. Follow your doctor's recommendations about supplementation during pregnancy.
- *Older people.* Older people with vitamin B_{12} deficiencies may also have elevated homocysteine levels, which increases the risk of cardiovascular disease. Folic acid and vitamins B_6 and B_{12} help to regulate homocysteine levels.
- *Individuals taking prescription drugs should be aware of possible drug interactions.* Many prescription medicines affect the body's ability to absorb vitamin B_{12}. If you are being treated for any medical condition, be sure to discuss your nutritional requirements with your doctor.

Vitamin C (Ascorbic Acid)

Vitamin C (ascorbic acid) is a water-soluble nutrient essential for good health. Many mammals can manufacture their own vitamin C, but humans must get their supply from foods. Vitamin C is an amazing nutrient, required for many of the body's functions. Vitamin C enhances the absorption of iron supplements and nonheme iron when taken at the same time. A potent antioxidant, vitamin C appears to help other antioxidants in the body, such as vitamin E, to regenerate.

Necessary For

Vitamin C is well known for preventing scurvy, warding off colds, enhancing the immune and nervous systems, promoting wound and peptic ulcer healing, cell protection, healthy teeth and gums, lowering high blood pressure, and reducing the risk of cataracts. Vitamin C is a natural antioxidant, fighting heart disease and cancer and preventing accelerated aging. It activates liver detoxification systems and enhances the ability of white blood cells to destroy bacteria.

RECOMMENDED DIETARY ALLOWANCES

		MG PER DAY	UPPER LIMITS**
Infants (assumes breastfeeding)	0–6 months	40 mg*	N/A
	7–12 months	50 mg*	N/A
Children	1–3 years	15 mg	400 mg
	4–8 years	25 mg	650 mg
	9–13 years	45 mg	1,200 mg
Males	14–18 years	75 mg	1,800 mg
	19 years and up	90 mg	2,000 mg
Females	14–18 years	65 mg	1,800 mg
	19 years and up	75 mg	2,000 mg
Pregnancy	Up to 18 years	80 mg	1,800 mg
	19 years and up	85 mg	2,000 mg
Nursing	Up to 18 years	115 mg	1,800 mg
	19 years and up	120 mg	2,000 mg

*Adequate intake

**No adverse effects shown below these levels

Notes: A normal diet provides an adequate amount of vitamin C.

> Many experts recommend taking daily supplements of 250–500 mg in addition to a diet rich in vitamin C.
>
> Vitamin C is best absorbed when taken in several doses throughout the day.

Food Sources

Vitamin C is obtained from plant sources such as acerola fruit, alfalfa, asparagus, blackberries, blueberries, broccoli, Brussels sprouts, cabbage, cauliflower, currants, grapefruit, honeydew melon, hot red and green peppers, kale, kiwifruit, lemons, limes, mangoes, mustard greens, oranges, parsley, raspberries, romaine lettuce, rose hips, spinach, strawberries, sweet red and green peppers, sweet potatoes, tangerines, tomatoes, tomato juice, turnip greens, watercress, and white potatoes.

Note: Cooking destroys vitamin C.

Note: Chewable vitamin C supplements may stay on the teeth and can dissolve tooth enamel. Brush or rinse after chewing.

Vitamin C Deficiency Risks

The primary risk of vitamin C deficiency is scurvy, a condition not usually seen in America today, but which was quite common in the past. It was especially common in sailors whose long voyages limited their opportunities to eat fresh fruits and vegetables. Captain James Cook is credited with preventing scurvy in his crews by providing them with limes, a fruit that holds up well in storage.

Symptoms of scurvy include loose teeth, swollen and bleeding gums, hemorrhaging blood vessels, tender and painful arms and legs, slow wound healing, weakness, confusion and fatigue, dry eyes and mouth, anemia, anorexia, diarrhea, and lung and kidney disorders.

Vitamin C Overdosing Risks

Most people don't need to worry about taking in too much vitamin C. However, the results include nausea, flatulence, and diarrhea at quantities of more than 1,000 mg per day.

Who Should Take Special Note of Their Intake?

The following individuals should be particularly aware of their intake:

- *Those who have a history of kidney stones or renal insufficiency.* In this case, you should take care not to exceed the RDA for vitamin C.
- *Smokers.* Smokers should be aware that cigarette smoke destroys vitamin C in the body. Smokers need at least 100 mg (one cup of orange juice, for example) per day. Exposure to secondhand smoke increases the need for vitamin C as well.
- *Alcoholics and those who drink alcohol regularly.* Alcohol depletes all of the body's stores of water-soluble vitamins. Anyone who drinks more than a moderate amount of alcohol (commonly considered to be one drink daily for women or two drinks for men) should discuss the need for supplements with a doctor.
- *Individuals with hemochromatosis.* This is the most common inherited condition in the United States. It affects roughly 1 in 200, especially descendents of northern Europeans, including those with Scandinavian, Welsh, Irish, Scottish, or English ancestry.

Hemochromatosis is an overabundance of iron in the blood and can be fatal. People with this condition should carefully monitor the amount of vitamin C they ingest, as it can increase the amount of iron absorbed by the body. Discuss your situation with your doctor. A simple blood test can determine if you have this condition. People of South African heritage may inherit sub-Saharan African hemochromatosis, as well.

- *Individuals with the inherited conditions thalassemia, sideroblastic anemia, sickle-cell anemia, and G-6-PD deficiency.*
- *Premature infants.* Premature infants may become predisposed to hemolytic anemia if they receive large doses of vitamin C during infancy.
- *Individuals taking prescription drugs should be aware of possible drug interactions.* Many prescription medicines affect the body's ability to absorb vitamin C. If you are being treated for any medical condition, be sure to discuss your nutritional requirements with your doctor.

Vitamin D (Calciferol)

Vitamin D (calciferol) is a fat-soluble vitamin found in food. It can be manufactured by the body after exposure to ultraviolet rays (sunlight). Vitamin D is converted to an active hormone form by the liver and kidneys.

Sunlight is a very important source of vitamin D, but prolonged exposure to ultraviolet rays can be dangerous and may lead to skin cancer. Luckily, the body can get all of the vitamin D it needs from the sun in fifteen to twenty minutes, so use sunblock when you will be outdoors longer than that. An SPF (sun protection factor) of 8 or higher will block the rays needed to produce vitamin D.

Where you live can prevent you from getting enough exposure to the sun. Smog, clouds, and the angle of the sun in the winter all cause problems. In such cases, be sure to include good food sources of vitamin D in your diet.

Necessary For

Vitamin D is required for normal blood levels of calcium and phosphorus, absorption of calcium, and teeth and bone formation. It prevents rickets in children and skeletal diseases in adults. It is also important in insulin and prolactin secretion, muscle function, immune system and stress response, melanin synthesis, and cellular differentiation, and is vital for kidney and parathyroid function. Vitamin D has anticancer properties. Laboratory studies of vitamin D have shown that it stimulates cell differentiation and/or inhibits the rapid growth and spread of some types of cancer cells.

ADEQUATE INTAKES			
		MCG PER DAY	UPPER LIMITS*
Infants (assumes breastfeeding)	0–6 months	5 mcg	25 mcg
	7–12 months	5 mcg	25 mcg
Children	1–3 years	5 mcg	50 mcg
	4–8 years	5 mcg	50 mcg
	9–13 years	5 mcg	50 mcg
Males/Females	14–49 years	5 mcg	50 mcg
	50–70 years	10 mcg	50 mcg
	70 years and up	15 mcg	50 mcg
Pregnancy/Nursing	All ages	5 mcg	50 mcg

*No adverse effects shown below these levels

Notes: 1 microgram or mcg = 40 IU of vitamin D

More than 1 gram of vitamin D per day can contribute to kidney stones.

Never exceed the adequate intake without the advice of a doctor.

Food Sources

Animal sources of vitamin D include beef liver, cod liver oil, eel, liver and fat from seals and polar bears, mackerel, margarine (fortified), milk (fortified), pudding mix (when made with fortified milk), salmon, sardines, and whole eggs (vitamin D is in the yolk if chickens have been given fortified feed). Plant sources include avocado, breakfast cereal (fortified), and cereal grain bars (fortified).

Few foods naturally contain high levels of vitamin D. Milk in the United States routinely has been fortified with vitamin D since the 1930s, contributing to the almost total disappearance of rickets in this country. This disease is still a problem in many developing nations, however. Four cups of fortified milk approximate the RDA for both adults and children. Dairy products made from milk, such as ice cream, cheese, and yogurt, are not usually fortified.

Vitamin D Deficiency Risks

Rickets, leading to skeletal deformities, is the major vitamin D deficiency problem for children. In adults, vitamin D deficiency leads to osteomalacia—muscle weakness and weak bones—as well as tooth decay and retention of phosphorus in the kidneys.

Vitamin D deficiency can be caused by inadequate dietary intake, limited exposure to sunlight, kidney malfunction, or the inability of the body to absorb vitamin D from the gastrointestinal tract.

Who May Be At Increased Risk?

- Children without access to fortified foods
- Women whose religious customs require full body coverage
- People living in northern climates
- People confined to their homes by illness
- People who work primarily indoors
- Older people whose gastrointestinal functions are slowing and whose skin is losing the ability to convert sunlight to vitamin D
- People who don't drink milk or whose diets exclude fortified dairy products
- People with dark skin, as dark skin reduces the body's ability to synthesize vitamin D from sunlight

Vitamin D Overdosing Risks

It is hard to ingest too much vitamin D from food, unless one routinely takes a lot of cod liver oil. *A more common source of toxicity comes from taking too many supplements and greatly exceeding the recommended dietary allowance.*

The primary risk of taking in too much vitamin D is hypercalcemia. Symptoms of excess vitamin D include nausea, vomiting, poor appetite, constipation, weakness, weight loss, confusion, and heart rhythm abnormalities. Possible consequences of ingesting too much vitamin D include brain or liver damage, jaundice, red blood cell destruction, headaches, dry mouth, sleepiness, and muscle pain.

Who Should Take Special Note of Their Intake?

The following individuals should be particularly aware of their intake:

- ***People with fat-absorption medical conditions.*** Such conditions as Crohn's disease, pancreatic enzyme deficiency, cystic fibrosis, sprue, liver disease, surgical removal of some or all of the stomach, and small bowel disease cause vitamins to be eliminated before they are absorbed. This is important because vitamin D is a fat-soluble vitamin and is stored in the body until needed.

- **Breastfed babies.** Breastfed babies may not get sufficient vitamin D in their mother's milk and may need supplements if they cannot get good exposure to sunlight. Consult your pediatrician. Formulas are routinely fortified.
- **People on steroids.** These individuals should consult their doctor about a possible need to increase vitamin D intake, because steroidal medicines decrease calcium absorption.
- **People with Alzheimer's disease.** These individuals are at risk of vitamin D deficiency because a lack of mobility may reduce exposure to sunlight, increasing the risk of hip fractures.
- **Postmenopausal women.** Estrogen stimulates the cells that build bones, so when estrogen production declines at menopause, bones are at an increased risk of fracture. Women can greatly reduce this risk (without HRT) by increasing the amount of vitamin D in their diets, or by taking supplements.
- **Individuals taking prescription drugs should be aware of possible drug interactions.** Many prescription medicines affect the body's ability to absorb vitamin D. If you are being treated for any medical condition, be sure to discuss your nutritional requirements with your doctor.

Vitamin E (Tocopherol)

The National Institutes of Health describes vitamin E (tocopherol) as follows:

> Vitamin E exists in eight different forms. Each form has its own biological activity, the measure of potency or functional use in the body. Alpha-tocopherol is the most active form of vitamin E in humans, and is a powerful biological antioxidant. Antioxidants such as vitamin E act to protect your cells against the effects of free radicals, which are potentially damaging by-products of the body's metabolism.
>
> Free radicals can cause cell damage that may contribute to the development of cardiovascular disease and cancer. Studies are underway to determine whether vitamin E might help prevent or delay the development of those chronic diseases.

Vitamin E is a fat-soluble vitamin. Absorption is considerably lower on an empty stomach. Vitamin E works with selenium to prevent free radicals from oxidizing lipids (fat molecules).

Necessary For

Vitamin E protects against the oxidation of vitamin A during digestion, reduces the risk of cataracts, and can help stop early neurological problems associated with cystic fibrosis and liver disease. It is needed for antibody production, burn healing, improved sexual function, and cell protection. Vitamin E is a natural antioxidant, detoxifying free radicals, fighting heart disease and cancer, and preventing accelerated aging. It strengthens capillary walls, protects red blood cells, prevents and dissolves blood clots, reduces leg cramps, and supports the body's use of beta-carotene.

RECOMMENDED DIETARY ALLOWANCES		MG PER DAY	UPPER LIMITS**
Infants (assumes breastfeeding)	0–6 months	4 mg*	N/A
	7–12 months	5 mg*	N/A
Children	1–3 years	6 mg	200 mg
	4–8 years	7 mg	300 mg
	9–13 years	11 mg	600 mg
	14–18 years	15 mg	800 mg
Males/Females	19 years and up	15 mg	1,000 mg
Pregnancy	Up to 18 years	15 mg	800 mg
	19 years and up	15 mg	1,000 mg
Nursing	Up to 18 years	19 mg	800 mg
	19 years and up	19 mg	1,000 mg

*Adequate intake

**No adverse effects shown below these levels

Note: 1 mg alpha-tocopherol equivalent = 1.5 IU

Most people get an adequate amount of vitamin E in their diets. But many experts advise adults to take 20–40 mg daily.

Food Sources

Animal sources of vitamin E are beef, chicken, dairy products, fish, mayonnaise (made with the appropriate oils), and whole eggs. Plant sources include almonds (dry, roasted), asparagus, broccoli, brown rice, cabbage, dandelion greens, dark green leafy vegetables, kiwifruit, lima beans, mangoes, oats, oils (canola, corn, cottonseed, olive, safflower, and soybean), peanuts, pistachios, sesame seeds, spinach, sunflower seeds, sweet potatoes, turnip greens, and whole-grain wheat.

Vitamin E Deficiency Risks

The major disease caused by vitamin E deficiency is peripheral neuropathy (nerve damage). This is usually the result of malabsorption problems, where vitamin E is excreted from the body instead of being stored.

Symptoms of vitamin E deficiency include greasy stools, chronic diarrhea, capillary ruptures, reproductive difficulties, abnormal fat deposits in muscle tissue, dry skin, and degeneration of the heart tissues. Symptoms in adults may take years to appear, and the neurological damage may be irreversible. Children may be treated successfully if their symptoms are recognized in time.

What May Increase Your Risk?

- Low-fat diets
- Medical conditions, such as Crohn's disease, that limit the ability to absorb fats
- Premature delivery with a very-low-birth weight
- Removal of all or part of the stomach
- Genetic abnormalities such as a-TTP and lipoprotein synthesis defects
- Pancreatic and intestinal disorders

Vitamin E Overdosing Risks

Although studies have not shown serious health risks associated with large doses of vitamin E from food sources, exceeding the tolerable upper limits established by the Food and Nutrition Board is not advisable. Excessive use of vitamin E is especially *not* advised for individuals with bleeding disorders or those taking anticoagulants.

Symptoms of overdose include blurred vision, dizziness, diarrhea, headache, nausea, stomach cramps, exhaustion, and fatigue.

Who Should Take Special Note of Their Intake?

The following individuals should be particularly aware of their intake:

- *Individuals with cystic fibrosis.* These patients have a very hard time absorbing fat, and therefore are at increased risk of vitamin E deficiency. See your doctor about the need for supplements.

- *Individuals with abetalipoproteinemia.* This rare inherited disorder of fat metabolism results in poor absorption of dietary fat and vitamin E. The deficiency associated with this disease causes problems such as poor transmission of nerve impulses, muscle weakness, and degeneration of the retina that can cause blindness. Individuals with abetalipoproteinemia may need special vitamin E supplements (by prescription) to treat this disorder.

- *People with blood coagulation problems.* Vitamin K deficiency may interfere with the blood's ability to coagulate, and high doses of vitamin E can exacerbate this problem. Anyone using anticoagulants should also be careful not to take too much vitamin E.

- *Those with blood type O.* These individuals have the "thinnest" blood of the different types and need to be cautious when taking vitamin E or aspirin, as bleeding problems may result.

- *People taking mineral oil.* Use of mineral oil may decrease absorption of vitamin E. This is not a problem with infrequent use.

- *Anyone with bleeding disorders.* Extreme caution should be taken by anyone with a risk of hemorrhagic stroke, or who has bleeding ulcers, hemophilia, and any other inherited bleeding disorders.

- *Surgery patients.* Some doctors advise that patients discontinue vitamin E supplementation prior to surgery to minimize the risk of bleeding.

- *People with retinitis pigmentosa.* Progression of this condition may be accelerated by too much vitamin E in supplement form. Discuss this with your doctor.

- *Individuals taking prescription drugs should be aware of possible drug interactions.* Many prescription medicines affect the body's ability to absorb vitamin E. If you are being treated for any medical condition, be sure to discuss your nutritional requirements with your doctor.

Vitamin K

Vitamin K is a fat-soluble vitamin that is essential to the blood-clotting process. In fact, the "K" designation comes from the German word "koagulation" (coagulation). A precursor to vitamin K, phylloquinone, is found naturally in some plants. Bacteria that live in our gastrointestinal tracts synthesize phylloquinone into vitamin K when we consume those plant foods. Coagulation factors are stored in the liver. Vitamin K works with vitamins A and D to build bone protein.

Necessary For

Vitamin K is an important factor in blood clotting and maintaining bone strength as we age.

ADEQUATE INTAKES

		MCG PER DAY*
Infants (assumes breastfeeding)	0–6 months	2.0 mcg
	7–12 months	2.5 mcg
Children	1–3 years	30 mcg
	4–8 years	55 mcg
	9–13 years	60 mcg
	14–18 years	75 mcg
Males	19 years and up	120 mcg
Females	19 years and up	90 mcg
Pregnancy/Nursing	Up to 18 years	75 mcg
	19 years and up	90 mcg

*No upper limits have been established for vitamin K

Food Sources

Vitamin K is found in mayonnaise (from the oils) and in plant sources such as broccoli, Brussels sprouts, cabbage, canola oil, carrots, cauliflower, cereals, collard greens, cottonseed oil, kale, leaf lettuce, margarine, olive oil, parsley, peas, spinach, soybeans, soybean oil, Swiss chard, tomatoes, and watercress. It is also found in fortified bread and cereals.

Vitamin K Deficiency Risks

The primary consequence of vitamin K deficiency is impaired blood clotting, which is not common in healthy adults and occurs primarily when the body is unable to absorb the vitamin.

Symptoms include easy bruising, nosebleeds, bleeding gums, bloody urine, blood in the stool, and heavy menstruation. Of course, all of these symptoms may indicate other health problems as well, so it is best to discuss your symptoms with a doctor before self-medicating.

Who May Be At Increased Risk?

- People with severe liver disease
- Infants and young children who are fed nothing but breast milk
- Nursing infants whose mothers are taking anticoagulants
- People with malabsorption conditions such as Crohn's disease and sprue

Note: Excessive amounts of vitamins A and E may inhibit the absorption of vitamin K.

Vitamin K Overdosing Risks

No adverse effects have been reported from overconsumption of vitamin K from food or supplements.

Who Should Take Special Note of Their Intake?

The following individuals should be particularly aware of their intake:

- ***People taking anticoagulant therapy.*** Because vitamin K affects blood clotting, anyone on anticoagulant therapy should be careful concerning vitamin K consumption.

- ***Newborns.*** The American Academy of Pediatrics advises that all newborns should be given a dose of vitamin K, orally or by injection, to prevent hemorrhagic disease of the newborn, a potentially fatal bleeding disorder.

- ***Individuals taking prescription drugs should be aware of possible drug interactions.*** Many prescription medicines affect the body's ability to absorb vitamin K. If you are being treated for any medical condition, be sure to discuss your nutritional requirements with your doctor.

Biotin

Biotin, sometimes known as vitamin H, is a water-soluble nutrient generally classified with the B vitamins. The majority of biotin in the body is found in the liver, kidneys, and muscle tissue. It is known that bacteria in the large intestine are capable of manufacturing biotin, but science doesn't yet know if we can absorb our own biotin. Biotin is found in many foods, however.

Necessary For

Biotin is required for the proper utilization of proteins, folic acid, pantothenic acid, and vitamin B_{12}. It helps in the synthesis of fat, glycogen, and amino acids, and the growth of healthy hair and nails.

ADEQUATE INTAKES		
		MCG PER DAY*
Infants (assumes breastfeeding)	0–6 months	5 mcg
	7–12 months	6 mcg
Children	1–3 years	8 mcg
	4–8 years	12 mcg
	9–13 years	20 mcg
Males/Females	14–18 years	25 mcg
	19 years and up	30 mcg
Pregnancy	All ages	30 mcg
Nursing	All ages	35 mcg

*No upper limits have been established for biotin

Food Sources

Animal sources of biotin include Camembert cheese, cheddar cheese, chicken, egg yolk, kidneys, liver, milk, pork, and salmon. Plant sources are artichokes, avocado, barley, brewer's yeast, cauliflower, raspberries, soy, wheat bran, and yeast.

Biotin Deficiency Risks

Biotin deficiency is not a common hazard. Symptoms include extreme exhaustion, sleepiness, muscle pain, appetite loss, depression, hair loss, loss of hair color, a grayish tinge to the skin, and rashes around the eyes, nose, mouth, and genitals.

What May Increase Your Risk?

- Eating large quantities of raw egg whites over many days
- Receiving extended IV feedings, if biotin has not been added to the fluid
- Having any of four hereditary disorders: biotinidase deficiency, holocarboxylase synthetase deficiency, multiple carboxylase deficiency or propionic-CoA carboxylase deficiency (In these cases, biotin deficiency can be fatal if it is not treated.)
- Liver disease
- Pregnancy
- Seborrheic dermatitis in infants
- Surgical removal of the stomach
- Malabsorption syndromes, such as Crohn's disease or sprue

Biotin Overdosing Risks

It is very hard to overdose on biotin, so overdosing on this vitamin is not a common concern.

Who Should Take Special Note of Their Intake?

The following individuals should be particularly aware of their intake:

- *IV patients.* Those on IVs are at risk for a condition called "biotin deficiency facies" identified by the development of a unique facial appearance resulting from the redistribution of fat cells in the face and the presence of a red, scaly rash around the eyes, nose, and mouth. This condition is easily prevented by the addition of biotin to the IV fluid and is not a problem for short-term or partial IV use.
- *Pregnant women.* Inadequate amounts of biotin in the diet during pregnancy can put the baby at risk for birth defects. Talk to your doctor about supplement requirements.
- *Individuals taking prescription drugs should be aware of possible drug interactions.* Many prescription medicines affect the body's ability to absorb biotin. If you are being treated for any medical condition, be sure to discuss your nutritional requirements with your doctor.

Choline

Choline, an essential nutrient, is usually classified as a vitamin. Humans can synthesize small amounts of choline, but we get most of what we need from the foods we eat. Choline helps to ensure normal fetal brain development.

Necessary For

Choline is an important nutrient for cell membrane structure, the nervous system, transporting fats from the liver, controlling fat and cholesterol levels, memory functions, and properly functioning kidneys and gallbladder.

ADEQUATE INTAKES		MG PER DAY	UPPER LIMITS*
Infants (assumes breastfeeding)	0–6 months	125 mg	N/A
	7–12 months	150 mg	N/A
Children	1–3 years	200 mg	1,000 mg
	4–8 years	250 mg	1,000 mg
	9–13 years	375 mg	2,000 mg
Males	14–18 years	550 mg	3,000 mg
	19 years and up	550 mg	3,500 mg
Females	14–18 years	400 mg	3,000 mg
	19 years and up	425 mg	3,500 mg
Pregnancy	Up to 18 years	450 mg	3,000 mg
	19 years and up	450 mg	3,500 mg
Nursing	Up to 18 years	550 mg	3,000 mg
	19 years and up	550 mg	3,500 mg

*No adverse effects shown below these levels

Food Sources

Animal sources of choline include beef liver and egg yolks. Plant sources are cauliflower, iceberg lettuce, peanuts, soybean oil, and wheat germ.

Choline Deficiency Risks

The risk of choline deficiency is largely absent in diets that are adequate in protein. Symptoms include cirrhosis and fatty degeneration of the liver, hardening of the arteries, cardiac distress, high blood pressure, bleeding kidneys, memory problems, and poor muscle coordination.

Choline Overdosing Risks

Too much choline in the diet (from food or supplements) can result in fishy body odor, sweating, excess salivation, hypotension, and liver toxicity.

What May Increase Your Risk?

- Depression
- Liver disease
- Parkinson's disease
- Renal (kidney) disease
- Trimethylaminuria, a rare genetic metabolic disorder

Who Should Take Special Note of Their Intake?

The following individuals should be particularly aware of their intake:

- *Individuals taking prescription drugs should be aware of possible drug interactions.* Many prescription medicines affect the body's ability to absorb choline. If you are being treated for any medical condition, be sure to discuss your nutritional requirements with your doctor.

Folic Acid (Folate)

Folic acid and folate are part of the water-soluble B-vitamin family. Folate is the natural form found in food; folic acid is the synthetic form used in supplements. It is sometimes called vitamin B_9. Folate (folic acid) works with vitamins B_{12} and C in the metabolism and synthesis of proteins, and works with vitamins B_6 and B_{12} to lower homocysteine levels. Unlike many other nutrients, absorption of folic supplements is slightly reduced when taken with food.

Necessary For

Folate is important in the blood-forming process, cell replacement (manufacture of DNA and RNA), fetal development (especially for prevention of spina bifida), preventing heart disease and some forms of cancer, including breast cancer, and preventing pregnancy-related anemia.

RECOMMENDED DIETARY ALLOWANCES

		MCG PER DAY	UPPER LIMITS**
Infants (assumes breastfeeding)	0–6 months	65 mcg*	N/A
	7–12 months	80 mcg*	N/A
Children	1–3 years	150 mcg	300 mcg
	4–8 years	200 mcg	400 mcg
	9–13 years	300 mcg	600 mcg
	14–18 years	400 mcg	800 mcg
Males/Females	19 years and up	400 mcg	1,000 mcg
Pregnancy	Up to 18 years	600 mcg	800 mcg
	19 years and up	600 mcg	1,000 mcg
Nursing	Up to 18 years	500 mcg	800 mcg
	19 years and up	500 mcg	1,000 mcg

*Adequate intake

**No adverse effects shown below these levels

Notes: 1 microgram or mcg of food folate = 0.6 mcg of folic acid from supplements and fortified foods

Do not exceed the recommended amounts except under a doctor's supervision.

Food Sources

Animal sources of folate are beef liver and whole egg. Plant sources include arugula, asparagus, avocado, bananas, black-eyed peas, bok choy, bran, bread (enriched), breakfast cereal (fortified), brewer's yeast, broccoli, Brussels sprouts, cantaloupes, cauliflower, chard, chicory, dandelion greens, egg noodles (enriched), escarole, garbanzo beans (chickpeas), great northern beans, green peas, iceberg lettuce, kale, kidney beans, lentils, lima beans, mache, mung beans, mustard greens, oranges, orange juice, papayas, peanuts, pigeon peas, pinto beans, potatoes, radicchio, romaine lettuce, soybeans, spinach, sunflower seeds, tomato juice, turnip greens, watercress, wheat germ, white beans, and white rice.

Folate Deficiency Risks

The primary risk of folate deficiency is megaloblastic anemia, which is similar to that caused by vitamin B_{12} deficiency.

Symptoms of folate deficiency include diarrhea, loss of appetite, weight loss, weakness, sore tongue, headaches, heart palpitations, irritability, behavioral disorders, premature graying, fatigue, cramps, and depression.

Because folate is a water-soluble vitamin, little is stored in the body and it needs to be replenished daily. Any condition such as pregnancy and breastfeeding that depletes your folate supply puts you at risk of deficiency. Another risk factor is taking medication that interferes with folate utilization.

What May Increase Your Risk?

- Alcoholism
- Anemia
- Being of childbearing age (see "Who Should Take Special Note of Their Intake" on the next page)
- Certain anticonvulsant medications
- Certain diuretics
- Chronic hemodialysis or peritoneal dialysis
- Kidney dialysis
- Liver disease
- Malabsorption conditions such as Crohn's disease, sprue, or amyloidosis
- Removal of all or part of the stomach or intestines
- Sickle-cell disease
- Some drugs used to treat Crohn's disease or ulcerative colitis

- Some genetic disorders
- Some medications used in treating diabetes

Folate Overdosing Risks

The risk of becoming ill from overdosing on folate is low. However, exceeding the recommended limits increases the risk that vitamin B_{12} deficiency symptoms will be hidden.

Who Should Take Special Note of Their Intake?

The following individuals should be particularly aware of their intake:

- *Women of childbearing age.* Any woman old enough to menstruate is theoretically old enough to have children, and she should be taking daily amounts of folate or folic acid supplements. Failure to have adequate amounts of folate in your system when you become pregnant puts your baby at a severe risk for birth defects, including malformations of the skull and brain, and spina bifida. *Note: Some studies suggest that the father's supply of folate at conception is equally important.*

   Girls need to start getting the recommended dietary allowance of folate as teenagers, even if it will be years before they become mothers. If the diet is sketchy, take folic acid supplements. Don't take chances with your (future) baby's health! If you already have had a child with a neural tube defect, your doctor will probably advise you to increase your dosage of folate or folic acid.

- *Alcoholics.* Alcoholics are at risk of folate insufficiencies, because alcohol interferes with folate absorption and increases the amount of folate excreted by the kidneys. Also, alcoholics often have poor diets and probably are not getting enough folate in the foods they eat.

- *Older people.* Older people who may be at risk of anemia from a vitamin B_{12} deficiency should not take folic acid supplements without advice from a physician. Often, taking folic acid will mask symptoms of vitamin B_{12} deficiency. You will feel better, but the underlying problem is still there and getting worse.

   If you are over fifty, have a complete blood count done at your annual physical and make sure you are not anemic before taking folic acid supplements.

- **Individuals taking prescription drugs should be aware of possible drug interactions.** Many prescription medicines affect the body's ability to absorb folate and folic acid. If you are being treated for any medical condition, be sure to discuss your nutritional requirements with your doctor.

Pantothenic Acid

Pantothenic acid, also known as vitamin B_5, is a water-soluble essential nutrient. It is a component of coenzyme A, which is necessary for a number of chemical reactions that convert food to energy. Bacteria in the large intestine are able to synthesize pantothenic acid but only in small quantities. Fortunately, pantothenic acid is found in a variety of foods.

Necessary For

Pantothenic acid is important to the immune system, the adrenal glands, antibody production, the central nervous system, growth, and reproduction. Pantothenic acid helps the body to use vitamins, helps with cell building and energy production, and synthesizes fat, cholesterol, hormones, and hemoglobin.

ADEQUATE INTAKES		MG PER DAY*
Infants (assumes breastfeeding)	0–6 months	1.7 mg
	7–12 months	1.8 mg
Children	1–3 years	2 mg
	4–8 years	3 mg
	9–13 years	4 mg
Males/Females	14 years and up	5 mg
Pregnancy	All ages	6 mg
Nursing	All ages	7 mg

*No upper limits have been established

Food Sources

Animal sources of pantothenic acid include beef, chicken, egg yolk, kidneys, liver, lobster, milk, and yogurt. Plant sources are avocado, brewer's yeast, broccoli, brown rice, Brussels sprouts, cashews, cereals (enriched), fava beans, filberts (hazelnuts), ginkgo nuts, green peas, lentils, mushrooms, oats, peanuts, pigeon peas, potatoes, royal jelly, soybeans, split peas, sunflower seeds, sweet potatoes, tomato products, whole grains, and yeast.

Pantothenic Acid Deficiency Risks

A pantothenic acid deficiency is very rare and is seen only in cases of extreme malnutrition.

Deficiency can result in stomach upset, nausea, vomiting, cramps, burning and tingling in the feet, fatigue, insomnia, and skin irritation.

Pantothenic Acid Overdosing Risks

There is no known risk of taking too much pantothenic acid.

Note: High doses of pantothenic acid may interfere with biotin absorption.

Who Should Take Special Note of Their Intake?

The following individuals should be particularly aware of their intake:

- *Women taking oral contraceptives.* Women who use birth control pills containing estrogen and progestin may have a greater need for pantothenic acid. Talk to your physician.

- *Individuals taking prescription drugs should be aware of possible drug interactions.* Prescription medicines may affect the body's ability to absorb pantothenic acid. If you are being treated for any medical condition, be sure to discuss your nutritional requirements with your doctor.

MINERALS

Calcium

Calcium is a mineral vital to the manufacture of bone and teeth. It is not stored in the body and needs to be taken daily because calcium is lost through feces, urine, and sweat. The body uses 99 percent of any available calcium for the bones and teeth. The blood and the body's soft tissues use the remaining 1 percent. Calcium will be taken from the bones when it is needed for critical body functions. The body builds bones until the late twenties, with rapid growth in the teens.

Calcium is available in food and in supplement form. Calcium in supplement form is most efficiently absorbed when taken in amounts of 500 mg or lower. The body can absorb only so much calcium at a time; divide doses throughout the day. Vitamin D and protein assist with calcium absorption, so try to take them together. Calcium carbonate and calcium phosphate supplements are absorbed more readily when taken with food.

Necessary for

Calcium is important to muscle health, the nervous system, strong bones and teeth, consistent heart rhythm, blood clotting, energy production, glandular secretions, and immune system health.

ADEQUATE INTAKES			
		MG PER DAY	UPPER LIMITS**
Infants (assumes breastfeeding)	0–6 months	210 mg*	N/A
	7–12 months	270 mg	N/A
Children	1–3 years	500 mg	2,500 mg
	4–8 years	800 mg	2,500 mg
Males/Females	9–18 years	1,300 mg	2,500 mg
	19–50 years	1,000 mg	2,500 mg
	51 years and up	1,200 mg	2,500 mg
Pregnancy/Nursing	All ages	1,200 mg	2,500 mg

*Breast milk provides about 320 mg of calcium per liter
**No adverse effects shown below these levels

Food Sources

Animal sources of calcium are canned salmon and sardines (requires eating the bones), milk, and other dairy products. Plant sources are bok choy, broccoli, calcium-fortified foods, collard greens, dandelion greens, fava beans, kale, lime-processed tortillas, mustard greens, nuts, okra, rutabagas, seaweeds, sesame seeds, soybeans, and sunflower seeds. Some calcium is found naturally in water.

Be Aware!

If you are prone to calcium oxalate kidney stones, you may want to limit your intake of the following foods and beverages: spinach, chard, sorrel, beet greens, rhubarb, wheat bran, nuts, chocolate, colas, coffee, strawberries, and tea. Also, the phytates or oxalates in these foods bind to calcium and keep it from being properly absorbed. Take supplements two hours before or after meals containing these foods.

Calcium Deficiency Risks

The most significant risk resulting from insufficient calcium intake is osteoporosis, and this is a serious risk, indeed. The older we get, the more the rate of calcium absorption slows. Currently, 25 million American women and 5 million American men suffer some degree of bone loss. In many cases, the damage isn't known until a fragile bone breaks—even a handshake can wreak havoc. Women are at a significant risk after menopause, when estrogen levels plummet, because estrogen is a key factor in bone production. Men who have low levels of testosterone also are at risk of osteoporosis.

Other calcium deficiency symptoms include abnormal heartbeat, dementia, muscle spasms, and convulsions.

Note: Iron interferes with calcium, so take these supplements at different times.

Calcium Overdosing Risks

It is hard to take too much calcium because the body

excretes any it doesn't use. However, it is best to keep intake below 2,000 mg per day as too much calcium may interfere with kidney function. Too much calcium may interfere with iron absorption and cause constipation, tissue calcification, and magnesium deficiency.

Calcium supplements not taken with food increase the risk of kidney stones for women, and possibly also for men.

Who Should Take Special Note of Their Intake?

The following individuals should be particularly aware of their intake:

- *Pregnant women.* Women who are pregnant need more calcium than they do otherwise. The growing baby uses calcium from the mother's body as it builds its bones. Follow your doctor's advice about calcium supplements while you are pregnant and if you breastfeed.

    On the plus side, researchers now believe that the extra calcium also helps to maintain normal blood pressure during pregnancy, minimizing the risk of toxemia.

- *Menopausal women.* Women who no longer produce large amounts of estrogen need to be especially careful of their osteoporosis risk. Extra calcium is recommended, especially if you don't use estrogen replacement therapy (ERT).

- *People with hypercalcemia.* These patients may be advised not to take calcium supplements. Talk to your doctor if you have a medical condition that puts you at risk of hypercalcemia.

- *People with certain medical conditions.* Talk to your doctor before you take calcium supplements if you have sarcoidosis or any disease of the kidneys, heart, intestines, or stomach.

- *Individuals taking prescription drugs should be aware of possible drug interactions.* Many prescription medicines affect the body's ability to absorb calcium. If you are being treated for any medical condition, be sure to discuss your nutritional requirements with your doctor

Magnesium

Magnesium is an essential mineral used by almost all of the body's components. Half of the body's stores of magnesium are found in the soft tissues and organs, the other half combines with calcium and phosphorus in the bones, and 1 percent is found in the blood supply.

Necessary For

Magnesium is vital for more than 300 biochemical reactions. It activates some 100 enzymes and helps to maintain normal muscles and nerves, heart rhythm, blood pressure, and bones. The body also uses magnesium to convert food to energy.

RECOMMENDED DIETARY ALLOWANCES

		MG PER DAY	UPPER LIMITS**
Infants (assumes breastfeeding)	0–6 months	30 mg*	N/A
	7–12 months	75 mg*	N/A
Children	1–3 years	80 mg	65 mg
	4–8 years	130 mg	110 mg
	9–13 years	240 mg	350 mg
Males	14–18 years	410 mg	350 mg
	19–30 years	400 mg	350 mg
	31 years and up	420 mg	350 mg
Females	14–18 years	360 mg	350 mg
	19–30 years	310 mg	350 mg
	31 years and up	320 mg	350 mg
Pregnancy	Up to 18 years	400 mg	350 mg
	19–30 years	350 mg	350 mg
	31 years and up	360 mg	350 mg
Nursing	Up to 18 years	360 mg	350 mg
	19–30 years	310 mg	350 mg
	31 years and up	320 mg	350 mg

*Adequate intake

**No adverse effects shown below these levels

Notes: The upper limits shown are based on consumption of magnesium from supplements and do not include the amounts normally found in food.

Studies suggest that many Americans do not get enough magnesium in their diets. However, try to improve the diet instead of taking supplements.

Food Sources

Animal sources of magnesium include seafood, such as shrimp. Plant sources include almonds, avocado, bananas, beans, bran, broccoli, chocolate, golden raisins, kiwifruit, lentils, nuts, peanut butter, potatoes, pumpkin seeds, soybeans, spinach, wheat and oat cereals, and wheat germ. "Hard" water contains magnesium, as does "soft" water, but in smaller amounts.

Magnesium Deficiency Risks

A number of studies have indicated that inadequate levels of magnesium can contribute to high blood pressure, heart attacks, strokes, osteoporosis, preeclampsia, eclampsia, and diabetes.

Symptoms of deficiency include confusion, disorientation, loss of appetite, depression, muscle contractions and cramps, tingling, numbness, abnormal heart rhythms, coronary spasm, nausea, vomiting, diarrhea, and seizures.

What May Increase Your Risk?

- Chronically low magnesium intake
- Disorders of the gastrointestinal tract that cause magnesium loss or limit absorption
- Excessive loss of magnesium in urine
- Hyperthyroidism
- Taking magnesium and phosphate (phosphorus) supplements together, which may decrease the absorption of each
- Treatment with diuretics, which cause greater urination

Magnesium Overdosing Risks

It is almost impossible to ingest too much magnesium, but it is possible to develop a problem with diarrhea from consuming too much magnesium in laxatives.

If the kidneys are unable to remove excess magnesium, kidney failure is another dangerous consequence. Older people are at risk of this complication because kidney function declines with age and their use of magnesium-rich laxatives and antacids may increase.

Symptoms of magnesium overdose include confusion, nausea, diarrhea, loss of appetite, muscle weakness, extremely low blood pressure, and irregular heartbeat.

Who Should Take Special Note of Their Intake?

The following individuals should be particularly aware of their intake:

- *People taking medications.* Certain medications can result in excessive urination. These include diuretics, cancer treatments, and some common antibiotics. Your doctor will monitor your magnesium levels if you are routinely taking any of these drugs.

- *Diabetics.* Poorly controlled diabetes could put you at risk of magnesium deficiency by increased loss through urination. If you have diabetes, be sure to follow your treatment regimen and see your doctor regularly.

- *Alcoholics.* Alcohol abuse puts one at a very high risk of magnesium deficiency. Low levels of magnesium are found in 30 to 60 percent of alcoholics and 90 percent of people undergoing alcohol withdrawal.

- *People with chronic gastrointestinal disorders.* Disorders such as Crohn's disease, gluten intolerance, and enteritis can lead to magnesium deficiency through excessive diarrhea or malabsorption problems.

- *People with low blood levels of calcium and potassium.* This indicates a strong possibility that magnesium levels are also low.

- *People with myasthenia gravis.* These individuals should talk to their doctors before taking magnesium supplements.

Phosphorus

Phosphorus is an essential mineral used by every cell in the body, although 85 percent of the body's store is found in the bones and teeth. Efficiently absorbed by the small intestine, excess phosphorus is excreted in the urine. The body carefully monitors and regulates levels of phosphorus and calcium and increases one or decreases the other to maintain a balance.

Necessary For

Phosphorus is needed for healthy bones and teeth, muscle contraction, kidney function, regular heartbeat, nerve conduction, and cell membrane health.

RECOMMENDED DIETARY ALLOWANCES

		MG PER DAY	UPPER LIMITS**
Infants (assumes breastfeeding)	0–6 months	100 mg*	N/A
	7–12 months	275 mg*	N/A
Children	1–3 years	460 mg	3,000 mg
	4–8 years	500 mg	3,000 mg
Males/Females	9–18 years	1,250 mg	4,000 mg
	19–50 years	700 mg	4,000 mg
	51–70 years	1,200 mg	4,000 mg
	70 years and up	1,200 mg	3,000 mg
Pregnancy	Up to 18 years	1,250 mg	3,500 mg
	19 years and up	700 mg	3,500 mg
Nursing	Up to 18 years	1,250 mg	4,000 mg
	19 years and up	700 mg	4,000 mg

*Adequate intake
**No adverse effects shown below these levels

Note: Most diets provide sufficient phosphorus. Generally speaking, if you eat the right foods to meet your calcium and protein requirements, you are also getting enough phosphorus.

Food Sources

Phosphorus is found primarily in animal sources such as fish, meat, milk, and poultry. Small amounts are found in whole eggs and in plant sources, including cabbage, collard greens, corn, dried beans and peas, kale, lentils, lima beans, millet, pumpkin seeds, romaine lettuce, soybeans, spinach, squash seeds, sunflower seeds, wheat bran, and wheat germ.

Phosphorus Deficiency Risks

Phosphorus deficiencies are very rare. Symptoms include bone loss, weakness, anorexia, malaise, cardiac arrhythmias, muscle atrophy, and general pain.

What May Increase Your Risk?

- Taking phosphorus and magnesium supplements at the same time, which may decrease the absorption of both
- Malabsorption syndromes, such as Crohn's disease and sprue (celiac disease)
- Chronic alcoholism

Phosphorus Overdosing Risks

If there is too much phosphorus in the diet, the excess combines with calcium, preventing the body from using the calcium.

Who Should Take Special Note of Their Intake?

The following individuals should be particularly aware of their intake:

- *Small premature infants.* Those fed only breast milk may not get enough phosphorus and thus develop rickets.
- *People using aluminum hydroxide antacid products.* Extended use results in an increased risk of phosphorus deficiency because aluminum hydroxide binds with phosphorus, preventing its absorption by the body.
- *Vegans.* People whose diets do not include any animal products may be at risk of phosphorus deficiency and should take care to supplement their diets appropriately.
- *Individuals taking prescription drugs should be aware of possible drug interactions.* Many prescription medicines affect the body's ability to absorb phosphorus. If you are being treated for any medical condition, be sure to discuss your nutritional requirements with your doctor.

Potassium

Potassium is one of the essential minerals needed by the body. It works with sodium to regulate the fluid balance inside and outside cell walls.

Necessary For

Potassium regulates the heartbeat, maintains fluid balance, and helps with muscle contraction, nerve conduction, and energy production.

ADEQUATE INTAKES		
		MG PER DAY*
Infants (assumes breastfeeding)	0–6 months	500 mg
	7–12 months	700 mg
Children	1 year	1,000 mg
	2–5 years	1,400 mg
	6–9 years	1,600 mg
	10–18 years	2,000 mg
Males/Females	19 years and up	2,000 mg

*No upper limits have been established

Notes: A typical diet provides at least 2,000 mg/da of potassium.

Studies have shown that increasing food-sourced potassium to 3,500 mg/day can help to reduce hypertension.

Eating more fruits and vegetables high in potassium has been found to reduce the risk of stroke.

The best way to increase your potassium levels is by eating potassium-rich foods.

Food Sources

Animal sources of potassium are flounder, salmon, and sardines. Plant sources are acorn squash, almonds, apricots (especially dried), artichokes, avocado, bananas, broccoli, celery, chard, peas, kale, lima beans, molasses, parsley, potatoes (especially the skins), prunes, prune juice, oranges, orange juice, raisins, raisin bran cereal, spinach, sunflower seeds, tomatoes, and tomato juice.

Potassium Deficiency Risks

Potassium deficiency is a condition known as hypokalemia. Symptoms include fatigue, weakness, muscle pain, bloating, and constipation. In severe cases this can lead to muscular paralysis or abnormal heart rhythms.

What May Increase Your Risk?

- Excessive vomiting
- Excessive use of diuretics
- Kidney disease
- Metabolic malfunctions
- Alcoholism
- Severe bouts of diarrhea
- Overuse or abuse of laxatives
- Anorexia or bulimia
- Magnesium deficiency
- Congestive heart failure

Note: Regularly eating lots of real (not flavored) black licorice can trigger hypokalemia, because a compound found in licorice increases the urinary excretion of potassium.

Potassium Overdosing Risks

The condition known as hyperkalemia occurs when there is more potassium in the body than can be excreted by the kidneys. It may also happen when blood cells rupture or when there is major tissue damage from trauma or burns.

Symptoms include tingling of hands and feet, muscle weakness, temporary paralysis, and abnormal heart rhythm. Certain prescription drugs, including cardiac and high blood pressure medications, increase this risk. Talk to your doctor about your nutritional and supplement requirements.

Who Should Take Special Note of Their Intake?

The following individuals should be particularly aware of their intake:

- ***People with medical conditions.*** These individuals can be affected by potassium supplements, which should be taken only with a doctor's approval.

    Talk to your doctor if you have Addison's disease, severe dehydration, diabetes mellitus, kidney disease, chronic diarrhea, heart disease, intestinal or esophageal blockage, or stomach ulcers.

- ***Individuals taking prescription drugs should be aware of possible drug interactions.*** Many prescription medicines affect the body's ability to absorb potassium. If you are being treated for any medical condition, be sure to discuss your nutritional requirements with your doctor.

Sodium

Sodium is an essential mineral absorbed in the small intestine. It is important for the absorption of water and other nutrients.

According to J. V. Higdon, "Sodium and chloride (sodium + chloride = salt) are electrolytes that contribute to the maintenance of the concentration and charge differences across cell membranes. Potassium is the positively charged ion inside the cells, and sodium is the principal ion outside cells." Maintenance of this balance is crucial to health.

Necessary For

Sodium is essential for cell membrane health. It is vital for nerve impulse transmission, muscle contraction, and optimum cardiac function, and it helps determine blood volume and blood pressure.

RECOMMENDED DIETARY ALLOWANCES

		SODIUM MG/DAY	CHLORIDE MG/DAY
Infants (assumes breastfeeding)	0–5 months	100 mg	180 mg
	6–11 months	200 mg	300 mg
Children	1 year	225 mg	350 mg
	2–5 years	300 mg	500 mg
	6–9 years	400 mg	600 mg
	10–18 years	500 mg	750 mg
Males/Females	19 years and up	500 mg	750 mg
Pregnancy	All ages	569 mg	877 mg
Nursing	All ages	635 mg	979 mg

Note: Most average diets provide much more salt than the RDA, which is the equivalent of about a teaspoon of salt. Estimates are that 75 percent of salt consumption comes from processed foods.

Food Sources

There is no problem in locating foods containing sodium; instead, it is important to know which foods are high in salt so they can be limited in the diet. High-salt foods include canned chicken noodle soup, canned macaroni and cheese, canned tomato juice, corn dogs, corned beef hash, dill pickles, ham, hot dogs, potato chips, and pretzels, to name only a few. Most fast foods and canned foods have high levels of salt.

Be Aware!

Eating large amounts of salted, smoked, and pickled foods increases the risk of stomach cancer. Also, increased salt intake increases the amount of calcium excreted in the urine, increasing the risk of osteoporosis.

Sodium Deficiency Risks

Because sodium is so prevalent naturally, it is hard to become deficient through inadequate intake. However, low concentrations of sodium can result from increased fluid retention. In other words, if you drink lots of fluids, and don't excrete them, your salt/fluid balance will be affected—too little salt in the mix.

Symptoms of salt deficiency include headaches, nausea, vomiting, muscle cramps, fatigue, disorientation, and fainting. This condition may be fatal without prompt medical attention.

Sodium Overdosing Risks

Too much salt can lead to hypernatremia, which is often caused by extreme fluid loss, leaving too much salt in the system.

Symptoms of hypernatremia include dizziness, fainting, low blood pressure, and diminished urine production. In severe cases symptoms include edema, hypertension, rapid heart rate, difficulty breathing, convulsions, coma, and death. The high blood pressure that is caused by this condition damages the heart, the kidneys, and blood vessels.

Eating too much salt rarely causes this. It is usually caused when the balance of salt/fluid is thrown out of kilter—the reverse of the deficiency situation.

What May Increase Your Risk?

- Participation in athletic events requiring extreme endurance, such as marathons, triathlons, and so on.

- Any activity that causes excessive sweating. Always maintain or even increase your normal fluid intake to replace the water lost through perspiration.

Who Should Take Special Note of Their Intake?

The following individuals should be particularly aware of their intake:

- *People with diets high in smoked and salted foods.* They usually have diets that are low in fruits and vegetables, so vital nutrients are not being consumed.

- *People who are more sensitive to the effects of salt on their blood pressure.* This includes those who are obese and insulin-resistant and older black women with high blood pressure.

TRACE ELEMENTS

Chromium

Chromium (trivalent) is an essential trace element. It is stored primarily in the bones, kidneys, liver, and spleen. Chromium is not produced by the body and must be obtained from food. Scientists are still evaluating the many functions of this mineral.

Necessary For

Chromium is needed for the metabolism of fats and carbohydrates and for regulating blood sugar. It is also important for cholesterol synthesis, and it activates several enzymes.

ADEQUATE INTAKES		
		MCG PER DAY*
Infants (assumes breastfeeding)	0–6 months	0.2 mcg
	7–12 months	5.5 mcg
Children	1–3 years	11 mcg
	4–8 years	15 mcg
Males	9–13 years	25 mcg
	14–50 years	35 mcg
	51 years and up	30 mcg
Females	9–13 years	21 mcg
	14–18 years	24 mcg
	19–50 years	25 mcg
	51 years and up	20 mcg
Pregnancy	Up to 18 years	29 mcg
	19 years and up	30 mcg
Nursing	Up to 18 years	44 mcg
	19 years and up	45 mcg

*No upper limits have been established

Note: Although no upper limits have been established, drastically exceeding the adequate intakes is not advised. Most multivitamin supplements contain 60–120 mcg, which is still considered to be within a safe range.

Food Sources

The best source of chromium is brewer's yeast. Animal sources include beef, butter, chicken, liver, oysters, turkey, and whole eggs. Plant sources are apples, bananas, beer, black pepper, broccoli, brown sugar, coffee, grape juice, green beans, green peppers, molasses, mushrooms, orange juice, potatoes, spinach, tea, thyme, wheat germ, and wine.

Note: Chromium uptake improves when taken in conjunction with vitamin C.

Chromium Deficiency Risks

Impaired glucose tolerance is one sign of chromium deficiency.

What May Increase Your Risk?

- Diabetes mellitus (non-insulin dependent)
- Infants suffering from protein-calorie malnutrition

Note: Taking the recommended amount of chromium will help patients manage these health conditions, but this should not be used to replace a physician's treatment.

Chromium Overdosing Risks

It is hard to overdose on chromium because the body normally absorbs so little and so much is excreted.

Who Should Take Special Note of Their Intake?

The following individuals should be particularly aware of their intake:

- *Individuals with hereditary hemochromatosis.* Chromium deficiency may result from the iron overload disease and may be a contributing factor in the diabetes often found in those with hemochromatosis.

- *Hypoglycemics, hyperglycemics and those with diabetes mellitus.* These individuals should talk to their doctors before taking chromium supplements.

Copper

Copper is an essential trace element that is found in every tissue of the body. It helps the body use iron to make hemoglobin. According to historians, Hippocrates was treating diseases with copper compounds as far back as 400 B.C., but scientists are still making new discoveries about the ways the body uses this mineral.

Necessary For

Copper is important in the body's search-and-destroy efforts against free radicals. Copper also is needed for healthy nerves and bones, immune system, heart and blood vessels, hair, skin, and eye pigmentation, normal infant development, brain development, and cholesterol metabolism.

RECOMMENDED DIETARY ALLOWANCES

		MCG PER DAY	UPPER LIMITS**
Infants (assumes breastfeeding)	0–6 months	200 mcg*	N/A
	7–12 months	220 mcg*	N/A
Children	1–3 years	340 mcg	1,000 mcg
	4–8 years	440 mcg	3,000 mcg
	9–13 years	700 mcg	5,000 mcg
Males/Females	14–18 years	890 mcg	8,000 mcg
	19 years and up	900 mcg	10,000 mcg
Pregnancy	Up to 18 years	1,000 mcg	8,000 mcg
	19 years and up	1,000 mcg	10,000 mcg
Nursing	Up to 18 years	1,300 mcg	8,000 mcg
	19 years and up	1,300 mcg	10,000 mcg

*Adequate intake
**No adverse effects shown below these levels

Food Sources

Animal sources of copper are clams, crab, and oysters. Plant sources are beans, black pepper, broccoli, cocoa, collard greens, kale, kidneys, liver, nuts, potatoes, prunes, romaine lettuce, seeds, spinach, whole grains, and yeast.

Copper Deficiency Risks

Copper deficiency is seldom seen in adults. Menkes' disease, a very rare congenital condition that affects boys, can result from a problem with copper metabolism. Symptoms of Menkes' disease include anemia, skeletal defects, and defects of the nervous system. Otherwise, copper deficiency is seen most often as a result of IV feedings.

Symptoms of copper deficiency include anemia (not associated with iron), reduced white blood cell counts, osteoporosis, hypercholesterolemia, arthritis, heart disease, arterial disease, and loss of pigmentation. Other conditions, however, may also contribute to copper deficiency (see below).

What May Increase Your Risk?

- Being a premature, low-birth-weight baby
- Conditions that diminish gastric or intestinal absorption of nutrients
- Cystic fibrosis
- Diets high in fructose
- Large amounts of foods containing phytates (beans, nuts, whole grains, seeds)
- Large amounts of molybdenum
- Large amounts of nonheme iron
- Lengthy bouts of diarrhea in infants
- Malnourishment in infants and children
- Too much vitamin C (more than 1,500 mg daily)
- Too much zinc

Copper Overdosing Risks

Copper can be toxic in very large amounts. This is usually seen only in a rare hereditary condition known as Wilson's disease that causes the body to store too much copper in the brain, liver, and other organs, leading to kidney and neurological problems, and hepatitis.

Symptoms of copper overdose are pain in the stomach and esophagus, nausea, vomiting, and diarrhea.

Who Should Take Special Note of Their Intake?

- *Babies.* Babies fed exclusively with cow's milk will not get enough copper in their diet.

Fluoride

Fluoride is a trace element not considered to be essential for growth or the maintenance of life itself, but it plays a key role in the prevention of tooth decay, and thus contributes vastly to the quality of life. Eighty percent of the fluoride used by children is found in the teeth and the bones. Fluoride is absorbed in the small intestine and stomach and is found in almost all soil, water sources, plants, and animals.

Necessary For

Fluoride strengthens bones and tooth enamel and protects against cavities.

ADEQUATE INTAKES			
		MG PER DAY	UPPER LIMITS*
Infants (assumes breastfeeding)	0–6 months	0.01 mg	0.7 mg
	7–12 months	0.5 mg	0.9 mg
Children	1–3 years	0.7 mg	1.3 mg
	4–8 years	1 mg	2 mg
	9–13 years	2 mg	10 mg
Males	14–18 years	3 mg	10 mg
	19 years and up	4 mg	10 mg
Females	14 years and up	3 mg	10 mg
Pregnancy/Nursing	All ages	3 mg	10 mg

*No adverse effects shown below these levels

Food Sources

Fluoride is found in almost everything we eat or encounter, especially chicken, salt-water fish (if the bones are consumed), and tea. And most city water supplies are treated with fluoride. However, if you have well water, talk to your dentist about using prescription fluoride pills.

Be Aware!

- The fluoride content of foods can be increased sevenfold by using fluoridated water for cooking.
- Using aluminum cookware decreases the fluoride content of foods.
- Fluoride absorption is reduced when taken with calcium supplements and antacids that contain aluminum. Wait two hours between taking these products and fluoride for maximum effectiveness.

Fluoride Deficiency Risks

Not getting enough fluoride will manifest itself in an increased amount of cavities, as well as unstable bones and teeth.

Note: The lower your salt intake, the more fluoride will be retained by your body. The more salt you consume, the more fluoride will be excreted in your urine.

Fluoride Overdosing Risks

Although fluoride can be toxic if consumed to excess, the amounts necessary to make anyone sick would be far greater than those typically consumed by Americans. No studies have ever shown fluoride to cause a risk of cancer.

However, too much fluoride can cause the teeth to become dull and pitted, although usually cavity-free. The bones may become brittle and chalky at very high amounts of fluoride (more than 20 mg per day) over an extended period of time.

Note: If your water supply has fluoride and you also use fluoridated pills, gels, rinses, and toothpastes, you may be at risk of ingesting too much fluoride. Ask your local board of health or water department about the level of fluoridation. If the level is 0.6 ppm (parts per million) or greater, ask your dentist if you should be using fluoridated products.

Who Should Take Special Note of Their Intake?

The following individuals should be particularly aware of their intake:

- ***Young children.*** Young children often swallow toothpaste while brushing, and this can cause them to ingest more fluoride than they should. While not dangerous to their health, this amount of fluoride can eventually cause permanent white specks on their teeth. It is a good idea for parents to supervise toothbrushing of children under age six, and to limit the amount of paste used. Just a dot is sufficient!

- ***Individuals taking prescription drugs should be aware of possible drug interactions.*** Some prescription medicines affect the body's ability to absorb fluoride. If you are being treated for any medical condition, be sure to discuss your nutritional requirements with your doctor.

Iodine

Iodine is an essential trace element found in food and water as iodide. Iodine is quickly absorbed by the body and sent to the thyroid gland, the kidneys, and the salivary and gastric glands. A key benefit of iodine is the protection it provides against the toxic effects of radiation.

Necessary For

Iodine is a key component in thyroid hormones and necessary for brain development.

RECOMMENDED DIETARY ALLOWANCES

		MCG PER DAY	UPPER LIMITS**
Infants (assumes breastfeeding)	0–6 months	110 mcg*	N/A
	7–12 months	130 mcg*	N/A
Children	1–3 years	90 mcg	200 mcg
	4–8 years	90 mcg	300 mcg
	9–13 years	120 mcg	600 mcg
Males/Females	14–18 years	150 mcg	900 mcg
	19 years and up	150 mcg	1,100 mcg
Pregnancy	Up to 18 years	220 mcg	900 mcg
	19 years and up	220 mcg	1,100 mcg
Nursing	Up to 18 years	290 mcg	900 mcg
	19 years and up	290 mcg	1,100 mcg

*Adequate intake
**No adverse effects shown below these levels

Note: Most people consume enough iodine in a typical diet.

Food Sources

Animal sources of iodine are beef, chicken, dairy products, seafood, turkey, and whole eggs (where iodine has been added to animal feed). Plant sources are navy beans, potatoes, and seaweed. Iodine also is found in iodized table salt and fortified foods.

Be Aware!

Some foods contain substances called goitrogens that block iodine use by the body. Consumption of these foods can result in goiter (enlargement of the thyroid gland), but only when eaten in enormous quantities or if there is already a problem with iodine deficiency.

These goitrogens are found in cassava, some types of millet, cabbage, broccoli, cauliflower, Brussels sprouts, rutabaga, and two soy isoflavones, genistein and daidzein.

Note: Goiter has almost never been seen in seacoast residents.

Iodine Deficiency Risks

Iodine deficiency is the most common cause of preventable brain damage worldwide.

Symptoms of deficiency include severe cretinism, mental retardation, goiter (enlargement of the thyroid gland), hypothyroidism, chronic fatigue, apathy, dry skin, intolerance to cold, weight gain, and abnormal growth and development.

What May Increase Your Risk?

- Deficiencies of selenium, vitamin A, and iron, which may exacerbate iodine deficiencies because the body requires all of these nutrients in order to produce thyroid hormone
- A diet that excludes iodized salt, animal products, fish and/or seaweed

  Note: Radiation-induced thyroid cancer from exposure, for instance, to radioactive material, is a particular risk for iodine-deficient individuals.

  Note: medications containing iodine are meant for the topical (surface) treatment of skin wounds and are toxic when ingested. Don't even think about drinking iodine!

Iodine Overdosing Risks

Iodine overdose is very rare. Symptoms include skin rashes, burning of the mouth, throat and stomach, fever, nausea, vomiting, a thready pulse, and coma.

What May Increase Your Risk?

- Children with cystic fibrosis, who may have problems with excess iodine in their systems
- Excessive use by children of povidone iodine as a cleanser, which may result in too much iodine being absorbed by the skin

Who Should Take Special Note of Their Intake?

The following individuals should be particularly aware of their intake:

- *Pregnant women.* Women who get inadequate iodine during pregnancy put the developing baby at risk of congenital hypothyroidism (cretinism)—irreversible mental retardation. Too much iodine is equally dangerous. Make sure you follow your doctor's recommendations for nutritional supplements during pregnancy.
- *Newborns.* Babies who received an adequate amount of iodine from their mothers during pregnancy are still at risk of abnormal brain development unless they get enough iodine as infants. Nursing mothers need to be sure to follow their doctor's advice about supplements.
- *Individuals with iodine allergies.* Exercise caution with iodine-containing foods and supplements if you have an iodine allergy.
- *Older people.* Older people with goiters are at risk of hyperthyroidism from too much iodine in the diet.

Iron

Iron is an essential trace element and an important component of proteins involved in oxygen transport and metabolism. Almost two-thirds of the iron in the body is found in hemoglobin, the protein in red blood cells that carries oxygen to the body's tissues. Smaller amounts of iron are found in myoglobin, a protein that helps supply oxygen to muscles, and in enzymes that assist biochemical reactions in cells.

About 15 percent of the body's iron is stored for future needs and mobilized when dietary intake is inadequate. The remainder is found in the body's tissues as part of proteins that help the body function. Iron helps to reduce the risks of stomach and esophageal cancer in those being treated for Plummer-Vinson syndrome, and works with vitamin A in red blood cell production and maintaining the health of the immune system. (*Source:* National Institutes of Health)

Necessary For

Iron is needed for blood cell formation and function, immune system health, DNA synthesis, and respiration functions.

RECOMMENDED DIETARY ALLOWANCES		MG PER DAY	UPPER LIMITS**
Infants (assumes breastfeeding)	0–6 months	0.27 mg*	40 mg
	7–12 months	11 mg	40 mg
Children	1–3 years	7 mg	40 mg
	4–8 years	10 mg	40 mg
	9–13 years	8 mg	40 mg
Males	14–18 years	11 mg	45 mg
	19 years and up	8 mg	45 mg
Females	14–18 years	15 mg	45 mg
	19–50 years	18 mg	45 mg
	51 years and up	8 mg	45 mg
Pregnancy	All ages	27 mg	45 mg
Nursing	Up to 18 years	10 mg	45 mg
	19 years and up	9 mg	45 mg

*Adequate intake. Normal full-term infants are born with a supply of iron that lasts for four to six months. Infants very easily absorb iron in breast milk. In fact, studies show that babies are able to use more than 50 percent of the iron in breast milk, compared with less than 12 percent of the iron in formula.

**No adverse effects shown below these levels

Notes: The RDA assumes that 75 percent of the iron is heme iron.

Exceeding the RDA is not recommended without the supervision of a doctor.

Food Sources

There are two kinds of iron: *heme* and *nonheme*.

Heme iron is found in beef, chicken, chicken liver, clams, crab, halibut, oysters, pork, shrimp, tuna, and turkey. The body absorbs this kind of iron very easily.

Nonheme iron is not as easily absorbed. Nonheme iron is found in amaranth (a grain), blackstrap molasses, cashew nuts, cereals (fortified), dark rye, dried beans, firm tofu, flours (fortified), grain products (fortified), kidney beans, lentils, millet, parsley, pigeon peas, potatoes with skins, prunes, prune juice, pumpkin seeds, raisins, sesame seeds, sorghum syrup, squash seeds, sunchokes, sunflower seeds, and wild rice.

Except for women of childbearing age, pregnant women, and those who are nursing, most adults get the recommended amount of iron in their diets.

Note: The body absorbs less than 7 percent of the nonheme iron you eat, but you can improve this rate by combining foods. For instance, eating meat products with beta-carotene-rich foods and vitamin-C-rich foods will increase the nonheme-iron absorption rate. However, calcium, polyphenols, the tannins in tea, and phytates (found in plants such as beans, rice, and grains) will decrease nonheme-iron absorption.

Generally speaking, a good diet will provide the necessary amount of iron, both heme and nonheme. If you know that you have iron-absorption problems—too much or too little—adjusting your meal plans should help.

Iron Deficiency Risks

A lack of iron causes the condition called iron deficiency anemia, which is defined as a major decrease in red blood cells. This is a global concern. The World Health Organization considers it to be the number-one nutritional disorder on the planet, affecting more than 30 percent of the total population.

Symptoms include feeling tired and weak, decreased work and school performance, slow cognitive and social development during childhood, difficulty maintaining body temperature, decreased immune function, rapid heartbeat, heart palpitations, brittle nails, and sore tongue.

It is caused by poor nutrition, excessive dieting, insufficient intestinal absorption, and excessive blood loss.

What May Increase Your Risk?

- Childbearing age
- Chronic blood loss due to infection
- Dark juices, such as red grape juice, which contain antioxidant compounds that block iron absorption (Prune juice is an exception. No research was done on cranberry juice.)
- Dialysis
- Gastrointestinal bleeding
- High doses (above 1,500 mg/day) of calcium supplements taken with iron at a single meal
- Infancy, young childhood, and adolescence
- Ingesting iron with antacids containing aluminum or magnesium
- Ingesting iron at the same time as zinc
- Insufficient consumption of vitamin A
- Insufficient consumption of copper
- Pregnancy
- Uterine bleeding in women on hormone replacement therapy

Notes on Iron Deficiency:

- *If your physician suggests iron supplementation, you will find it comes in two forms, ferrous and ferric. Ferrous iron is more easily absorbed and the kind usually prescribed. Because some other nutrients (such as zinc) are depleted when iron supplements are taken, be sure to take the iron with food and not at the same time as other supplements.*
- *Some medications interfere with iron absorption if taken at the same time. Be sure to tell your doctor about all medications you use, including over-the-counter drugs and vitamins.*
- *Adult men and postmenopausal women lose very little iron except through bleeding. Women with heavy monthly periods can lose a significant amount of iron. The body usually maintains normal iron status by controlling the amount of iron absorbed from food.* (Source: National Institutes of Health)

Iron Overdosing Risks

Iron overdosing is a serious concern. Individuals not at risk of iron deficiency should not take extra iron without a doctor's advice. *Children especially should not be given access to iron supplements.*

Excess iron is found in the blood and stored in the liver, heart, pancreas, skin, brain, and eyes, where it can cause major damage.

What May Increase Your Risk?

- Frequent blood transfusions (You may receive iron-rich blood from donors.)
- Having a non-iron-deficiency anemia that is misdiagnosed and treated with iron supplements
- Light-colored juices (pear, white grape, grapefruit, apple, orange), which increase iron absorption (This may not be a problem unless you already have high levels of iron.)

Who Should Take Special Note of Their Intake?

The following individuals should be particularly aware of their intake:

- *Infants.* Infants benefit much more from the iron in breast milk than they do from the iron in formula. Cow's milk is low in iron, which is poorly absorbed by infants anyway. Because cow's milk can cause gastrointestinal distress and bleeding in infants, the little iron they might get from the milk is usually lost. The American Academy of Pediatrics recommends that babies who are not fed breast milk instead receive an iron-fortified formula.
- *Pregnant women.* Pregnant women are at risk of iron deficiency anemia, which in turns puts their babies at risk of premature delivery and low birth weight. Physicians routinely prescribe vitamins with iron for their pregnant patients.
- *Vegetarians.* People who exclude all animal products, including dairy, also exclude the best sources of heme iron, the kind most easily absorbed by the body and useful for the absorption of nonheme iron. As a result, their diets should be even richer in nonheme iron foods, and they should consider consuming foods rich in vitamin C with the nonheme foods. The recommended dietary allowance for vegetarian diets is 14 mg per day for adult men and postmenopausal women; 33 mg per day for premenopausal women and 26 mg per day for teenage girls.
- *Women with heavy menstrual bleeding.* This is a common risk factor for iron deficiency anemia. Blood loss of any kind is accompanied by a depletion of the body's iron stores. Women who use IUDs often experience heavy menstrual bleeding.
- *Athletes.* Intense exercise performed on a regular basis can quickly deplete the body's iron stores. Talk to your doctor about the possible need for iron supplements, but don't assume you need them.
- *Individuals taking prescription drugs should be aware of possible drug interactions.* Many prescription medicines affect the body's ability to absorb iron. If you are being treated for any medical condition, be sure to discuss your nutritional requirements with your doctor.
- *Individuals with hereditary hemochromatosis.* This genetic disease affects some 1 in 200 Americans of northern European descent, especially those with Scandinavian, English, Irish, Scottish, or Welsh ancestry. People with this disease absorb iron too efficiently and can rapidly build up too much iron in various organs, leading to cirrhosis of the liver or heart failure. A simple blood test can tell if you are at risk of hemochromatosis.

  Sub-Saharan African hemochromatosis appears to result from a high iron intake along with an as-yet-unidentified genetic factor. Although seen primarily in South Africa where iron cooking pots are used, African Americans who are diagnosed with iron overload may have inherited the genetic mutation.
- *Adult men and postmenopausal women.* People who eat a healthful diet including meat are most likely not at risk of being iron deficient. Please don't assume you are iron deficient just because you have some of the symptoms. Talk to your doctor before taking iron supplements. A CBC (complete blood count) will give you the necessary information about your iron levels.

Manganese

Manganese is an essential mineral that is required for many key body functions. Derived from the Greek word for "magic," manganese's various effects on the body are still being studied. Excess iron, calcium, and magnesium reduce manganese absorption and vice versa.

Necessary For

Manganese protects the body's mitochondria from oxidants; activates enzymes for the metabolism of carbohydrates, amino acids, and cholesterol; and assists with glucose production, liver functions, bone formation, and wound healing.

ADEQUATE INTAKES		MG PER DAY	UPPER LIMITS*
Infants (assumes breastfeeding)	0–6 months	0.003 mg	N/A
	7–12 months	0.6 mg	N/A
Children	1–3 years	1.2 mg	2 mg
	4–8 years	1.5 mg	3 mg
Males	9–13 years	1.9 mg	6 mg
	14–18 years	2.2 mg	9 mg
	19 years and up	2.3 mg	11 mg
Females	9–13 years	1.6 mg	6 mg
	14–18 years	1.6 mg	9 mg
	19 years and up	1.8 mg	11 mg
Pregnancy	Up to 18 years	2.0 mg	9 mg
	19 years and up	2.0 mg	11 mg
Nursing	Up to 18 years	2.6 mg	9 mg
	19 years and up	2.6 mg	11 mg

*No adverse effects shown below these levels

Food Sources

Manganese is found in plant sources including almonds, brown rice, lima beans, navy beans, oatmeal, peanuts, pecans, pineapple (raw), pineapple juice, pinto beans, raisin bran cereal, spinach, sweet potato, tea (green and black), and whole wheat.

Manganese Deficiency Risks

Symptoms of manganese deficiency include growth, reproductive, and skeletal abnormalities, and impaired glucose tolerance.

What May Increase Your Risk?

- Osteoporosis in women
- Diabetes mellitus
- Epilepsy
- Taking antacids and laxatives containing magnesium while eating manganese-rich foods
- Taking tetracycline while eating manganese-rich foods
- Eating foods rich in phytates and oxalates—beans, whole grains, nuts, spinach, chard, sorrel, beet greens, parsley, rhubarb, and sweet potatoes—which may interfere with manganese absorption (This should not be a problem in an otherwise healthful diet.)

Overdosing Risks

The highest risk of overdose comes from inhaling manganese dust during manganese-mining operations. The possible consequences include Parkinson's disease, with symptoms of tremors, difficulty walking, and muscle spasms.

What Else May Increase Your Risk?

- Chronic liver disease
- Being newborn, with an immature liver

Note: The Food and Nutrition Board does not know enough about possible toxicity from manganese supplements, so it is advisable to stay below the upper limits. However, there is no evidence to suggest that eating normal quantities of manganese-rich foods poses any hazards.

Who Should Take Special Note of Their Intake?

The following individuals should be particularly aware of their intake:

- ***Individuals taking prescription drugs should be aware of possible drug interactions.*** Many prescription medicines affect the body's ability to absorb manganese. If you are being treated for any medical condition, be sure to discuss your nutritional requirements with your doctor.

Molybdenum

Molybdenum is an essential trace element required by all living things on earth. It works with a number of key enzymes that stimulate chemical activities in carbon, nitrogen, and sulfur processes. These three processes are essential to the body's functions.

Necessary For

Molybdenum works with several enzymes, including those used for alcohol detoxification, formation of uric acid, and sulfur metabolism.

RECOMMENDED DIETARY ALLOWANCES		MCG PER DAY	UPPER LIMITS*
Infants (assumes breastfeeding)	0–6 months	2 mcg	N/A
	7–12 months	3 mcg	N/A
Children	1–3 years	17 mcg	300 mcg
	4–8 years	22 mcg	600 mcg
	9–13 years	34 mcg	1,100 mcg
Males/Females	14–18 years	43 mcg	1,700 mcg
	19 years and up	45 mcg	2,000 mcg
Pregnancy/Nursing	Up to 18 years	50 mcg	1,700 mcg
	19 years and up	50 mcg	2,000 mcg

*No adverse effects shown below these levels

Food Sources

Molybdenum occurs naturally in most water supplies. It is also found in milk, and in the plant foods beans, peas, nuts, and enriched breads and cereals.

Molybdenum Deficiency Risks

Although it is rare in healthy people, a lack of sufficient molybdenum in the diet can be seen in sulfite toxicity.

Symptoms of deficiency include increased heart rate, shortness of breath, headache, confusion, nausea, and vomiting.

Insufficient molybdenum also is thought to be a factor in some cancers.

What May Increase Your Risk?

- Total parenteral nutrition
- Deficiency of the molybdenum cofactor, an inherited condition

Molybdenum Overdosing Risks

Overdosing with molybdenum is not a common enough occurrence to be considered a concern.

Selenium

Selenium is an essential trace element. A number of enzymes require selenium for chemical processes that form proteins. Selenium works with iodine to synthesize thyroid hormone.

Necessary For

Selenium is required for normal growth and development, the immune system, healthy sperm cells, the prostate, and the thyroid gland. It is an important component of the antioxidant enzymes that combat free radicals.

RECOMMENDED DIETARY ALLOWANCES

		MCG PER DAY	UPPER LIMITS*
Infants (assumes breastfeeding)	0–6 months	15 mcg	45 mcg
	7–12 months	20 mcg	60 mcg
Children	1–3 years	20 mcg	90 mcg
	4–8 years	30 mcg	150 mcg
	9–13 years	40 mcg	280 mcg
Males/Females	14 years and up	55 mcg	400 mcg
Pregnancy	All ages	60 mcg	400 mcg
Nursing	All ages	70 mcg	400 mcg

*No adverse effects shown below these levels

Food Sources

Animal sources of selenium are beef, beef liver, cheddar cheese, chicken, cod, cottage cheese, tuna, turkey, and whole eggs. Plant sources are black walnuts, Brazil nuts, noodles (enriched), oatmeal, rice, and white and whole-wheat breads (enriched).

Note: Selenium is naturally found in the soil and is absorbed by the plants grown in that soil. Within the United States selenium is very high in the soil of northern Nebraska and the Dakotas.

Selenium Deficiency Risks

Symptoms of selenium deficiency, sometimes known as Keshan disease, include an enlarged heart and diminished heart function. Selenium deficiency also has been linked to thyroid problems and an increased risk of several cancers. A lack of selenium may exacerbate iodine deficiency symptoms.

What May Increase Your Risk?

- Severe gastrointestinal disorders, which adversely affect nutrient absorption by the stomach and intestines

Selenium Overdosing Risks

Selenium is highly toxic, but while it is possible to ingest too much selenium, this is rare in the United States. Most cases have been connected to industrial accidents.

Symptoms include hair loss, fingernail changes, fatigue, nausea, garlic breath, and vomiting.

Who Should Take Special Note of Their Intake?

The following individuals should be particularly aware of their intake:

- *IV patients.* Total parenteral nutrition is a way of providing certain nutrients through intravenous tubes. Patients who receive all of their nourishment this way may be at risk of selenium deficiency if care is not taken to add the mineral to the fluid.

- *Individuals taking prescription drugs should be aware of possible drug interactions.* Many prescription medicines affect the body's ability to absorb selenium. If you are being treated for any medical condition, be sure to discuss your nutritional requirements with your doctor.

Zinc

Zinc is an essential trace element necessary for all forms of life on the planet. In humans, zinc is found in almost every cell in the body. Zinc deficiency is increasingly recognized as a serious health issue, particularly in underdeveloped parts of the world. Although zinc is found in many different foods, it is most readily available in animal products. Zinc supplements are best absorbed on an empty stomach.

Necessary For

Zinc is an important trace element involved in stimulating the activity of some 100 enzymes, supporting a healthy immune system, wound healing, cell membranes, metabolism, digestion, maintaining the senses of taste and smell, DNA synthesis, sperm production, testosterone metabolism, night vision, insulin use, and normal growth and development during pregnancy, childhood, and adolescence.

RECOMMENDED DIETARY ALLOWANCES

		MG PER DAY	UPPER LIMITS*
Infants (assumes breastfeeding)	0–6 months	2 mg	4 mg
	7–12 months	3 mg	5 mg
Children	1–3 years	3 mg	7 mg
	4–8 years	5 mg	12 mg
	9–13 years	8 mg	23 mg
Males	14 years and up	11 mg	34 mg
Females	14–18 years	9 mg	34 mg
	19 years and up	8 mg	34 mg
Pregnancy	Up to 18 years	12 mg	34 mg
	19 years and up	11 mg	34 mg
Nursing	Up to 18 years	13 mg	34 mg
	19 years and up	12 mg	34 mg

*No adverse effects shown below these levels

Food Sources

Animal sources of zinc are beef, cheddar cheese, chicken, crab, flounder, milk, mozzarella cheese, oysters, pork, sole, Swiss cheese, turkey, and yogurt. Plant sources are almonds, black walnuts, breakfast cereals (fortified), cashews, garbanzo beans (chickpeas), green peas, kidney beans, navy beans, oatmeal, peanuts, and pecans.

Zinc Deficiency Risks

Zinc deficiency can be a severe problem for people born with a genetic disorder called acrodermatitis enteropathica, an impaired ability to uptake and transport zinc. At one time this condition resulted in death in infancy, but now it is successfully treated with oral zinc therapy. It is possible to develop a zinc deficiency for other reasons, however, such as those listed below.

Symptoms of zinc deficiency include growth retardation, hair loss, diarrhea, delayed sexual maturation, impotence, lesions of the eyes and skin, loss of appetite, immune system problems, hypogonadism, anorexia, neural tube defects in fetuses, and miscarriages. Weight loss, slow-healing wounds, night blindness, taste abnormalities, and mental lethargy may also occur.

The immune system is severely affected by any amount of zinc deficiency.

What May Increase Your Risk?

- A vegetarian diet
- Acrodermatitis enteropathica
- Alcoholism
- Being above age sixty
- Chronic dieting
- Digestive diseases that might inhibit zinc absorption, or cause a loss of zinc through diarrhea
- Severe burns
- Sickle-cell anemia
- Taking the following substances together with zinc: iron, phosphate, calcium, coffee, tea, caffeinated beverages, and phytate and oxalate foods
- Total parenteral nutrition
- Too much calcium (For instance, people who eat a lot of tortillas made with lime—calcium oxide—are at risk of zinc deficiency.)

Zinc Overdosing Risks

Too much zinc increases the risk of low copper status in the body, stomach upset, modified iron function, reduced immune system function, and lower levels of HDL (good cholesterol).

Who Should Take Special Note of Their Intake?

The following individuals should be particularly aware of their intake:

- *Vegetarians.* Vegetarians need to know that the body absorbs more zinc from a diet high in animal protein than one high in plant proteins. In fact, phytates, found in whole-grain breads and other plant products, actually can decrease zinc absorption. You may need as much as 50 percent more zinc than non-vegetarians. Talk to your doctor about your intake and possible need for supplementation.

- *Unborn children of mothers with a zinc deficiency.* There is a risk of slow fetal growth. If you are pregnant, be sure to follow your doctor's advice about diet and vitamin and mineral supplements.

- *Nursing infants.* Babies between seven and twelve months of age cannot get enough zinc from breast milk and will need zinc-rich foods appropriate for their ages.

- *Nursing mothers.* Women who are nursing will deplete their zinc stores faster than usual and should take care with their diets and supplements.

- *Alcoholics.* Alcoholics are at risk of zinc insufficiency because alcohol decreases the ability of the body to absorb zinc and increases the loss of zinc through the urine. Also, alcoholics often have poor diets and are not getting the zinc they need in the food they eat.

- *Iron-deficiency anemics.* Those who take more than 25 mg of supplemental iron are at risk of zinc deficiency.

- *Pregnant women.* Those women who take supplemental iron may inadvertently decrease the amount of zinc their bodies can absorb. Talk to your doctor about your need for supplemental nutrition.

- *Postmenopausal women.* These women should discuss the amount of zinc they need because calcium intake affects zinc absorption.

- *Older Americans.* These individuals are at risk of absorption problems because they are more likely to have prolonged illnesses or conditions requiring medications that increase the excretion of zinc.

PART FIVE
DISEASE PREVENTION GUIDE

At the moment of conception, you are imbued with a number of characteristics that will affect your health for the rest of your life. These include gender, ethnicity or ancestry, blood type, and family history. The fact that you are a woman, for instance, automatically puts you at risk for diseases affecting the female reproductive organs. Men are automatically at risk for prostate conditions. Blacks, unlike whites, have a potential risk of sickle-cell disease; Japanese with blood type A have a potentially higher risk than Italians for stomach cancer. Family history is a tremendous predictor of risk, and you are born with a possible risk for any health condition experienced by your ancestors, going back thousands of years.

Other factors that could increase your risk for specific diseases include your workplace, living conditions, and personal medical history. Your workplace may expose you to chemicals, allergens, or pollutants that might exacerbate an existing health problem. Living in a city might cause problems for those who don't handle stress well or who have respiratory conditions. And if you have a medical condition such as diabetes, your risk for other health problems goes up dramatically. This is because the body consists of dozens of intricately connected systems and parts. What goes wrong in one system *must* affect others.

Thus, you are born with characteristics—risk factors—that you cannot change. Does this mean that if you are a hypertensive black male whose father died of heart failure, you will have a heart attack? Not necessarily. But your risk is greater than that of a young white woman with low blood pressure.

So, the bad news is that you are at risk for a serious heart problem. The good news is that you can do something about it. *If you know your risk factors for a specific condition, you can take steps to minimize the risks.* Proactive things that you can do include learning as much as possible about your family medical history. Make sure your doctor knows your family and personal medical histories. Find out about checkups, tests, and screenings available for your condition. Track the results in Part Two.

Another important step you can take is to examine your lifestyle. Are you inadvertently or deliberately engaging in behavior that increases your risk for a specific health condition? For instance, if heart disease runs in your family and you smoke cigarettes, your risk of heart attack goes up significantly. Simply quitting will increase the odds in your favor immediately.

The Disease Prevention Guide is organized alphabetically by body part. Each section includes an illustration of the specific part, its key components, its location within the body, and the following sections, where applicable:

Function

Keeping [the body part] Healthy

Beneficial Foods and Nutrients

Other Tips

What Can Go Wrong

Medical Conditions That Can Affect [the body part]

Risky Behavior and Possible Consequences

It is important to note that the Disease Prevention Guide is not meant to be a diagnostic tool. You will not find descriptions of symptoms or suggested treatments for specific conditions. Instead, the focus is on learning what the average person needs to do to keep that part of the body healthy. When specific diseases or conditions are mentioned, it is for the purpose of identifying factors that may put you at risk of developing that disease. Some of the factors are immutable—in other words, unchangeable—because you were born with certain characteristics. Some factors are lifestyle choices and *can* be changed to minimize the risk. It is up to you. (See "Risk Factors" on page 3.)

The more you know about your own health, your personal history, your family history, and your risk factors for certain diseases, the more control you can take over your life, lifestyle, and well-being.

Part Five Contents

The Bladder, 187

The Blood Supply, 190

The Bones, 197

The Brain, 202

The Breasts, 207

The Cervix, 210

The Circulatory System, 212

The Ears, 217

The Esophagus, 220

The Eyes, 222

The Gallbladder, 228

The Hands, 229

The Heart, 231

The Hormones, 235

The Immune System, 238

The Intestines, 243

The Joints, 248

The Kidneys, 251

The Liver, 254

The Lungs, 259

The Lymphatic System, 263

The Mouth, 265

The Muscles, 267

The Nervous System, 269

The Nose, 272

The Ovaries, 274

The Pancreas, 277

The Penis, 280

The Prostate, 282

The Rectum, 284

The Skin, 287

The Spine, 290

The Stomach, 293

The Teeth, 296

The Testicles, 299

The Throat, 301

The Thyroid, 303

The Urinary Tract, 305

The Uterus, 308

The Vagina, 310

The Bladder

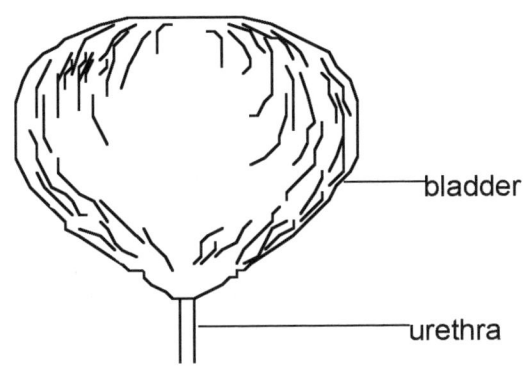
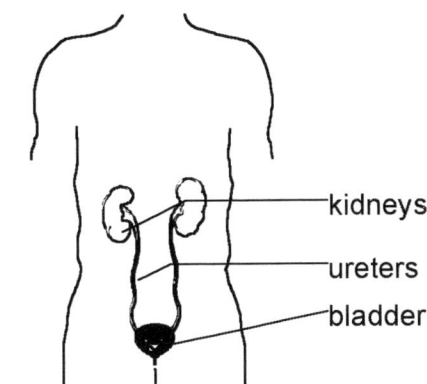

Function

The bladder is a hollow organ located in the lower part of the abdomen, just below the navel. It collects and stores urine, which is delivered to the bladder from the kidneys by way of hollow tubes called ureters. Powerful sphincter muscles keep the bladder closed until you are ready to urinate. The average adult passes about a quart and a half of urine daily.

Keeping the Bladder Healthy

What You and Your Doctor Should Know

- Family history of bladder cancer
- Any other existing medical conditions that may affect your bladder

Preventive Maintenance

- Drink six to eight glasses of water or other fluids daily. This keeps the whole urinary tract system adequately flushed and diluted. Urine should be pale or straw colored.
- Urinate when you feel the urge. Holding back can be painful as the bladder fills and, if you have a urinary tract infection, allows bacteria to breed to very unhealthy levels.

Beneficial Foods and Nutrients

See Part Four, The Importance of Nutrients, for a list of foods containing the vitamins mentioned in this section.

Cranberry Juice

An excellent preventative, this juice contains acids that have been shown to combat the bacteria that cause urinary tract infections.

Green Tea

Green tea contains polyphenols, which may help to reduce the risk of bladder cancer.

Vitamin A

Vitamin A may have a protective effect against bladder cancer.

Vitamin C (Ascorbic Acid)

Vitamin C is a natural antioxidant that may help to protect against bladder cancer.

Other Tips

- Wear protective clothing if your work environment exposes you to chemicals.
- Don't let your children use playground equipment made of pressure-treated wood. The arsenic used in the treatment process will get on your children's hands and into their mouths. This increases their risk of bladder cancer later in life.

Women:

- If you wear pads during your period, change them at least twice a day. The warm, moist environment provides a perfect breeding ground for bacteria that cause bladder infections.

See "The Urinary Tract" for more information on keeping the urinary system healthy.

What Can Go Wrong

Bladder Cancer

Bladder cancer is the fourth most common type of cancer for men, and the eighth most common for women. Each year new cases are diagnosed in 38,000 men and 15,000 women. The following conditions increase your risk of developing bladder cancer.

Age. The risk increases over age forty. The median age at diagnosis is sixty-eight.

Blood type. Type B has a higher risk, types A and AB moderate risk, and type O has a lower risk. Non-secretors of all blood types have a higher risk. Rh-positive individuals have more invasive tumors of the upper urinary tract.

Ethnicity/ancestry. White men have twice the risk of black and Hispanic men, but black men are more likely to die of bladder cancer than other groups, probably due to delayed diagnoses.

White women have a higher risk than black women, and black women have a higher risk than Hispanic women. Like black men, black women have the highest mortality rate of all the groups. Asians have the lowest risk.

Family history. An incident of bladder cancer in one's family increases the risk to the individual.

Gender. Men are three to four times as likely as women to develop bladder cancer.

Genetic factors. Mutations of various genes have been associated with bladder cancer.

Habitat. Living in certain geographic areas can increase risk of bladder cancer.
- Tropical areas (not in the United States) with common parasites that can infect the bladder
- Living in industrialized countries (United States, Canada, France, Denmark, Italy, Spain)

Medical conditions. These conditions are risk factors:
- Frequent bladder and kidney infections
- Persistent inflammation from bladder stones and/or extended use of catheters

Medications. Cyclophosphamide and arsenic, sometimes used for medical purposes, increase the risk of bladder cancer.

Personal history. Having these conditions increases risk:

- Anyone who has had bladder cancer has a risk of redeveloping the condition
- Exposure to radiation through x-rays, workplace, or medical treatment, especially for cervical cancer.
- Use of playground equipment made of pressure-treated wood

Workplace. Those who work with carcinogens in certain industries are at increased risk: hairdressers, machinists, metal workers, printers, painters, textile workers, truck drivers, dry cleaners, paper manufacturers, rope and twine makers, and other workers using dyes, rubber, chemicals, and leather. The risk increases with exposure to substances called aromatic amines (arylamines).

What you can do: Know your family and personal history. Minimize your controllable risks. Although there are no effective screening methods for detecting bladder cancer in individuals with no history of the disease, cystoscopy can be used to detect new cases in patients with a history of bladder cancer. For more information, type BLADDER CANCER into an Internet search engine.

Congenital Risks

Exstrophy of the Bladder

This surgically reparable malformation occurs during fetal development in about 1 in every 40,000 births.

Family history. A family history increases the risk.

Gender. Boys are more likely to be born with this condition.

Vesicoureteral Reflux

This is a congenital condition in which urine backs up from the bladder into the ureters toward the kidneys. This condition occurs in about 4 of 1,000 people.

Ethnicity/ancestry. Whites have ten times the risk of blacks, and children with red hair are at an increased risk.

Family history. Although this condition may not be inherited, if one child is diagnosed with reflux, doctors usually will want to check the other children in the family.

Gender. Girls are twice as likely as boys to be born with this condition.

Medical conditions. Urinary tract infections (UTIs) may be an indication of this condition, because about one in three children with UTIs are found to have reflux.

Bladder Conditions That Tend to Run in Families

These conditions have no known genetic links:
- Enuresis (bed-wetting)
- Recurrent cystitis

Medical Conditions That Can Affect Bladder Health

It is important to properly treat any medical condition with which you are diagnosed, because the condition may affect other parts of your body. The body's organs and systems are inextricably connected to one another, so what goes wrong in one part may create problems in another. The following conditions can affect bladder health.

- *Bladder infection (cystitis)*—risk factors are:
  - Bladder stones
  - Blood types B and AB
  - Diabetes
  - Enlarged prostate (benign prostatic hypertrophy)
  - Infections from salmonella and *E. coli* (*Escherichia coli*) bacteria
  - Parkinson's disease
  - Pregnancy
  - Risk increases with age, especially for the elderly
  - Spinal cord injury

- *Bladder stones*—risk factors are:
  - Bladder diverticulum
  - Bladder outlet obstruction
  - Cushing's disease
  - Enlarged prostate (95 percent of all bladder stones develop in men)
  - Foreign matter in the bladder
  - Hyperparathyroidism
  - Increase in calcium levels in the urine
  - Neurogenic bladder
  - Urinary tract infection

- *Neurogenic bladder* is indicated by abnormal emptying of the bladder—too often or too seldom. Risk factors include:
  - Acute infections
  - Congenital nerve problems
  - Diabetes mellitus
  - Heavy metal poisoning
  - Herpes zoster (shingles)
  - Multiple sclerosis
  - Tumor of the nervous system
  - Trauma to the brain or the spinal cord

- *Urinary incontinence* is an uncontrollable emptying of the bladder or leakage. Risk factors include:
  - Childbirth
  - Constipation
  - Neurological diseases, such as Parkinson's disease and multiple sclerosis
  - Pelvic surgery in women
  - Postmenopause
  - Pregnancy
  - Prostate surgery
  - Shy-Drager syndrome
  - Spinal cord injuries
  - Urinary tract infections
  - Use of certain medications
  - Weakened sphincter muscle

Risky Behavior and Possible Consequences

RISKY BEHAVIOR	POSSIBLE CONSEQUENCES
Cigarette smoking*	Bladder cancer Urinary incontinence
Exposure to radiation	Bladder cancer
Alcoholism	Bladder cancer
Consuming stimulants such as caffeine and spicy foods	Incontinence
Rectal intercourse	Bladder infections (cystitis)
Use of spermicides or non-lubricated condoms	Bladder infections (cystitis)
Use of a diaphragm	Bladder infections (cystitis)
Not drinking enough fluids	Urinary tract infections
Routinely holding back when you need to urinate	Urinary tract infections
Untreated gonorrhea in pregnancy	Babies born with gonococcal ophthalmia
Untreated chlamydia infection in pregnancy	Babies born with eye infections and pneumonia
Unprotected sexual intercourse	Gonococcal urethritis caused by gonorrhea Nongonococcal urethritis caused by chlamydia
Obesity	Urinary incontinence

*Increases the risk by five times over nonsmokers. Pipe and cigar smokers also have a higher risk than nonsmokers.

Visit www.healthwatchguide.com for updates on the bladder.

The Blood Supply

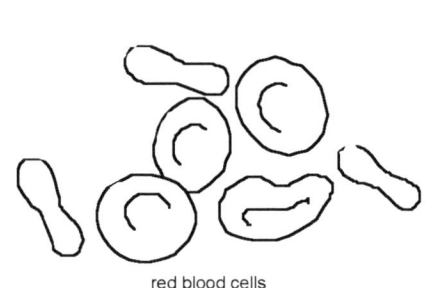
red blood cells

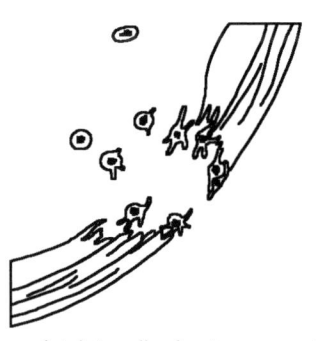
platelets adhering to a wound site

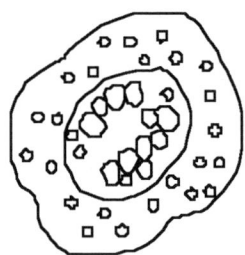
white blood cell

Function

Most blood cells are produced in the marrow of your bones. An average adult has four to six quarts of blood. The blood consists of red blood cells, white blood cells, platelets, and plasma. Red blood cells contain hemoglobin, which helps the cells pick up oxygen in the lungs and carry it to the other organs of the body. They also remove carbon dioxide from the cells and take it to the lungs. Thirty to 40 billion white blood cells fight infection, and platelets help the blood to clot after an injury. The liquid part of the blood is called plasma. Plasma picks up dissolved food from the intestines and liver and delivers it throughout the body. Plasma also collects and transports wastes for removal from the body.

Definitions of Terms

Antibodies—Antibodies are specialized chemicals produced by the immune system to fight intruder antigens (germs, cells, viruses, and so forth). The response to foreign blood antigens is the most potent immune mechanism in the human body. These antibodies agglutinate (clump) foreign blood cells for removal from the body. Transfusion of the wrong blood type results in huge amounts of clumped cells, which can block the arteries of filtration devices in the kidneys and lead to death.

Type O produces antibodies against A, B, and AB antigens, and therefore cannot receive transfusions of these blood types. Type A produces antibodies against B antigens, and cannot receive transfusions of B or AB. Type B produces antibodies against A antigens, and cannot receive transfusions of A or AB. Type AB produces no antibodies, so it can receive transfusions of A, B, AB, and O. Type O produces no antigens, so it can donate to any of the other groups.

Blood Types—Blood has four types: A, B, AB, and O.

Blood types are inherited from parents, with each parent contributing a gene. Genes for types A and B are dominant and will always be expressed (appear). Type O is recessive.

A child who inherits one A gene and one O gene will be type A with a recessive O, shown as Ao. Both genes may be passed on by children to their children. Similarly, a child who inherits one B and one O gene will be type Bo. If both an A and a B gene are passed on, a child will be type AB. A child who receives type A from both parents will be type AA.

Only a child who inherits one O gene from each parent can be type oo. Thus, type A or B children with an O parent will have the recessive gene for O, which may be expressed (appear) in their children.

The following table shows the inheritance patterns.

PARENTS' BLOOD TYPES	POSSIBLE BLOOD TYPES IN CHILDREN
Both A	A or O (O is possible only if both parents have the recessive gene for O)
Both B	B or O (O is possible only if both parents have the recessive gene for O)
Both AB	A, B, or AB
Both O	O
One A and one B	A, B, AB, or O (O is possible if both parents have passed on a recessive O)
One A and one O	A or O (O is possible only if the A parent has passed on a recessive O)
One A and one AB	A, B, or AB
One B and one O	B or O (O is possible only if the B parent has passed on a recessive O)
One B and one AB	A, B, or AB
One AB and one O	A or B (a child will inherit either the A or the B, both of which are dominant to the recessive O)

Source: D'Adamo, Peter J.

Complete Blood Count (CBC)—A CBC measures the number of red blood cells (RBC) and white blood cells (WBC). It also includes a hematocrit (HCT) reading, calculates the total amount of hemoglobin (HGB), and measures the size of the red blood cells. A platelet count is usually included in a CBC.

	NORMAL READINGS
RBC:	Men—4.7–6.1 million cells per microliter (mcL)
	Women—4.2–5.4 million cells per mcL
WBC:	4,500–10,000 million cells per mcL
HGB:	Men—13.8–17.2 grams per deciliter (gm/dL)
	Women—12.1–15.1 gm/dL
HCT:	Men—40.7 to 50.3%
	Women—36.1 to 44.3%
Platelets:	150,000–400,000 mm$_3$

Hematocrit (HCT)—An HCT is a test that measures the ratio of red blood cells to fluid in the blood.

Hemoglobin (HGB)—Hemoglobin is a protein that carries oxygen in red blood cells. Variations from the norm in the hemoglobin count can indicate abnormalities in the red blood cells or the presence of disease.

Rh Factor—All blood types may contain a factor called Rh after the rhesus monkey in whose blood it was first identified in 1946. Rh-positive blood has the Rh antigen; Rh-negative blood does not. Rh-negative mothers who carry Rh-positive babies (regardless of blood type) will be exposed to the baby's blood during delivery. The mother's blood will then make antibodies to the Rh factor. These antibodies will attack the blood cells of any subsequent Rh-positive babies, which may also lead to the death of the mother. Only Rh-negative women need to worry about this. A vaccine has been developed that is given to Rh-negative mothers after the delivery of their first child and again after every future birth. The first child is never in danger.

Note: Rh-negative mothers need to tell their doctors about any abortions or miscarriages before the birth of the first full-term baby.

Secretors and Nonsecretors—The blood type of a secretor (approximately 80 percent of the population) can be found in body fluids such as saliva, mucus, and semen. Nonsecretors, who represent about 20 percent of the population, are far more vulnerable to immune system disorders. (*Source:* D'Adamo, Peter J.)

Keeping the Blood Supply Healthy

What You and Your Doctor Should Know

- Family history of blood disorders
- Blood type

- Hematocrit
- Hemoglobin count
- Rh factor
- Secretor status

Beneficial Foods and Nutrients

See Part Four, The Importance of Nutrients, for a list of foods containing the vitamins and minerals mentioned in this section.

Vitamin A and Beta-Carotene
These vitamins assist with red blood cell development and provide antioxidant protection.

The B Vitamins
Several of the B vitamins are essential for red blood cell production: vitamin B_2 (riboflavin), vitamin B_6 (pyridoxine), and vitamin B_{12} (cobalamin).

Vitamin C (Ascorbic Acid)
Vitamin C is a natural antioxidant that helps to protect the blood cells.

Vitamin E (Tocopherol)
Vitamin E protects red blood cells.

Vitamin K
Vitamin K is vital to enhancing the blood's ability to clot.

Iron
Iron supplements may be needed in the event of iron deficiency.

Folic Acid (Folate)
Folate is needed to produce enough red blood cells.

Calcium
Calcium helps the blood to clot.

Other Tips

If you have blood type O or B (the thinnest blood types), be wary of blood-thinning products, like aspirin, and minimize your opportunities to bleed, such as tooth extraction or surgery.

What Can Go Wrong

Leukemia
Leukemia is cancer of the blood cells. Each year more than 27,000 adults and 2,000 children are diagnosed with leukemia. The following factors increase your risk of developing leukemia.

Age. Age is a risk factor for these forms of leukemia:
- Acute lymphocytic leukemia (ALL)—young children, and adults over age sixty-five
- Acute myeloid leukemia (AML)—all ages
- Chronic lymphocytic leukemia (CLL)—usually adults over age fifty-five
  - Incidence—two in 100,000 people
  - Specific ethnicity/ancestry risks—Jews of Russian or Eastern European heritage are most at risk
- Chronic myeloid leukemia (CML)—mainly occurs in adults, rarely in children (This disease is caused by a chromosomal defect. It can be aggravated by exposure to ionizing radiation and benzene.)
- Hairy cell leukemia—adults over age fifty-five (It is extremely rare; men are five times more at risk than women. There is no known cause.)

Blood types. Types A and AB have a higher risk, type B has a moderate risk, and type O has a moderate risk. However, more type O males are affected than females.

Ethnicity/ancestry. In descending order of risk within age categories:
- Adults—white non-Hispanics, blacks, Hispanics, Asians, Pacific Islanders, Native Americans, and Alaska Natives.
- Children—Filipinos, white Hispanics, white non-Hispanics, blacks

Family history. Individuals are more likely to develop acute lymphocytic leukemia (ALL) if it is present in a sibling.

Gender. Men have a much greater risk for acute leukemia than women.

Medical conditions. These medical conditions are risk factors:
- Down syndrome (for ALL)
- Blood disorders (for AML)

Workplace. These working conditions place a person at risk:
- Exposure over long periods of time to chemicals such as benzene (for ALL, AML, and CML)
- Exposure to high levels of radiation (for ALL, AML, and CML)

What you can do: There is no known cause of leukemia, except in CML, which is a chromosomal defect that can be determined by a blood test. Know your risk factors and minimize the controllable ones. Have regular medical checkups and maintain a healthful diet-and-exercise routine. For information on symptoms, type LEUKEMIA into an Internet search engine.

Multiple Myeloma

This cancer affects the white blood cells (plasma cells). There are 8,500 new cases diagnosed in the United States annually. The following factors increase your risk of developing multiple myeloma.

Age. Individuals between fifty and seventy are most likely to get this cancer.

Ethnicity/ancestry. In descending order of risk: blacks, whites, Hispanics, Native Americans, Alaska Natives, Asians, and Pacific Islanders.

Family history. Having first-degree relatives (parents, siblings, children) with multiple myeloma increases your risk.

Gender. Men have a greater risk than women.

Workplace. The following working conditions can put a person at risk:

- Farmers and petroleum workers exposed to certain chemicals
- Exposure to radiation

What you can do: Know your risk factors, and make sure your doctor knows your family history. Minimize your controllable risks. For more information, type MULTIPLE MYELOMA into an Internet search engine.

Anemia

Anemia is an insufficiency of red blood cells. There are many different types of anemias, some of which are caused by chromosomal defects (see "Hereditary Conditions" in Part One), others by vitamin insufficiency, and still more by other medical conditions. Some conditions run in families, so it is important to know your family health history. Other factors that may put you at risk of anemia include the following.

Blood types. Types A and AB have an increased risk of iron deficiency (especially vegetarians) and an increased risk of pernicious anemia (insufficiency of vitamin B_{12}), especially type A.

Medical conditions. These medical conditions are risk factors:

- In pregnancy, the fetus can deplete the mother's store of iron, contributing to iron deficiency anemia.
- AIDS, cancer, liver disease, kidney failure, rheumatoid arthritis, bacterial endocarditis, osteomyelitis, rheumatic fever, chronic renal failure, chemotherapy, and chronic inflammatory diseases, such as Crohn's disease, can affect the production of red blood cells, leading to chronic anemia.
- Hepatitis and certain medications can lead to aplastic anemia.
- Some blood diseases, inherited diseases (such as sickle-cell anemia), autoimmune disorders, and certain medications can destroy red blood cells, resulting in hemolytic anemia.

Personal history. Certain individual factors may place one at risk of anemia:

- Heavy menstruation, which can lead to iron deficiency and iron deficiency anemia
- Hookworm infection (a risk only if you come into direct contact with soil containing human feces).

Workplace. Exposure to toxic chemicals can be a factor in developing anemia.

What you can do: Know your risk factors. If you are at risk of anemia, talk to your doctor about getting regular blood counts and recommended treatments, including supplements. Minimize your controllable risks. For more information, type ANEMIA into an Internet search engine.

Warning! Don't assume that because you are tired you must be anemic. Get a blood test from your doctor before taking any supplements.

Anemia of Vitamin B_{12} Deficiency

This type of anemia is due to a decrease in the number of red blood cells, resulting from an insufficiency of vitamin B_{12}. This anemia can result in serious, irreversible neurological complications. Some 2 in 1,000 people have this anemia. The following factors increase your risk of developing vitamin B_{12} deficiency anemia.

Age. This form of anemia can affect any age. Breast-fed infants of mothers with vitamin B_{12} deficiency are especially vulnerable.

Blood types. Type A has a higher risk, type AB has a moderate risk, and types B and O have a lower risk.

Ethnicity/ancestry. All groups are at the same risk level.

Family history. The tendency for developing this anemia can run in families.

Gender. Both men and women are affected.

Medical conditions. These medical conditions are risk factors:

- Crohn's disease
- Intestinal malabsorption conditions
- Intestinal or abdominal surgery
- Pernicious anemia
- Tapeworm infestation

Personal history. Some factors that can lead to vitamin B_{12} deficiency anemia:

- Following a strict vegan diet (excluding dairy, fish, eggs, meat—the only food sources of vitamin B_{12})
- Low levels of intrinsic factor (a protein secreted by the stomach)

What you can do: Make sure your diet contains enough vitamin B_{12}. If you eat a vegan diet, or your stomach doesn't produce enough intrinsic factor to process the B_{12} from beef, talk to your doctor about vitamin supplements or vitamin B_{12} injections. Vitamin B_{12} is not stored in the body, so the supply needs to be constantly replenished. See the section "Vitamin B_{12}" in Part Four for more information, or type ANEMIA OF VITAMIN B12 DEFICIENCY into an Internet search engine.

Iron Deficiency Anemia

Iron deficiency anemia results from a decrease in the number of red blood cells caused by insufficient iron. It is seen in approximately 20 percent of women, 50 percent of pregnant women, and 3 percent of men. The following factors increase your risk of developing iron deficiency anemia.

Age. Growing children and women of childbearing age are at higher risk of iron deficiency anemia.

Blood types. Type A has a higher risk, and types B, AB, and O have a lower risk.

Ethnicity/ancestry. All groups have the same risk level.

Family history. A tendency for iron deficiency anemia may run in families, but this is a universal condition.

Gender. Women have the greater risk due to blood loss through menstruation and the increased need for iron during pregnancy and nursing. Men are at risk largely through dietary insufficiency or contributing medical conditions.

Medical conditions. These medical conditions are risk factors:

- Gastrointestinal blood loss caused by ulcers
- Aspirin use
- NSAID (nonsteroidal anti-inflammatory drug) use
- Colon cancer

Personal history. The following factors create a higher risk:

- Heavy menstrual bleeding
- A strict vegan diet or a diet low in meat or eggs
- Lead poisoning

What you can do: A simple blood test can tell you if you need to increase the iron in your diet or take supplements. Too much iron can be hazardous to your health, so never assume that you need extra iron. Talk to your physician. See the section "Iron" in Part Four for more information, or type IRON DEFICIENCY ANEMIA into an Internet search engine.

Folate Deficiency Anemia

This form of anemia is the result of a decrease in the number of red blood cells that is caused by an insufficiency of folate. It occurs in 4 out of 100,000 people. The following factors increase your risk of developing folate deficiency anemia.

Medical conditions. The following medical conditions are risk factors:

- Malabsorption diseases; for instance, celiac disease and sprue
- Use of certain medications

Personal history. The following factors place one at risk:

- Poor diet, especially one low in fruits and vegetables
- Pregnancy

What you can do: Ensure that your diet is rich in foods containing folate. Take supplements if needed, as folate is not stored in the body and needs to be replenished daily. This is especially important for any woman who may become pregnant, as inadequate folic acid in the mother's body early in the pregnancy can result in spina bifida and other neurological damage to the baby. *The damage is done before the mother even knows she is pregnant, and is irre-*

versible. That is why it is important to begin eating a diet high in folate or taking adequate folic acid supplements when a girl begins to menstruate, so that her body is ready when she starts her family. See the section "Folic Acid" in Part Four, for more information, or type FOLATE DEFICIENCY ANEMIA into an Internet search engine.

Pernicious Anemia

This form of anemia is caused by the lack of intrinsic factor, a substance produced by the gastrointestinal tract and used by the body to extract vitamin B_{12} from foods. Some 2 percent of all Americans over the age of sixty are affected. The following factors increase your risk of developing pernicious anemia.

Age. Usually not seen before age thirty, although a juvenile form does exist. Average age at diagnosis is sixty.

Blood types. Type A has a higher risk, type AB has a moderate risk, and types B and O have a lower risk.

Ethnicity/ancestry. Scandinavians or northern Europeans have the highest risk, though all groups are susceptible.

Family history. This form of anemia runs in families.

Gender. Women are slightly more at risk than men.

Medical conditions. Pernicious anemia is often seen in conjunction with:
- Addison's disease
- Chronic thyroiditis
- Type I diabetes
- Graves' disease
- Hypoparathyroidism
- Hypopituitarism
- Myasthenia gravis
- Secondary amenorrhea
- Testicular dysfunction
- Vitiligo

Pernicious anemia may result from:
- Inflammatory bowel diseases such as Crohn's disease and sprue
- Removal of all or part of the stomach or intestines
- Chronic gastritis

What you can do: Know your family history and your personal risk factors. If you are at risk, see your doctor to be tested for a possible lack of intrinsic factor. The condition is easily treated. For more information, type PERNICIOUS ANEMIA into an Internet search engine.

Sickle-Cell Anemia

Sickle-cell anemia is a condition in which red blood cells are curved like crescent moons, causing small clots to form and resulting in painful events. Sickle-cell trait is present in about 8 percent of African Americans. The following factors increase your risk of developing sickle-cell anemia.

Age. Symptoms usually appear after four months of age.

Ethnicity/ancestry. African Americans have the greatest risk.

Family history. This is an autosomal recessive trait and is caused by a genetic defect passed down from parent to child. Both parents must contribute a defective gene.

Gender. Both men and women are at risk.

What you can do: Know your family history. This is a treatable condition, and untreated sickle-cell disease can lead to other complications. For more information, type SICKLE-CELL ANEMIA into an Internet search engine.

Hemochromatosis

This is a condition in which the blood contains too much iron. The excess iron is stored in the heart, the liver, the pancreas, the eyes, and the skin and can have serious, even fatal consequences on other organs. It affects 1 in 200 to 250 Americans. The following factors increase your risk of developing hemochromatosis.

Age. Although this is commonly diagnosed between the ages of thirty and fifty, symptoms may develop earlier.

Ethnicity/ancestry. The following groups are at higher risk:
- It is most often seen in people of English, Scottish, Irish, Welsh, and northern European ancestry.
- Another form of this disease, sub-Saharan African hemochromatosis, is seen most often in parts of South Africa where iron cooking pots are used, but some Americans with African ancestry have the condition as well, so it may be hereditary.

Family history. This is an autosomal recessive condition, so it does run in families.

Gender. Men have five times the risk of women.

Medical conditions. Hemolytic anemia is a risk factor.

Personal history. The following factors place individuals at higher risk:
- Frequent blood transfusions
- Excessive oral intake of iron supplements

What you can do: Know your family and personal histories. Has your doctor ever advised you to give blood because you have too much iron? You may have hemochromatosis. This condition is treatable! For more information, type HEMOCHROMATOSIS into an Internet search engine.

Blood Clotting Disorders

Many kinds of hereditary conditions are linked to blood clotting disorders. The most well known is hemophilia, in which the blood fails to clot properly with potentially life-threatening consequences. Knowing your family history regarding these disorders is crucial.

Note: Bacteria from periodontitis can cause blood clotting problems.

Blood types. Certain blood factors carry risk of blood clotting disorders:
- Clotting factors—type A is highest risk, followed by type AB with types O and B at lowest risk.
- Nonsecretors have a higher risk than secretors.
- Blood types A and AB have a high risk for clots in leg veins following hip replacement surgery.

Examples of clotting disorders:
- Congenital antithrombin III deficiency
- Congenital protein C or S deficiency
- DIC (disseminated intravascular coagulation)
- Drug-induced immune thrombocytopenia
- Factor II deficiency
- Factor V deficiency
- Factor VII deficiency
- Factor X deficiency
- Factor XII deficiency
- Hemophilia A
- Hemophilia B
- Idiopathic thrombocytopenic purpura (ITP)
- Platelet function defects
- Thrombotic thrombocytopenic purpura
- Von Willebrand's disease (types I and II)

Blood Conditions That Tend to Run in Families

These conditions have no known genetic links:
- Chronic lymphocyte leukemia
- Chylomicronemia syndrome
- Congenital spherocytic anemia
- Multiple myeloma
- Pernicious anemia
- Various other anemias

Medical Conditions That Can Affect the Blood Supply

It is important to properly treat any medical condition with which you are diagnosed, because the condition may affect other parts of your body. The body's organs and systems are inextricably connected to one another, so what goes wrong in one part may create problems in another. This is especially true of the blood supply. Knowing your family history and taking good care of yourself are two of the best things you can do to keep this important component healthy.

Risky Behavior and Possible Consequences	
RISKY BEHAVIOR	**POSSIBLE CONSEQUENCES**
A diet low in iron and vitamins	Anemia
Smoking	Leukemia
Exposure to high levels of radiation or long-term exposure to benzene	Leukemia
Exposure to high levels of radiation before pregnancy	Having a baby who develops leukemia
Chronic alcohol abuse	Anemia or vitamin B_{12} deficiency
	Folate deficiency anemia
	Hemochromatosis

Visit www.healthwatchguide.com for updates on the blood supply.

The Bones

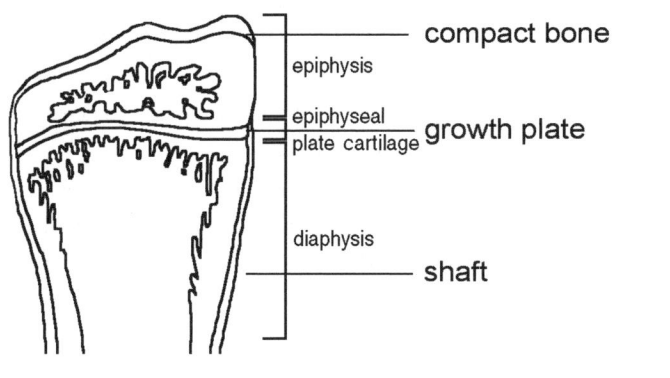
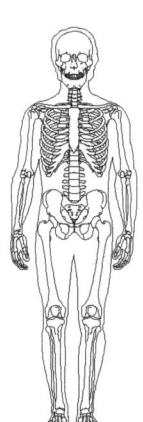

Function

The human body has some 206 individual bones, forming the skeleton. The skeleton gives shape to the body, provides protection for the soft organs, and allows the body to move, using a leverage system controlled by muscles and tendons. Bones store marrow, some of which produces red blood cells. The bones also store calcium and phosphorus, releasing these minerals as needed.

Keeping the Bones Healthy

Bone is built and stored very efficiently until age thirty, under normal circumstances. After that age it begins to break down faster than it is restored. Postmenopausal women are at special risk of osteoporosis (loss of bone) because they no longer produce estrogen, an important hormone for preventing bone loss. Important steps for preventing bone loss include exercise, daily exposure to sunlight, and having bone density tests.

Exercise

Exercise builds bone mass at any age. Weight training can help to improve the bone strength of older women; even light weight training has significant benefits. High-impact activities, such as running, jumping, soccer, and volleyball, are most beneficial. Walking, stretching, swimming, bicycling, hiking, stair climbing, dancing, tennis, badminton, and golf are all good activities for strengthening the bones.

Sunlight
Daily exposure to fifteen to twenty minutes of sunlight (without sunblock) allows the body to produce the amount of vitamin D required by the bones.

Recommended Tests and Evaluations
- Women should have a baseline bone density test at the onset of menopause. The frequency of future testing depends on the results of the first test.
- Men with low levels of testosterone should have a baseline bone density test at age fifty.

Beneficial Foods and Nutrients
See Part Four, The Importance of Nutrients, for a list of foods containing the vitamins and minerals mentioned in this section.

Tea (Green or Black)
Green and black tea strengthen bone when consumed daily for ten or more years.

Animal Protein
Animal-based protein improves bone density. The diet should derive 15 to 20 percent of the calories from animal protein to achieve this improvement.

Vitamin A
Vitamin A is necessary for bone growth.

Vitamin D
Vitamin D increases calcium absorption in the gastrointestinal tract. Men and women should have at least 400 IU, but not more than 800 IU daily (400 IU is the equivalent of one quart of milk).

Vitamin K
Vitamin K helps to maintain bone strength as we age.

Calcium
Although other parts of the body need calcium, it is an essential nutrient for bone health. Bones store 99 percent of the body's calcium. If the amount of calcium lost during normal activity is not replaced through vitamins or food, the body takes calcium from the bones. This weakens the bones and can lead to osteoporosis.

Magnesium
Magnesium helps build strong bones.

Phosphorus
This mineral works with calcium for strong bones.

Copper
Copper is needed for healthy bones.

Fluoride
Fluoride helps strengthen the bones.

Manganese
Manganese assists with bone formation.

Other Tips
- Vitamin D is most readily available in direct sunlight.
- The more salt you eat, the more calcium your body excretes, increasing your calcium requirement.
- The oxalates in spinach, sweet potatoes, and rhubarb prevent the calcium in those foods from being absorbed by the body. Other foods containing calcium are not affected when eaten with the oxalate foods.
- Caffeine can reduce calcium absorption by a tiny amount. Add a little milk to your coffee, or make sure you get calcium elsewhere in your diet.
- Moderate use of alcohol by postmenopausal women can increase bone density.
- Calcium supplements can reduce the risk of bone fracture by 30 to 50 percent for menopausal women with low calcium intake.
- Gum disease and tooth loss are associated with bone loss.
- Elderly people who are homebound because of illness or extended periods of inclement weather risk bone fractures due to lack of sufficient sunlight and vitamin D.

What Can Go Wrong
Osteoporosis
Osteoporosis causes fragile, brittle bones. This disease currently affects about 10 million Americans with an additional 34 million showing low bone mass. The following factors increase your risk of developing osteoporosis.

Age. The risk increases with age.

Blood types. Types A and O have a higher risk; types B and AB have a moderate risk.

Body size. Small, thin-boned women have a greater risk.

Ethnicity/ancestry. In general, fair-skinned groups have a higher risk. Whites and Asians have the greatest risk, followed by blacks and Hispanics.

Family history. A family history of low mineral density is a risk factor, especially a mother with osteoporosis or vertebral or hip fractures.

Gender. The risk of osteoporosis increases with age for both men and women. Women have a greater risk, as they start with less bone tissue and lose bone rapidly after menopause. Menopausal women no longer produce significant quantities of estrogen, an essential hormone for bone health.

Medical conditions. These medical conditions are risk factors:

- Amenorrhea
- Anything that requires immobility
- Asthma (primarily because of corticosteroid use and avoidance of dairy products)
- Being thin or having a small frame
- Chronic bronchitis
- Chronic diseases of the heart, lungs, stomach, kidneys, or intestines
- Cushing's syndrome
- Early menopause
- Hypogonadism (in men)
- Hyperparathyroidism
- Hyperprolactinemia
- Hyperthyroidism
- Hysterectomy before menopause
- Kidney disease requiring dialysis
- Low levels of testosterone in men
- Low muscle mass
- Lupus
- Renal osteodystrophy
- Rheumatoid arthritis

Medications. Drugs that increase risk include antacids with aluminum or cortisone, some anticonvulsants, and large doses of thyroid hormones for extended periods of time.

Personal history. Having had a bone fracture not due to a serious accident or injury increases risk.

What you can do: Be sure to have bone density tests when appropriate. Know your risk factors and minimize your controllable risks. Beginning in childhood, develop the habit of getting enough sunlight, exercise, and calcium. For more information, type OSTEOPOROSIS into an Internet search engine.

Osteosarcoma

Osteosarcoma is an extremely rare cancer of new tissue in growing bones, and it is usually found in the upper arms, knees, and upper legs. There are about 900 new cases annually in the United States. The following factors increase your risk of developing osteosarcoma.

Age. Ages ten to twenty-five are at most risk of developing this disease.

Gender. Males during the late teen years are slightly more at risk than females.

Ethnicity/ancestry. Blacks have a higher risk than whites.

Personal history. Individuals with any of the following factors are at higher risk:

- Taller-than-average teens
- Prior treatment for other conditions with radiation and/or chemotherapy
- High doses of radium in adults

Medical conditions. These medical conditions are risk factors:

- Hereditary retinoblastoma
- Paget's disease
- Li-Fraumeni syndrome

What you can do: Know your risk factors, especially the medical conditions. For more information, type OSTEOSARCOMA into an Internet search engine.

Myeloma

Myelomas are tumors made of cells normally found in bone marrow. Some 14,000 new cases are diagnosed annually in the United States. The following factors increase your risk of developing myeloma.

Age. This disease usually affects those over fifty-five, though the age at inception is dropping.

Ethnicity/ancestry. Blacks have a greater risk than whites.

Family history. Having children or a sibling with myeloma increases your risk.

Gender. Men have a 150 percent greater risk than women.

Workplace. Ongoing research is investigating possible links between the petroleum industry and myeloma.

What you can do: This type of cancer seems to be increasing, but this may be due to better identification of new cases. Be aware of your risk factors and stay on top of your health. For more information, type MYELOMA into an Internet search engine.

Osteomalacia

Osteomalacia is a softening of the bones caused by a deficiency of vitamin D. The following factors increase your risk of developing osteomalacia.

Age. This disease is diagnosed in adulthood.

Gender. Osteomalacia affects men and women equally.

Medical conditions. These medical conditions are risk factors:

- Acquired disorders of vitamin D metabolism
- Hereditary disorders of vitamin D metabolism
- Kidney disease
- Malabsorption syndromes, such as Crohn's disease

What you can do: Make sure you get enough sunlight, calcium, and vitamin D. Under most circumstances, this is a preventable condition! For more information, type OSTEOMALACIA into an Internet search engine.

Rickets

Rickets is a childhood form of osteomalacia. Bones are formed with inadequate calcium or phosphorus intake and a deficiency of vitamin D. The following factors increase your risk of developing rickets.

Age. Rickets is seen in infancy through young childhood.

Blood types. Type A has a higher risk, type AB has a moderate-to-high risk, and types B and O have a moderate risk.

Family history. Hereditary rickets is an inherited, sex-linked disorder (other forms result from nutritional deficiencies or medical conditions).

Gender. Males have the greatest risk.

Medical conditions. These medical conditions are risk factors:

- Abnormal liver or kidney function that inhibits the body's ability to absorb and activate vitamin D
- Breastfeeding exclusively, without supplements, especially if the baby has inadequate exposure to sunlight
- Kidney disease
- Malabsorption syndromes, such as Crohn's disease

What you can do: During pregnancy, be careful to follow your doctor's advice regarding food, vitamins, and minerals. Make sure to get sufficient quantities of calcium, phosphorus, and vitamin D in your child's diet. Follow your doctor's advice if the child has stomach or bowel malabsorption syndromes. For more information, type RICKETS into an Internet search engine.

Bone Conditions That Tend to Run in Families

These conditions have no known genetic links:

- Osteitis fibrosa
- Osteoarthritis
- Osteosarcoma
- Russell-Silver syndrome

Medical Conditions That Can Affect Bone Health

It is important to properly treat any medical condition with which you are diagnosed, because the condition may affect other parts of your body. The body's organs and systems are inextricably connected to one another, so what goes wrong in one part may create problems in another. The following conditions and factors may increase risk.

- *Asthmatics* are at an increased risk for bone loss.
- *Cancer of the adrenal cortex* may lead to weakened bones.
- *Celiac disease, Crohn's disease, and colitis* interfere with calcium absorption.
- *Extended bed rest* can reduce bone density due to a lack of exercise.
- *Lactose intolerance,* a condition that is found in 75 percent of African Americans and Native Americans and 90 percent of Asian Americans, can keep people from getting enough calcium through dairy products.
- *Pregnancy and breastfeeding* can reduce the calcium levels in the mother's bones, leading to osteoporosis and dental problems.
- *Primary hyperparathyroidism* can contribute to excessive levels of blood calcium, calcium loss from bones, and excessive excretion of calcium from the kidneys.
- *Receiving radiation or chemotherapy* for other conditions increases the risk of developing bone cancer.
- *Some medications used to treat asthma* interfere with the body's ability to absorb calcium.

Risky Behavior and Possible Consequences

RISKY BEHAVIOR	POSSIBLE CONSEQUENCES
A low calcium diet in childhood	Reduces peak bone mass by 5 to 10 percent
	Increases the risk of hip fractures later in life
	Rickets
Weight loss	Bone mass is reduced as weight is lost
Heavy alcohol use	Interferes with the body's ability to use vitamin D
	In men, reduces the level of testosterone, which increases the risk of osteoporosis
	In premenopausal women, can result in irregular menstrual cycles, which increases the risk of osteoporosis
	Increases the risk of falling and fracturing bones
Menstrual cycle disruptions from excessive physical exercise	Significant bone loss, which may never be fully recovered
Smoking	Bone loss
Anorexia nervosa	Significant bone loss, which may never be fully recovered
An inactive lifestyle	Osteoporosis
Overtraining, especially with poor nutrition	Osteoporosis
An adult diet low in calcium	Osteoporosis
Steroid use	Osteoporosis
Inadequate exposure to the sun	Rickets, osteomalacia
Heavy use of strong sunblock	Osteomalacia
A vegan diet relying on vegetable protein sources instead of animal protein sources	Osteoporosis

Visit www.healthwatchguide.com for updates on the bones.

NOTES

The Brain

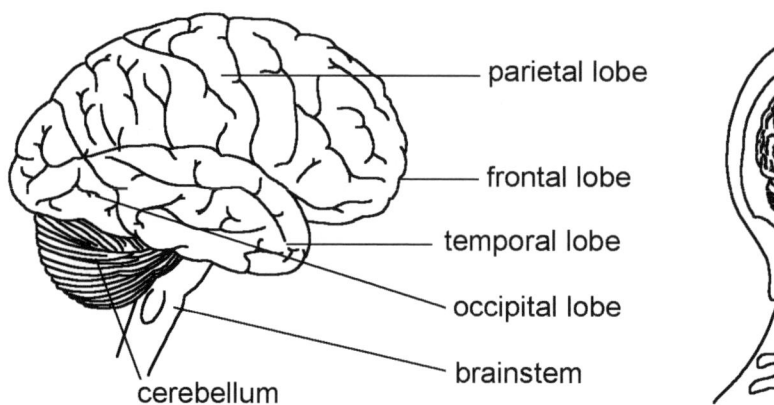 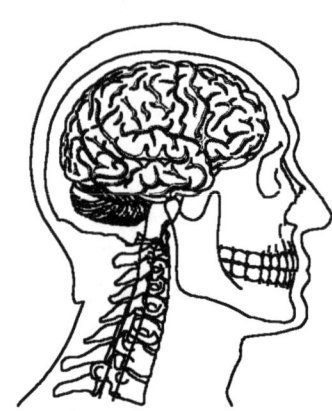

Function

The brain is the nerve center of the body. It sits on top of the spinal cord through which the brain's billions of nerve cells continuously receive information from inside and outside the body; it then sends signals to the various body parts on how to respond. The brain's ability to store and process information allows us to remember and reproduce what we learn. The brain is the source of our moods, thoughts, and emotions. It uses 20 percent of the oxygen used by the entire body at rest.

Keeping the Brain Healthy

The following immunizations help keep the brain healthy:
- Immunizations by the mother against rubella help protect against infections that could damage the baby's brain during pregnancy.
- HiB vaccine for children prevents one type of meningitis. The pneumococcal conjugate vaccine, which now is routinely given to all children, can prevent pneumococcal meningitis.

Beneficial Foods and Nutrients

See Part Four, The Importance of Nutrients, for a list of foods containing the vitamins mentioned in this section.

Vitamin B_{12}

B_{12} helps to protect against peripheral neuropathy (disorders of the peripheral nervous system).

Choline

Choline helps with memory functions and helps ensure normal fetal brain development.

Folic Acid (Folate)

Folic acid is required for the prevention of birth defects in a baby's brain. The recommended dosage is 400 micrograms or 0.4 mg daily. Women need to have enough folic acid in their systems before they become pregnant in order to protect their babies, so folic acid supplements should be taken daily as soon as girls reach their teenage years. Most multivitamins contain the recommended daily allowance of folic acid.

Alcohol

Research has shown that a moderate amount of alcohol daily (one drink for women, two for men) may keep the brain healthy and reduce the risk of stroke as we age.

Antioxidants

Antioxidants stop free-radical attacks on brain cells. They are found in red grapes, berries, ginkgo, alpha-lipoic acid, and green tea; the are also found in supplements of vitamins A, B, C, and E.

Other Tips

- Regular exercise and relaxation techniques help to reduce the frequency of tension-type headaches.
- Adequate exposure to sunlight during winter months helps reduce the symptoms of seasonal affective disorder (SAD).
- Use it or lose it! Keep the brain healthy by giving it lots of mental stimulation on a regular basis.
- Raccoon feces can transmit a form of encephalitis to humans. Raccoons are attracted to your yard by outside garbage cans, compost piles, pet food bowls, swimming pools, ponds, hot tubs, bird

feeders, and woodpiles. Wear gloves when picking up sticks that have fallen to the ground.
- Minimize your toddler's exposure to television, movies, and video games. The brain's circuitry is being "wired" during a child's first three years of life. Researchers suspect that the rapid on-screen movements condition the brain to respond to fast-paced stimulus, thus paving the way for hyperactivity. Your toddler will probably be much better off engaged in activities that develop motor skills, focus, and concentration. Bring out the blocks and coloring books!

What Can Go Wrong

Brain Tumor

Some 17,000 brain tumors are diagnosed annually in the United States. The following factors increase your risk of developing a brain tumor.

Age. Brain tumors are most commonly diagnosed in children ages three to twelve and adults aged seventy and older.

Blood types. Types A and AB have a higher risk, type B has a moderate risk, and type O has a lower risk.

Ethnicity/ancestry. In descending order of risk: whites, Hispanics, blacks, Asians, Pacific Islanders, Native Americans, and Alaska Natives.

Family history. Heredity is a factor in some tumors, such as neurofibromatosis.

Gender. Males have a higher overall risk. Women have a higher risk for a brain tumor called a meningioma.

Personal history. Radiation therapy for other forms of cancer increases risk of brain tumor.

Workplace. The following industries and professions are at higher risk:
- Plastic manufacturing because of vinyl chloride exposure and acrylonitrile exposure
- Embalmers and pathologists because of exposure to formaldehyde (Other professions using formaldehyde apparently are not at risk, however.)

What you can do: Know your risks and minimize your controllable risks. For more information, type BRAIN TUMORS into an Internet search engine.

Meningitis

Meningitis is an extremely serious infection affecting the fluids and membranes of the spinal cord and brain. There are two types: acute bacterial meningitis and viral meningitis. Bacterial meningitis is the more severe form and can be life threatening. Viral meningitis is much more common and not as dangerous, though avoidance is desirable. The following factors increase the risk of developing meningitis.

Age. The risk exists from infancy onward.

Blood types. Types A, B, AB, and O all have a moderate risk for bacterial meningitis. Nonsecretors of all types have a higher risk.

Exposure to infection. Schools, dormitories, barracks, day-care facilities, and other places where groups of children congregate are all possible points of infection.

Note: Most colleges and universities now require entering freshmen to be vaccinated against meningitis. Military recruits are routinely vaccinated against meningitis.

Medical conditions. These medical conditions are risk factors:
- Allergies to certain drugs
- Tumors

Workplace. Chemical irritation is a risk factor.

What you can do: Most infection occurs during the late summer and fall, coinciding with the start of the school year. Familiarize yourself with meningitis symptoms, and if your child has not been vaccinated, be alert for warnings of outbreaks in your child's school. For more information, type MENINGITIS into an Internet search engine.

Parkinson's Disease

Parkinson's disease causes damage to a part of the brain that controls movement. It affects 1 in every 500 people. The following factors increase the risk of developing Parkinson's disease.

Age. Affects the middle-aged to the elderly.

Blood types. Type A has a lower risk; types B and AB have a moderate risk. Type O seems to be most susceptible, because of its association with dopamine imbalances.

Environment. When certain pesticides and herbicides are mixed, they form a chemical compound that crosses the brain's membranes and may be a factor in Parkinson's disease. To be safe, thoroughly wash all produce before eating, or purchase only organically grown food.

Family history. Early onset Parkinson's disease (before age fifty) seems to run in families.

Gender. Men and women are at equal risk.

What you can do: Know your risk factors. Minimize your controllable risks. For more information, type PARKINSON'S DISEASE into an Internet search engine.

Schizophrenia

Schizophrenia is a serious brain disorder, affecting the ability to distinguish between the real and the imaginary and to function normally, whether emotionally or socially. There are five recognized forms. Schizophrenia appears to affect 1 percent of the world's population. The following factors increase the risk of schizophrenia.

Age. Initial onset of the condition is usually at age eighteen to twenty-five for men; age twenty-six to forty-five for women.

Blood types. Types A and O have a moderate-to-high risk, and types B and AB have a moderate risk. Rh incompatibility in a second or subsequent pregnancy is associated with an increased risk of schizophrenia in offspring. (*Source:* D'Adamo, Peter J.)

Family history. There is a genetic predisposition, and schizophrenia probably runs in families.

Gender. Men and women are at equal risk.

Medical conditions. Viral infections may be a cause. Pregnant women exposed to influenza in the second trimester are at risk of having babies affected by schizophrenia.

What you can do: Know your risks and your family history. Take care during pregnancy to protect your unborn child. For more information, type SCHIZOPHRENIA into an Internet search engine.

Stroke

A stroke is a brain attack. Stroke is the third most common cause of death and the number-one cause of disability in American adults. There are 750,000 episodes of stroke annually in the United States. The following factors increase your risk of suffering a stroke.

Age. The risk doubles with each decade over age fifty-five. Two-thirds of strokes occur over age sixty-five.

Blood types. Type A has a greater tendency toward blood clots in general, followed by type AB; these two types are at greatest risk of cerebral thrombosis (brain clot). Types O and B are at greater risk of strokes caused by cranial bleeding.

Ethnicity/ancestry. Blacks and Hispanics have a 60 percent higher risk than whites. Blacks also are 250 percent more likely to die of stroke.

Family history. Having a family member who has suffered a stroke significantly increases your risk.

Gender. Men have a 30 percent greater risk than women.

Medical conditions. These medical conditions are risk factors:
- Atherosclerosis
- Atrial fibrillation
- Diabetes mellitus (type II)
- Heart disease
- Hemophilia
- High blood pressure
- High levels of C-reactive protein in the blood, especially for men
- Hyperhomocysteinemia
- Lupus
- Periodontitis
- Transient ischemic attack (see below)

Personal history. Having had a stroke or transient ischemic attach (TIA) increases your risk of additional strokes.

What you can do: Make sure your doctor knows your risk factors, and get regular checkups. Ask your doctor about aspirin therapy. Modify your lifestyle if necessary and minimize your controllable risks. For more information, type STROKE into an Internet search engine.

Transient Ischemic Attack (TIA)

A TIA is often referred to as a mini-stroke. This attack causes a temporary decrease in the blood supply to the brain. These mini-strokes increase the risk of a full-blown stroke by ten times. The following factors increase your risk of having a TIA.

Age. The risk increases for each decade over age fifty.

Ethnicity/ancestry. Blacks have the highest risk, partly due to their increased risk of diabetes and high blood pressure. The next group at risk is Hispanics.

Family history. The risk increases if a parent or sibling has had a TIA or stroke.

Gender. Men have the greater risk, especially those over age sixty.

Medical conditions. These medical conditions are risk factors:

- Cardiovascular disease
- Diabetes
- Elevated cholesterol levels
- High blood pressure
- Lupus

What you can do: Make sure you know your family history, risk factors, and the warning signs for TIAs. Ask your doctor about aspirin therapy. Seek medical care immediately if you have any TIA symptoms. Minimize your controllable risk factors. For more information, type TRANSIENT ISCHEMIC ATTACK into an Internet search engine.

Brain Conditions That Tend to Run in Families

These conditions have no known genetic links:

- Alzheimer's disease (late onset) or senility
- Amyotrophic lateral sclerosis (ALS)—approximately 5 to 10 percent of people with ALS inherited it
- Attention deficit disorder
- Autism
- Bipolar affective disorder
- Dementia
- Epilepsy (either grand mal or petit mal)
- Febrile seizures
- Manic depression disorder
- Maple syrup urine disease
- Migraines with auras—women, especially younger women, are three times more likely to have migraines than men
- Olivopontocerebellar atrophy
- Parkinson's disease (early onset)
- Pick's disease
- Schizophrenia
- Selective mutism
- Sleepwalking

Medical Conditions That Can Affect the Brain

It is important to properly treat any medical condition with which you are diagnosed, because the condition may affect other parts of your body. The body's organs and systems are inextricably connected to one another, and what goes wrong in one part may create problems in another.

- *An inflammation of the brain from meningitis or encephalitis* may cause grand mal or febrile seizures.
- *Birth defects* may cause seizures.
- *Blood vessel disorders* and *strokes* may cause seizures.
- *Hemochromatosis* may lead to iron deposits in the brain.
- *Kidney or liver disease* may cause seizures.
- *Thyroid disease* can contribute to depression.

Note: Most patients with chronic conditions are at risk of depression.

Risky Behavior and Possible Consequences	
RISKY BEHAVIOR	**POSSIBLE CONSEQUENCES**
Eating foods, such as aged cheeses, containing tyramine. Also chocolate, MSG, alcohol, certain seasonings, aspartame, caffeine, red wine, and fermented, pickled, or marinated foods	May trigger migraines in susceptible people
Using drugs or chemicals	May cause seizures
Using addictive substances	May have long-term effects on brain chemistry
Repetitive motions, cramped positions, and toxic chemicals	May cause nerve damage
Drinking, smoking, or using drugs during pregnancy	May damage the fetal brain. Increased risk of children with attention deficit disorder
Pregnancy after age thirty-five	Increased risk of Down syndrome babies
Smoking, heavy drinking, illicit drug use, marijuana use	Increased risk of stroke, TIA
Maintaining a high cholesterol level	Increased risk of stroke, TIA

RISKY BEHAVIOR	POSSIBLE CONSEQUENCES
Exposure to lead or other heavy metals	Increased risk of attention deficit disorder
Exposure to rubella (German measles) during pregnancy	Possible birth of a child with mental retardation
Maintaining high blood pressure	Stroke, TIA
Stress	Stroke
Cardiovascular disease	Stroke, TIA
Diabetes	Stroke, TIA
Infection with genital herpes	Viral meningitis
Giving aspirin (and medications containing aspirin) to a child with chicken pox	Child develops Reye's syndrome (brain damage)
Cocaine use	Hemorrhagic stroke
Contracting syphilis	Stroke, TIA

Visit www.healthwatchguide.com for updates on the brain.

NOTES

The Breasts

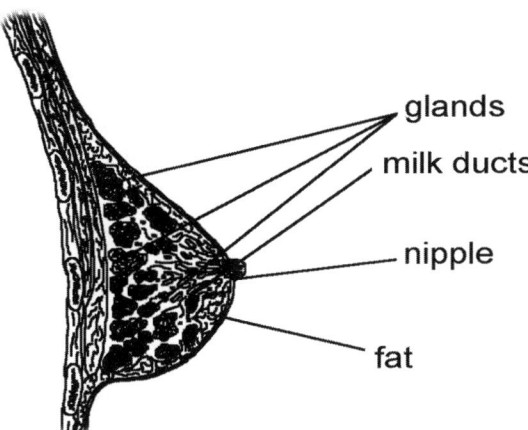
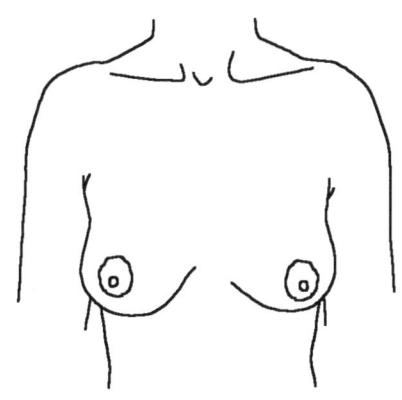

Function

The breast contains mammary glands, which in females produce milk for the nourishment of young. Humans have two breasts, normally small in males and various sizes in females. The breast consists mostly of fatty tissue and milk glands. Some women have additional breast tissue along the "breast line," which extends vertically down the abdomen from the breasts. In this extremely rare condition, women are born with extra nipples, which almost never pose a health risk and can be surgically removed.

Keeping the Breasts Healthy

What You and Your Doctor Should Know

Inform your doctor about any personal history of:
- Early menstruation (before age twelve)
- Late menopause (after age fifty-five)
- Not having had children
- Giving birth for the first time after age thirty
- Taking, or having a mother who took, diethylstilbestrol (DES) during pregnancy between 1940 and 1971
- Having dense breasts
- Having had uterine, colon, or ovarian cancer
- Breast cancer (personal and family history)

Recommended Tests and Evaluations

Regular exams can identify problems and other conditions in breast tissue and are a major factor in successful early detection and treatment of cancer.
- Breast lumps in women under age thirty are usually benign fibroadenomas or cysts.
- Cysts (fluid-filled sacs) often appear in women in their forties and fifties.
- Because breast cancer is sometimes detected in women who are pregnant or who have just given birth, breast examination should be part of prenatal care. The risk is greatest in women aged thirty-two to thirty-eight and occurs in one of every 3,000 pregnancies.
- Be sure to follow your doctor's recommendations concerning the best ways to breastfeed in order to minimize mastitis, inflammation of the mammary gland.

Note: There may be a connection between working at night and an increased risk of breast cancer. Bright light in dark hours may decrease melatonin levels and increase estrogen levels.

Mammograms. The American Cancer Society recommends that a woman have her first mammogram by age forty, followed by one every one to two years up to age forty-nine and yearly thereafter, unless you have a family history of breast cancer or other risk factors. If someone in your family has had breast cancer, begin mammograms at least ten years earlier than her age at diagnosis. Try to go to the same facility each time for better tracking of your history, and make sure that a report is sent to your ob/gyn. Scheduling your annual mammogram about a month before your ob/gyn visit will give your physician the latest test information. Many women schedule their annual mammogram on or near their birthday as a healthful present to themselves. *Note: Screening recommendations change with every new study on the subject. The best advice on your mammogram schedule will come from your ob/gyn.*

Breast self-exams. Self-exams are best done by all women over age twenty every month in the shower, after your period so the breasts are not swollen or painful. *Ninety percent of breast lumps are found through self-exams.*

Clinical breast exams. All women between the ages of twenty and thirty-nine should have a breast exam performed by a health professional such as a gynecologist or family physician at least every three years. Have an exam yearly after the age of forty.

Beneficial Foods and Nutrients

See Part Four, The Importance of Nutrients, for a list of foods containing the vitamins mentioned in this section.

Green Tea

Green tea contains polyphenols, which may help to reduce the risk of breast cancer.

Vitamin B_6 and Folic Acid (Folate)

These vitamins have been shown to reduce breast cancer risk significantly, especially for women who drink moderate amounts of alcohol.

Other Tips

- Breastfeeding appears to lower breast cancer risk.
- Regular exercise may lower the risk of breast cancer.
- Teenagers who eat an egg a day may lower their later risk of breast cancer.
- Oral contraceptives may reduce the risk of benign breast disease, such as fibrocystic disease, but may lead to an increased risk of breast cancer.

What Can Go Wrong

Breast Cancer

Breast cancer is the most common cancer for women. More than 200,000 new cases are diagnosed annually in the United States. The following factors increase the risk of developing breast cancer.

Age. Risk is present starting at age thirty-five; the risk increases dramatically after age fifty and is very high after age sixty.

Blood types. Types A and AB have a higher risk and types B and O have a moderate risk. Secretors of all types have a higher risk.

Ethnicity/ancestry. In descending order of risk: whites, Hawaiians, blacks, Asians, Pacific Islanders, Hispanics, Alaska Natives, and Native Americans. Black Americans are more likely to die of breast cancer, largely due to late diagnoses. Ashkenazi Jews have a high risk.

Family history. Having a mother, sister, or daughter with breast cancer increases your risk.

Genetic factors. BRCA1 and BRCA2 genes are risk factors. Other genes are being researched, including BARD1, p53, BRCA3, and Noey2.

Habitat. Living in cities or urban areas increases risk.

Medical conditions. These medical conditions are risk factors:
- Atypical hyperplasia
- Lobular carcinoma in situ

Medical treatments. Chest radiation increases risk, especially those given for childhood Hodgkin's disease.

Personal history. Lengthy exposure to estrogen increases the risk of breast cancer. (The longer you menstruate or take combined hormone therapy, the greater your risk of breast cancer.) Factors increasing an individual's risk include:
- A birth weight of more than ten pounds increases the risk of premenopausal breast cancer
- Early menstruation (before age twelve)
- Late menopause (after age fifty-five)
- Not having had children
- Giving birth for the first time after age thirty
- Taking, or having a mother who took, diethylstilbestrol (DES) during pregnancy between 1940 and 1971
- Having dense breasts
- Cancer in one breast, which increases the risk of developing cancer in the other breast
- Having had uterine, colon, or ovarian cancer

On the other hand, risk decreases with:
- Pregnancy before age eighteen
- Breastfeeding
- Having been breastfed
- Menopause before age fifty
- Removal of ovaries before age forty

What you can do: Know your family and personal history. Minimize your controllable risks. Learn the signs and symptoms of breast cancer. Perform monthly self-exams. See your doctor regularly for clinical breast exams. Have regular mammograms. For more information, type BREAST CANCER into an Internet search engine.

Male Breast Cancer

This is a rare cancer, accounting for 1 percent of all breast cancers. The following factors increase a man's risk of developing breast cancer.

Age. Risk is highest between the ages of sixty and seventy.

Ethnicity/ancestry. Blacks have the highest risk.

Family history. Higher risk is associated with:
- Having several female relatives with breast cancer
- Genetic mutations

Medical conditions. Anything that increases the amount of estrogen in your system increases risk, such as the following:
- Liver disease (such as cirrhosis)
- Klinefelter's syndrome

Medical treatments. Exposure to chest radiation increases risk.

Personal history. Cancer in one breast increases the risk of cancer in the other breast.

What you can do: Know your family and personal history. See your doctor if you notice a lump or thickening on your chest. For more information, type BREAST CANCER into an Internet search engine.

Genetic Risks

Cancer has been proven to be genetically linked.

Medical Conditions That Can Affect Breast Health

It is important to properly treat any medical condition with which you are diagnosed, because the condition may affect other parts of your body. The body's organs and systems are inextricably connected to one another, so what goes wrong in one part may create problems in another. The following condition can affect breast health.

- *Gynecomastia* involves breast enlargement in men, and is usually due to an excess of estrogen. Risk factors include:
  - Administration of estrogen in treatment of medical conditions or for sex-change procedures
  - Cirrhosis of the liver
  - Exposure to maternal hormones in newborns
  - Genetic defects
  - Kidney failure
  - Tumors
  - Uneven hormone production during adolescence
  - Use of androgens for bodybuilding
  - Use of certain medications. Some 125 commonly prescribed medications list male breast enlargement as a possible side effect. In most cases, the effect is temporary. You may want to discuss this issue with your doctor if gynecomastia runs in your family, or if you have other risk factors.

Risky Behavior and Possible Consequences

RISKY BEHAVIOR	POSSIBLE CONSEQUENCES
Birth control pills	May lead to a higher risk of breast cancer
Hormone replacement therapy	May lead to a higher risk of breast cancer
More than one alcoholic drink per day	Increased risk of breast cancer
Being overweight for both men and women	Increased risk of breast cancer
Using marijuana	Breast enlargement in males

Visit www.healthwatchguide.com for updates on the breasts.

NOTES

The Cervix

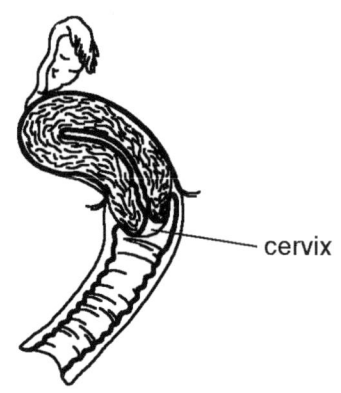
cervix

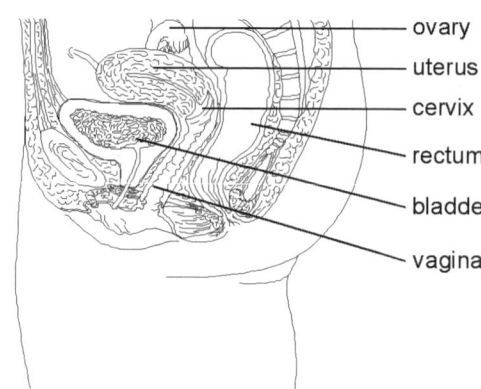
ovary, uterus, cervix, rectum, bladder, vagina

Function

The cervix is located at the bottom of the uterus, just above the vagina. It is the entrance to the womb and allows sperm to travel from the vagina to the uterus. The cervix also permits the passage of menstrual fluids and unborn children into the vagina from the uterus.

Keeping the Cervix Healthy

One of the best ways to avoid health problems with the cervix is by practicing safe sex. Infection with human papillomavirus (HPV) is the primary cause of cervical cancer and dysplasia. HPV causes genital warts, so avoid having sex with someone who has warts on his genitals or any kind of sexually transmitted disease. Know your partner and his sexual history before having intercourse.

What You and Your Doctor Should Know

- Your contraceptive history
- Your sexual history—how old you were when you began having intercourse, how many partners you have had, how many partners you currently have.
- Your medical history, especially any sexually transmitted diseases you may have contracted.

Recommended Tests and Evaluations

Pap smears. Every woman should have a first Pap smear at age twenty, or earlier if sexually active. You should have a Pap smear annually until age thirty-five unless:

- You have had three successive negative smears
- You have no sexual partner
- You have only one, committed sexual partner

If any of these three conditions apply, talk to your doctor about having a Pap smear every two or three years.

You should have a Pap smear annually if:

- You are eighteen or younger and sexually active
- You are older than eighteen and sexually active
- You are over age thirty-five
- You have multiple sexual partners
- You take birth control pills
- You have a history of genital warts or human papillomavirus (HPV)
- Your mother took diethylstilbestrol (DES) during her pregnancy with you.

Note: a vaccine against HPV may be available in the next few years, but that won't eliminate the risk of cervical cancer from other causes, so ask your doctor to advise you on your need for Pap smears.

What Can Go Wrong

Benign Polyps, Tumors, and Genital Warts

These are treatable growths on the cervix. They can be removed and usually do not return.

Cervical Cancer

About 12,200 new cases of cervical cancer are diagnosed each year in the United States.

Mortality rates for cervical cancer have declined dramatically in the last half century as women have more frequent gynecological checkups. The following factors increase your risk of developing cervical cancer.

Age. Most at risk of precancerous low-grade lesions are those of ages twenty-five to thirty-five. The rate of invasive cervical cancer increases over age forty.

Blood types. Types A and AB have a higher risk, types B and O have a moderate risk.

Ethnicity/ancestry. In descending order of risk: Vietnamese, Alaska Natives, Koreans, Hispanics, blacks, Japanese, Chinese, whites

Medical conditions. These medical conditions are risk factors:

- Organ transplants
- Compromised immune systems
- Infection with human papillomavirus (the primary risk factor)

Personal history. Most at risk are those born to a mother who, between 1940 and 1971, took diethylstilbestrol (DES) to prevent miscarriage during the pregnancy.

What you can do: Practice safe sex! Know your personal risk factors. Minimize your controllable risk factors. Be aware that cervical cancer often has no symptoms in its earliest, most treatable stage. Unless you have had a hysterectomy, you should have regular Pap tests and pelvic exams to catch any problems early. If you had a hysterectomy because of cervical cancer, you still need to have Pap smears taken.

There is no age limit for Pap smears—you are never too old, even after menopause. *The older you get, the greater the risk of developing cervical cancer.* (See the checkup schedule in Part Two under "Tests for Women." For more information, type CERVICAL CANCER into an Internet search engine.

Cervicitis and Cervical Erosion

Cervicitis is an inflammation of the cervix. Cervical erosion is the absense of surface tissue on the cervix. Risk factors for both include:

- Abrasion from objects inserted into the cervix, including pessaries, diaphragms, tampons, and so forth
- Allergic reactions to spermicides or latex condoms
- Vaginal infections

Risky Behavior and Possible Consequences

RISKY BEHAVIOR	POSSIBLE CONSEQUENCES
Infection with HPV	The primary risk for cervical cancer
Sexual intercourse before age 18	Cervical cancer, cervicitis
Multiple sexual partners	Cervical cancer, cervicitis, cervical erosion
A sexual partner who had intercourse before age 18	Cervical cancer
A sexual partner who has had multiple partners	Cervical cancer, cervicitis
Marriage to a man who was married to a woman who had cervical cancer	Cervical cancer
Never having had a Pap smear	Cervical cancer
Not having had a Pap smear for a number of years	Cervical cancer
Obesity	Cervical cancer
Use of birth control pills	Cervical cancer
Smoking	Cervical cancer
Infection from an STD	Cervicitis (infection of the cervix), cervical cancer
Use of deodorant douches, tampons, or sprays	Cervicitis, cervical erosion
Intercourse with a man who has urethritis	Cervicitis
Becoming infected with HIV or AIDS*	Cervical cancer
Having chronic chlamydia infections*	Cervical cancer
Becoming infected with syphilis*	Cervical erosion

*These conditions increase the risk of HPV infection

Visit www.healthwatchguide.com for updates on the cervix.

NOTES

The Circulatory System

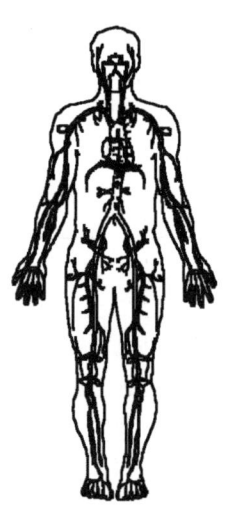
arterial system

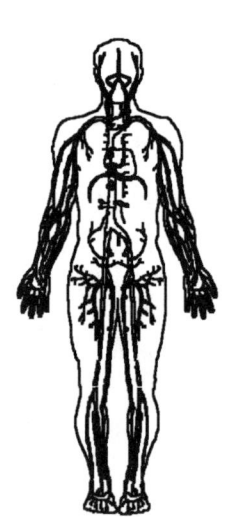
venous system

Function

The arteries and veins in your body comprise a system that is thousands of miles long. The arteries deliver nutrients and oxygen throughout the body and to all the cells. The veins pick up wastes and carbon dioxide from the lungs, kidneys, and liver. The heart is the pump that activates and maintains the system.

Keeping the Circulatory System Healthy

Understand Your Blood Pressure Reading

The blood pressure reading consists of two numbers, displayed one above the other. The upper number represents the maximum pressure in your arteries when the heart is pumping (pressure is greatest at this time). This is called the *systolic number*. The lower of the two numbers, called the *diastolic number*, shows pressure between heartbeats (when it is lowest).

A normal blood pressure reading is considered to be anything under 120/80; however, lower readings are better for your arteries.

Exercise

Regular exercise is one of the best ways to lower blood pressure and cholesterol! Men, especially, who exercise can lower their levels of C-reactive protein. The inflammation that contributes to heart disease causes C-reactive protein levels to rise. A reduction in C-reactive protein levels indicates a similar decline in the inflammation condition.

Understand Your Cholesterol Readings

A cholesterol reading measures different properties of cholesterol, including:

- LDL, or low-density lipoprotein—the bad kind of cholesterol that clogs your arteries
- HDL, or high-density lipoprotein—the good factor that takes excess cholesterol to the liver for excretion
- Triglycerides—compounds that move fatty acids through the body; high levels signal danger

Refer to "Cholesterol Screenings" in Part Two for more information on cholesterol numbers and ratios.

Keep Your Weight Under Control
Maintain a healthy weight and restrict fat consumption to no more than 30 percent of daily calories.

Don't Smoke
Don't smoke, or quit smoking. Avoid breathing in secondhand smoke.

Stress
Keep your life as stress-free as possible, or find good ways to decompress.

What You and Your Doctor Should Know
- Your family history
- Your blood pressure reading
- Your total cholesterol count

Beneficial Foods and Nutrients
In general, eat foods low in fat and high in fiber to maintain or improve blood cholesterol levels. Also, a moderate consumption of alcohol (one drink per day for women, two drinks per day for men) may help to raise the level of HDL (good) cholesterol. But nondrinkers should not start drinking, and people with a high level of triglycerides should avoid alcohol altogether.

See Part Four, The Importance of Nutrients, for a list of foods containing the vitamins and minerals mentioned in this section.

Green Tea
Studies have shown that regular consumption of green tea lowers cholesterol.

Prunes
Prunes contain soluble fiber, which helps lower cholesterol.

Soy Products
Soy products contain isoflavones that help to regulate cholesterol levels.

Omega-3 Fatty Acids
Foods high in omega-3 fatty acids, found in salmon, mackerel, herring, and flax seed, lower your triglyceride levels.

Vitamin B_3 (Niacin)
Niacin helps reduce blood cholesterol levels and lower high blood pressure.

Vitamins B_6, B_{12}, and Folic Acid (Folate)
These vitamins help to lower homocysteine levels.

Choline
Choline helps control cholesterol levels.

Pantothenic Acid
Pantothenic acid helps in the synthesis of cholesterol.

Magnesium
Magnesium helps to maintain normal blood pressure.

Potassium
Potassium helps to maintain cellular fluid balance.

Sodium
Sodium helps determine blood pressure and volume.

Other Tips
- Keep salt consumption below six grams of sodium a day. Check the labels of cans and food packages—sodium is a common additive for everything from baked goods to bacon and can add up in a hurry.
- Unfiltered, "French-press" style coffee can raise cholesterol levels. Espresso and Turkish coffees have a similar effect.

What Can Go Wrong
Aneurysm
During an aneurysm the wall of a blood vessel balloons, dangerously thinning the wall at that point. The blood vessel may burst if the aneurysm is left untreated. The following factors increase your risk of aneurysm.

Age. Individuals ages forty to seventy are at highest risk.

Blood types. Blood type A has a higher risk of abdominal aortic aneurysm; types B, AB, and O have a lower risk. Blood types B and O have a moderate-to-high risk of cerebral aneurysm; types A and AB have a low-to-moderate risk.

Family history. Having a close relative who has had an aneurysm increases your risk.

Gender. Men have the higher risk.

Medical conditions. These medical conditions are risk factors:
- Atherosclerosis
- Hypertension
- Inflammation or infection
- Pregnancy

Specific risk factors for cerebral aneurysm:
- Coarctation of the aorta
- Family history
- Polycystic kidney disease

Specific risk factors for abdominal aneurysm:
- Ehlers-Danlos syndrome
- Marfan syndrome

What you can do: Know your risk factors. Control your blood pressure. For more information, type ANEURYSM into an Internet search engine.

Atherosclerosis

Atherosclerosis is hardening of the arteries, caused by fatty deposits on the walls of the arteries. The following factors increase your risk of developing atherosclerosis.

Age. This condition is usually seen in people middle-aged or older, but age at onset is dropping as obesity rates in youngsters climb.

Blood types. Type A has a higher risk, type AB and nonsecretors of all groups have a moderate risk, type B has a low-to-moderate risk, and type O has a lower risk.

Ethnicity/ancestry. Blacks have a higher risk than whites.

Family history. The presence of heart disease in the family is a risk factor.

Gender. Men have a higher risk.

Medical conditions. These medical conditions are risk factors:
- Chronic low-grade infections that increase levels of C-reactive proteins, such as:
  - Chlamydia pneumonia
  - *H. Pylori*
  - Bronchitis
  - Dental infections
  - Gum disease
- Cerebrovascular disease
- Diabetes
- High blood cholesterol levels
- High blood pressure
- Kidney disease requiring dialysis
- Peripheral vascular disease

What you can do: Know your risk factors. Minimize your controllable risks, especially regarding weight, blood pressure, and cholesterol. Exercise, eat a sensible diet, and follow your doctor's advice concerning treatment for any other medical conditions you may have. For more information, type ATHEROSCLEROSIS into an Internet search engine.

Giant Cell Arteritis (GCA)

GCA is inflammation and damage to arteries, especially those extending out from the carotid. The following factors increase your risk of developing GCA.

Age. This condition usually affects individuals over the age of fifty.

Ethnicity/ancestry. Whites are more affected than any other group. This condition is very rare in blacks.

Family history. This condition can run in families.

Gender. Women are more at risk than men.

Medical conditions. The following conditions place one at higher risk:
- Chronic infections, such as rheumatoid arthritis and lupus
- Polymyalgia rheumatica
- Severe infections

What you can do: Know your risk factors. Find out if it runs in your family and tell your doctor if it does. Treat any medical conditions that can trigger GCA. For more information, type GIANT CELL ARTERITIS into an Internet search engine.

Hypertension (High Blood Pressure)

Hypertension is diagnosed when a patient's blood pressure reading is greater than 120/80 for sustained periods of time. Fifty-eight million Americans have high blood pressure. The following factors increase your risk of developing high blood pressure.

Age. Your risk of hypertension increases with age. Rates are higher for men than women until age sixty-five. Women are more at risk after age sixty-five.

Children under age ten are at risk of hypertension

from kidney disease, narrowing of the aorta, and adrenal gland disorders.

Blood types. Types A and AB have a moderate risk, types B and O and nonsecretors of all types have a lower risk.

Environment. Exposure to heavy metals through acid rain, for instance, is a factor.

Ethnicity/ancestry. Hypertension is more common in blacks than whites. The death rate from hypertension for black males is 356 percent greater than for white males. Black men with diabetes have a very high risk of hypertension. Japanese-American men over age seventy-one also have a very high risk of hypertension.

Family history. Hypertension tends to run in families.

Medical conditions. These medical conditions are risk factors:
- Acromegaly
- Arteriosclerosis
- Calcium deficiency
- Cancer of the adrenal cortex
- Coarctation of the aorta
- Cushing's syndrome
- Diabetes mellitus
- Food allergies or sensitivities
- Hemolytic uremic syndrome
- Henoch-Schönlein purpura
- Kidney disease
- Magnesium deficiency
- Perarteritis nodosa
- Potassium deficiency
- Radiation enteritis
- Renal artery stenosis
- Retroperitoneal fibrosis
- Sodium (salt) sensitivity
- Thyroid problems, both hyper and hypo
- Wilms' tumor

Medications. Cold medicines, diet aids, and some prescription drugs for migraine treatment can be risk factors.

Complications of high blood pressure. High blood pressure increases your risk of:
- Aortic dissection
- Heart attack
- Heart disease
- Irregular heartbeat
- Kidney failure
- Retinopathy
- Stroke

What you can do: Know your risk factors. Minimize your controllable risks. Make sure your doctor knows about any medications you are taking, especially if you are at high risk of hypertension, because many prescription drugs can elevate blood pressure. For more information, type HIGH BLOOD PRESSURE into an Internet search engine.

Peripheral Artery Disease

This disease causes reduced blood flow to the arms and legs and affects some 12 percent of the adult population. The following factors increase the risk of developing peripheral artery disease.

Age. People fifty years and older are at risk.

Blood types. Types A and AB have a higher risk; types B and O have a moderate risk.

Family and personal history. Individuals are at higher risk if there is a personal or family history of:
- Diabetes
- Heart disease
- High blood pressure
- Kidney disease requiring hemodialysis
- Stroke

Gender. Men are more greatly affected than women.

Medical conditions. Having high cholesterol or triglyceride levels are risk factors.

What you can do: Be sure to follow your doctor's advice regarding treatment of existing medical conditions. For more information, type PERIPHERAL ARTERY DISEASE into an Internet search engine.

Toxemia (Preeclampsia)

Preeclampsia causes dangerously high blood pressure in the final stage of pregnancy. This condition occurs in some 8 percent of pregnancies. The following factors increase your risk of developing toxemia.

Age. Most at risk are women thirty-five and older.

Blood types. Type O has a higher risk; types A, B, and AB have a moderate risk.

Ethnicity/ancestry. Blacks have a higher risk than other groups.

Medical conditions. These medical conditions are risk factors:
- Diabetes
- First pregnancy
- High blood pressure even before pregnancy begins
- Kidney disease
- Pregnant with multiple fetuses

What you can do: Before pregnancy, modify your diet and exercise regimen to lower blood pressure, and lose weight if necessary. During pregnancy, work with your obstetrician to monitor your blood pressure. Follow your obstetrician's advice! For more information, type TOXEMIA into an Internet search engine.

High Cholesterol
The following conditions are risk factors:
- Cirrhosis of the liver
- Diabetes (untreated)
- Diet high in cholesterol
- Familial hyperlipidemias
- Hypothyroidism
- Kidney disease
- Pregnancy
- Removal of the ovaries

Varicose Veins
This condition arises from poorly functioning valves in the veins, causing blood to pool in the veins instead of flowing properly. When blood pools, vein walls stretch and distend, causing discomfort, even pain. The following factors place individuals at higher risk:
- Family history of varicose veins
- Pregnancy
- Prolonged standing
- Gender—women are twice as likely as men to develop varicose veins

Circulatory System Conditions That Tend to Run in Families
These conditions have no known genetic links:
- Giant cell arteritis
- Hypertension
- Varicose veins

Medical Conditions That Can Affect the Circulatory System
It is important to properly treat any medical condition with which you are diagnosed, because the condition may affect other parts of your body. The body's organs and systems are inextricably connected to one another, so what goes wrong in one part may create problems in another. Conditions that may cause problems are:
- *Anemia*
- *Hormonal problems*
- *Stress,* which raises blood pressure

Risky Behavior and Possible Consequences

RISKY BEHAVIOR	POSSIBLE CONSEQUENCES
Eating foods high in fat	Coronary artery disease, atherosclerosis
Poor nutrition	Cold feet and hands
Smoking	Cold feet and hands, atherosclerosis, damage to the walls of blood vessels (making them vulnerable to plaque buildup), high blood pressure, abdominal aortic aneurysm, peripheral artery disease
High cholesterol levels	Atherosclerosis
Obesity	High blood pressure, atherosclerosis, peripheral artery disease, varicose veins
Standing in one position for long periods	Varicose veins
Inactivity	High blood pressure
Heavy alcohol consumption	High blood pressure
High stress levels	High blood pressure
A diet high in sugar	High blood pressure
Use of oral contraceptives	High blood pressure

Visit www.healthwatchguide.com for updates on the circulatory system.

The Ears

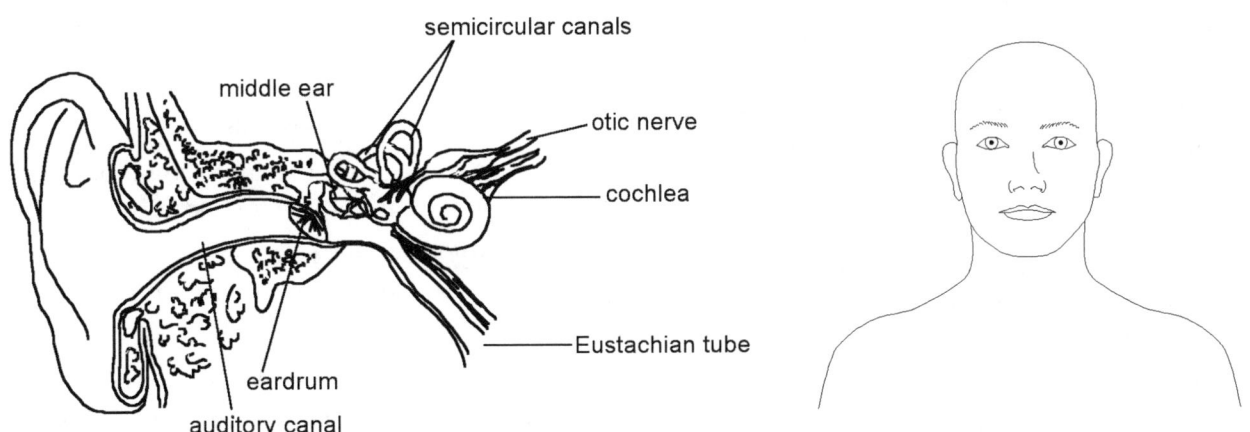

Function

Besides being the organ that lets us hear, the ear helps us keep our balance. Certain parts of the ear monitor our head movements and send signals to the brain to help keep the body and the head steady as we move.

Keeping the Ears Healthy

- Children who are breastfed for at least four months have a lower risk of ear infections.
- Avoid exposure to loud noises over long periods, and wear ear protection to reduce the risk of hearing loss.
- Avoid sudden changes in air pressure.
- Use earplugs or wear a cap to keep water out of the ears while swimming.
- Avoid putting your head underwater while swimming if you have a tendency to get ear infections.
- Don't swim in polluted water.
- Dry ears thoroughly after swimming or bathing.
- Avoid using swabs to clean the inside of the ear. This delicate area is easily irritated and swabbing

can lead to infection. Fingernails also can scratch and infect the ear canal. If you have wax buildup, see your doctor. Otherwise, allow the body to handle wax efficiently and safely.

Other Tips

- Pediatricians often prescribe the pneumococcal 7-valent conjugate vaccine (Prevnar) to protect against the seven most common subtypes of pneumococcal bacterium found in children.
- Some medications, including aspirin and certain antibiotics, can temporarily cause deafness when taken for long periods.
- Earlobe creases are extremely uncommon in children and young adults. If they exist, it often is an indication that the individual has a rare syndrome, which may be inherited. Some research has found that earlobe creases in the young indicate an elevated risk of heart attack.

What Can Go Wrong

Ear Infections, Acute Otitis Media (Inner Ear)

These are caused by a bacterial or viral infection of the fluid in the middle ear. The following factors increase the risk of developing ear infections.

Age. Ear infections are usually seen in infants and young children, but anyone can be affected. Babies who have otitis media in the first year have a greater risk of future ear infections.

Blood types. Type A has a very high risk, types B and AB have a high risk, and type O and nonsecretors of all types have a moderate risk. Children of type A mothers are extremely susceptible to ear infections.

Bottle fed. The risk of bottle feeding is partly to do with the angle at which the baby is held. It is also not a good idea to allow a baby to drink a bottle while lying on his back. Breastfeeding helps pass along immunities that prevent middle-ear infections, and the angle at which the baby is held during breastfeeding provides for better drainage of the Eustachian tubes.

Ethnicity/ancestry. Although all groups are at risk, Native Americans, Alaskan Eskimos, and Canadian Eskimos have particular risks.

Family history. The tendency to develop this infection runs in families.

Environment. The following environmental conditions place one at risk:
- Cold climate
- Congested or unsanitary living quarters
- Exposure to secondhand smoke
- High altitudes
- Those who attend day care

Gender. Boys have more ear infections than girls, but both are at risk.

What you can do: Don't ignore ear infections. Untreated ear infections can lead to *mastoiditis* (an inflammation of the mastoid process, a projection of the temporal bone behind the ear), especially in children, and *cholesteatoma*, a type of cyst located in the middle ear. Know your risk factors. Your baby may be producing mucus in response to an allergy to cow's milk (mucus is the body's way of trying to trap and get rid of allergens). Mucus in the mouth and nasal passages will flow back to the ears and contribute to ear infections. For more information, type EAR INFECTION into an Internet search engine.

Ménière's Disease

This disease affects the inner ear, disrupting balance and hearing. About 100,000 new cases are diagnosed annually. The following factors increase your risk of developing Ménière's disease.

Age. Ménière's disease most commonly develops between the ages of twenty and fifty.

Ethnicity/ancestry. This disease is found predominantly in those of northern European ancestry, blacks, and Asians.

Family history. This disease may have a genetic link.

Gender. Men and women are equally affected.

Medical conditions. These medical conditions are risk factors:
- Allergies
- Autoimmune disorders
- Fatigue
- Middle-ear infections
- Respiratory illness
- Viral infection

Medications. Avoidance of caffeine, aspirin, and medications containing aspirin is recommended for people with other risk factors for Ménière's disease.

Personal history. Individuals are more at risk if they have suffered a head injury.

What you can do: Know your risk factors. Ménière's disease cannot be cured, but may be controlled with treatment. If you know you have risk factors, take precautions—use helmets when advisable, treat illnesses promptly, and discuss medication side effects with your doctor. For more information, type MENIERE'S DISEASE into an Internet search engine.

Hearing Loss

The following conditions are risk factors for hearing loss:

- Advancing age
- Diseases affecting any of the three middle ear bones
- Excessive earwax (see your doctor for help in removing)
- Fetal exposure to German measles (rubella)
- Fetal exposure to mercury
- Fetal lack of iodine
- Fluid in the middle ear
- Measles
- Ménière's disease
- Meningitis
- Middle-ear infection
- Mumps
- Nerve damage
- Noise exposure
- Obstructions in the ear canal
- Paget's disease
- Perforations in the eardrum membrane
- Scarlet fever
- Skull fracture
- Some twenty genetic (inherited) disorders, such as osteogenesis imperfecta
- Toxic response to antibiotics

For more information, type HEARING LOSS into an Internet search engine.

Tinnitus (Ringing in the Ears)

The following conditions are risk factors for tinnitus:
- Anemia
- Aneurysm
- Cardiovascular disease
- Earwax buildup
- Hearing loss from excessive noise
- High blood pressure
- Malfunctioning thyroid
- Ménière's disease
- Misalignment of the jaw
- Some medications
- Some types of tumors
- Trauma to the head or neck

Ear Conditions That Tend to Run in Families

This condition has no known genetic link:
- Otosclerosis—surgery is usually helpful.

Medical Conditions That Can Affect Ear Health

It is important to properly treat any medical condition with which you are diagnosed, because the condition may affect other parts of your body. The body's organs and systems are inextricably connected to one another, so what goes wrong in one part may create problems in another. Conditions that may cause problems are:

- *Diabetes*—may cause malignant otitis externa
- *Neurofibromatosis type 2*—increased risk of acoustic neuromas

Risky Behavior and Possible Consequences	
RISKY BEHAVIOR	**POSSIBLE CONSEQUENCES**
Prolonged exposure to loud noise	Hearing loss, tinnitus
Excessive consumption of coffee, salt, or alcohol	Tinnitus, Ménière's disease
Stress	Tinnitus, Ménière's disease
Scratching, inserting objects, or allowing moisture to get into the ear canal	Otitis externa (swimmer's ear)
Using cotton-tipped applicators (or anything else to clean the ears of earwax)	Otitis externa
Swimming in dirty or contaminated water	Otitis externa
Becoming infected with syphilis	Ménière's disease
Smoking	Ménière's disease, tinnitus

Visit www.healthwatchguide.com for updates on the ears.

NOTES

The Esophagus

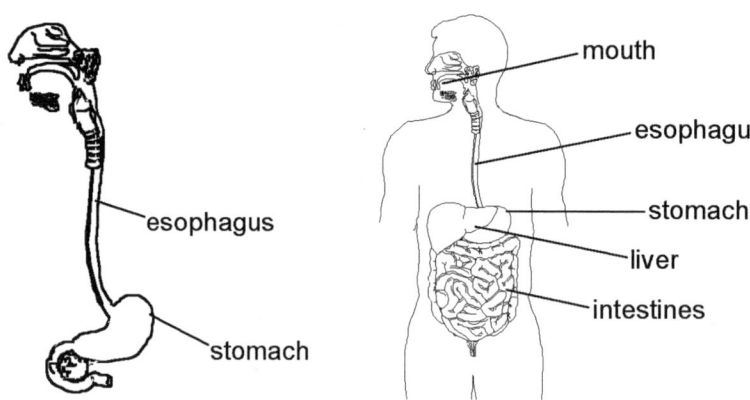

Function

The esophagus is a tube connecting the mouth to the stomach. Its muscular contractions help food travel to the stomach after chewing and swallowing. The lower esophageal sphincter provides an important secondary function of the esophagus—the prevention of reflux (the return of stomach contents to the esophagus).

Keeping the Esophagus Healthy

The esophagus is designed to stay healthy with a minimum of help from you. If GERD (gastroesophageal reflux disease) or heartburn runs in your family, avoiding troublesome foods may decrease your risk.

Beneficial Foods and Nutrients

A diet featuring fresh fruits and vegetables (especially raw) seems to help reduce the risk of developing esophageal cancer.

Green Tea

Green tea has been found to reduce the risk of esophageal cancer by 60 percent.

What Can Go Wrong

Barrett's Esophagus

Barrett's esophagus is a precancerous condition for both esophageal cancer and stomach cancer. The following conditions increase your risk of developing Barrett's esophagus.

Blood type. Type A, especially those with O subtype, have a higher risk. Types B, AB, and O have a moderate risk.

Gender. Men are more at risk than women.

Medical conditions. These medical conditions are risk factors:

- Gastroesophageal reflux disease (GERD)—20 percent of patients with chronic GERD, which is commonly known as heartburn, will develop Barrett's esophagus, with an increased risk of esophageal cancer. One half of one percent of Barrett's esophagus patients develop esophageal cancer.
- *H. pylori* infection

What you can do: If you frequently suffer from heartburn, seek medical treatment as early as possible. For more information, type BARRETT'S ESOPHAGUS into an Internet search engine.

Esophageal Cancer

There are two kinds of esophageal cancer—squamous cell esophageal carcinoma and adenocarcinoma. Some 13,000 people die of esophageal cancer annually in the United States. The following factors increase your risk of developing esophageal cancer.

Age. Most at risk are those over age fifty.

Blood types. Types A and AB have a higher risk. Types B and O have a moderate risk.

Ethnicity/ancestry. Blacks are at highest risk, followed by Hawaiians, Chinese, Japanese, whites, and Hispanics.

Gender. Men have three to five times the risk of women.

Medical conditions. These medical conditions are risk factors:

- Barrett's esophagus—a primary factor in adenocarcinoma
- Gastroesophageal reflux disease (GERD)—a primary factor in adenocarcinoma

Personal history. Having had other cancers of the head or neck places one at higher risk.

What you can do: Know your risk factors. Minimize your controllable risks and adjust your dietary habits as needed. For more information, type ESOPHAGEAL CANCER into an Internet search engine.

Gastroesophageal Reflux Disease (GERD)

Risk factors for GERD include:

- Dietary habits, including foods high in fat, and overuse of peppermint
- Hiatal hernia
- Pregnancy
- Prior surgery on the esophagus

Esophagus Conditions That Tend to Run in Families

These conditions have no known genetic links:

- Achalasia
- Plummer-Vinson syndrome

Risky Behavior and Possible Consequences	
RISKY BEHAVIOR	**POSSIBLE CONSEQUENCES**
Smoking	GERD, squamous cell esophageal cancer
Excessive alcohol consumption	GERD, squamous cell esophageal cancer
Excessive coffee consumption	GERD
Drug abuse	GERD
Obesity	GERD
Using smokeless (chewing) tobacco	Esophageal cancer
Swallowing caustic substances	Esophageal cancer
Excessive or prolonged vomiting	GERD

Visit www.healthwatchguide.com for updates on the esophagus.

NOTES

The Eyes

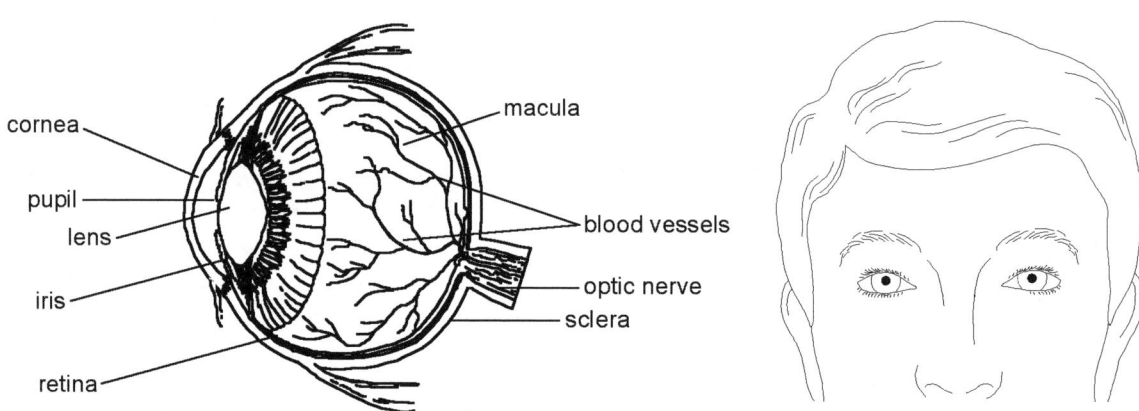

Function

The eye is an organ that collects light rays and sends them to the brain in the form of electronic messages, which are then converted into pictures.

Parts of the Eye

The **cornea** is a clear, curved tissue that covers the front of the eye.

The **iris** is the colored ring that surrounds the black pupil. The iris widens (dilates) the **pupil** to admit light, and shrinks it to keep light out.

The **lens** is found right behind the iris. It focuses light onto the **retina**, which is located at the back of the eye. Retinal tissue has millions of photoreceptors, also called rods and cones, which convert light into electrical signals.

These signals travel to the brain by way of the **optic nerve** and are converted to visual images. The sides of the retina control peripheral vision.

The **macula** is located in the center of the retina. It controls color vision and fine central vision, such as that needed for reading.

The **sclera** is the white part of the eye. It forms a strong protective barrier that gives the eye its shape and protects the internal components.

Eye Color

Eye color (the color of the iris) is inherited; each parent contributes an eye-color gene. The gene for blue eyes is recessive, while the gene for brown eyes is dominant, so a child born to parents with brown and blue eyes will have brown eyes. A child born to parents with blue eyes will probably have blue eyes (but if there is a brown eyes gene somewhere in the gene pool, the baby may have brown eyes).

Keeping the Eyes Healthy

What You and Your Eye Doctor Should Know

- Family history of vision problems
- Any medical conditions, as noted under "What Can Go Wrong" on the following page

Recommended Eye Exams

- *From birth to two years*—the pediatrician should do a basic eye exam at each checkup. Be sure to mention any family history of vision problems.
- *Age two to five years*—a more comprehensive exam at age three or as recommended for specific conditions.
- *Age six to forty years*—once every three years; once every eighteen months if corrective lenses are used.
- *Over age forty*—at least once every two years, including a glaucoma test. Glaucoma tests should be done more frequently for blacks or anyone with a family history of glaucoma; every eighteen months for contact lenses or glasses, or as recommended for specific conditions.

As You Age

- Keep a watch on your general health in order to treat other conditions that could affect your vision.
- See your eye doctor regularly—most vision problems can be easily treated.
- Adjust the lighting in your home or office, if necessary, if your eyesight has gotten weaker.

Beneficial Foods and Nutrients

See Part Four, The Importance of Nutrients, for a list of foods containing the vitamins, minerals, and trace elements mentioned in this section.

Vitamin A

Vitamin A is needed for normal and night vision. *Note: Vitamin A deficiency can lead to night blindness and the perception of glare and haze under normal light conditions. Serious vitamin A deficiency can lead to total blindness.*

Vitamin B_2 (Riboflavin)

Vitamin B_2 is necessary for normal eyesight.

Copper

Copper is a factor in the production of melanin, the substance that controls skin and eye color.

Omega-3 Fatty Acids

Fish and other dietary sources of omega-3 fatty acids are shown to reduce the risk of macular degeneration and dry eye syndrome (DES).

Other Tips

- Keep consumption of refined sugars to a minimum—this is healthier for the eyes.
- Avoid exposure to cigarette smoke and airborne pollutants, such as exhaust fumes.
- Give your eyes a five-minute rest every half hour when doing close, concentrated work.
- Blink regularly to lubricate the eye and minimize eyestrain from continuous focus.
- When you drive, glance away from the road (long distance) from time to time, and look at the steering wheel (near distance).
- Take a few minutes during the day to close your eyes and let them rest completely.

Definitions of Terms

Myopia—nearsightedness, where distant objects are blurry and close ones are clear.

Hyperopia—farsightedness, where close objects are blurry and distant ones are clear.

Astigmatism—a vision difficulty caused by a warping of the cornea of the eye. Often occurs with myopia or hyperopia. Prescription glasses correct astigmatism, but contact lenses are usually not an option.

Presbyopia—a decrease in the eye's ability to focus finely on small, near objects, such as newsprint. This is a natural part of the aging process, usually symptomatic around age forty-five.

Strabismus—deviations in alignment of the eyes in relation to each other; for instance, crossed eyes, squint-eyed, walleye.

- Wear sunglasses, *but during the day only.* Glasses that block 75 to 90 percent of the sun's visible light are best. This enhances the eyes' ability to adjust to lower light levels at night. Gray lenses are recommended (because they do not affect color perception), followed by green or brown tints. Avoid medium and dark blue lenses—these can seriously interfere with the ability of some people to distinguish traffic-signal colors. If you wear prescription glasses, talk to your eye-care specialist about prescription sunglasses.

- Wear sunglasses to avoid ultraviolet light damage from snow reflection, tanning-bed lamps, and welding equipment. But your eyes benefit from fifteen to twenty minutes of daily exposure to sunlight without sunglasses (but don't look directly at the sun!).

  Note: Children need sunglasses, too. Hats with a brim in addition to sunglasses offer real protection against sun and heat.

- Wash your hands frequently during cold-and-flu season and keep them away from your eyes.

What Can Go Wrong

Adult Cataracts

Cataracts are a clouding of the lens that affects 70 percent of those over age seventy-five. The following factors increase your risk of developing adult cataracts:

Age. Clouding usually begins after age sixty.

Family history. Cataracts may run in families.

Medical conditions. These medical conditions are risk factors:
- Diabetes
- Low serum calcium levels

Medications. Cortisone (steroid) use can increase risk.

Personal history. The following conditions place one at risk of cataracts:
- Eye injury
- Radiation exposure

What you can do: Know your risk factors. Minimize your controllable risks. Have regular eye exams. For more information, type CATARACTS into an Internet search engine.

Amblyopia (Lazy Eye)

About 5 percent of children have this condition. Left untreated, the eye will be permanently impaired. Risk factors include:
- Cataracts
- Crossed or wandering eyes
- Droopy eyelids
- Family history

What you can do: Seek treatment as soon as possible. For more information, type AMBLYOPIA into an Internet search engine.

Congenital Cataracts

Congenital cataracts are an inherited autosomal dominant trait. Risk factors include:
- Family history of cataracts
- Galactosemia—an inherited condition that causes cataracts in newborns
- Inherited metabolic disease
- Viral infection, such as German measles (rubella), of the mother during pregnancy

Glaucoma

Glaucoma is an increase of fluid in the eye, which puts pressure on the optic nerve. Glaucoma is the third most common cause of blindness in America. There are four forms of glaucoma: chronic, acute, secondary, and congenital.

Chronic glaucoma is the most common type of glaucoma. It results when channels in the eye that normally drain fluid become narrow. Pressure builds on the junction of the optic nerve and the retina, decreasing blood flow to the optic nerve and causing the death of optic nerve cells. This results in vision loss. The following factors increase your risk of developing chronic (open angle) glaucoma.

Age. Chronic glaucoma usually occurs after age forty.

Blood types. Types A, B, AB, and O have a moderate risk. Nonsecretors of all types have a higher risk. Rh-negative of all types have a lower risk.

Ethnicity/ancestry. Blacks over forty have four times the risk of whites. Also at risk are those of Irish, Russian, Japanese, Hispanic, and Scandinavian extraction.

Family history. A family history doubles the risk.

Gender. Men and women are affected equally.

Medical conditions. These medical conditions are risk factors:
- Diabetes

- Exfoliation syndrome (most common among those with European ancestry)
- High blood pressure

Personal history. These conditions place one at risk:
- Injuries to the eyes
- Nearsightedness

Acute glaucoma is more common in people who were born with a very small opening between the cornea and the iris. The iris might slide forward without warning and block the flow of fluids, causing a drastic increase in pressure. The following factors increase your risk of developing acute (narrow angle) glaucoma.

Age. Older people have the greatest risk.

Blood types. Types A, B, AB, and O have a moderate risk. Nonsecretors of all types have a higher risk, and Rh-negative of all types have a lower risk.

Ethnicity/ancestry. Asians have the greatest risk.

Family history. Acute glaucoma runs in families.

Personal history. The following conditions place one at risk:
- Farsightedness
- Use of dilation drops (if you are at risk of acute glaucoma, make sure to discuss this with your eye doctor)

Secondary glaucoma occurs as a result of other medical conditions, including eye diseases, diseases that affect the entire body, and the use of corticosteroids.

Congenital glaucoma is a condition present from birth. It results from a malformation of the eyes' fluid-release channels. Corrective surgery is required.

What you can do: Know your risk factors. Make sure you have your eyes checked as often as necessary. Many medications, both prescription and over-the-counter, exacerbate glaucoma. Avoid tight neckties and shirt collars, especially if you have a thick neck. If you are being treated for any medical condition, make sure your physician knows that you have glaucoma, and check medicine labels carefully. For more information, type GLAUCOMA into an Internet search engine.

Macular Degeneration

Macular degeneration (MD) is a degenerative vision disorder affecting the center of the retina. This condition affects some 15 percent of the population over age seventy-five. The following factors increase your risk of developing macular degeneration.

Age. Risk increases after age fifty.

Ethnicity/ancestry. Whites have the greatest risk.

Family history. A family history increases the risk. Early onset MD is an inherited condition.

What you can do: Know your risk factors. If you are at risk, be sure to get regular eye examinations and talk to your eye doctor about ways to cope. Some vitamin and mineral supplements have been found to be useful; discuss this option with your eye doctor. For more information, type MACULAR DEGENERATION into an Internet search engine.

Melanoma of the Eye

This is a cancerous tumor affecting the pigmented portion of the eye, which affects about 1,800 people in the United States annually. The following factors increase your risk of developing melanoma of the eye.

Ethnicity/ancestry. Fair-skinned, blue-eyed people have the greatest risk.

Personal history. Excessive exposure to the sun is a risk factor.

What you can do: Melanoma of the eye can begin in the eye, or it can spread there from another melanoma on the body. The precautions you take against skin cancer will also protect against melanoma of the eye, but don't forget to add sunglasses to the list. For more information, type MELANOMA OF THE EYE into an Internet search engine.

Night Blindness

Nightblindness is the inablility to see in dim light or at night. Risk factors include:
- Cataracts
- Liver disorder
- Myopia
- Retinitis pigmentosa
- Vitamin A deficiency

What you can do: If you are having trouble with your nighttime vision, make an appointment for a full eye exam. For more information, type NIGHT BLINDNESS into an Internet search engine.

Sarcoidosis

Sarcoidosis is an inflammation that can affect the eyes. The cause is unknown. The following factors increase your risk of developing sarcoidosis.

Age. People aged thirty to fifty years are at risk.

Blood types. Type A has a moderate-to-high risk for the most severe form of the disease. Types B, AB, and O have a low-to-moderate risk. Nonsecretors have a moderate-to-high risk.

Ethnicity/ancestry. At highest risk are those with African, northern European, Japanese, and Irish ancestry.

Family history. This inflammation may run in families.

Gender. Women have the greatest risk.

What you can do: Be aware of your risk factors. If it runs in your family, be sure to let your doctor know. For more information, type SARCOIDOSIS into an Internet search engine.

Age-Related Eye Disorders

- Cataracts—three-fourths of cataracts are caused by advancing age.
- Color vision deficiency
- Dry eyes
- Glaucoma
- Macular degeneration
- Retinal detachment—risk factors include:
  - Diabetes
  - Family history
  - Inflammation
  - Nearsightedness
  - Previous eye injury or surgery

Medical Conditions That Can Affect Eye Health

It is important to properly treat treat any medical condition with which you are diagnosed, because the condition may affect other parts of your body. The body's organs and systems are inextricably connected to one another, so what goes wrong in one part may create problems in another. The following conditions may cause problems.

- *Bell's palsy* usually causes temporary facial paralysis, but it can affect the ability to blink.
- *Diabetes* is a risk factor for:
  - Cataracts
  - Detached retinas
  - Diabetic retinopathy
  - Glaucoma
- *Graves' disease* can lead to Graves' eye disease (Graves' opthalmopathy).
- *Herpes simplex* (cold sore virus) can cause serious corneal infections.
- *Herpes zoster* (chicken pox and shingles virus) can damage the eyes or cause blindness.
- *High blood pressure* is a risk factor for:
  - Atrophy of the optic nerve, leading to blindness
  - Hemorrhages and scar tissue on the retina
- *Juvenile rheumatoid arthritis* can lead to vision problems or blindness.
- *Osteosarcoma* (bone cancer) has been linked to hereditary retinoblastoma.
- *Reiter's syndrome* can lead to blindness as a result of inflammation of the eyes.
- *Sickle-cell disease* is a risk factor for sickle-cell retinopathy, a progressive loss of vision leading to blindness.

Note: Diabetic retinopathy is the leading cause of blindness in the United States. Signs of diabetic retinopathy begin to appear within seven years of the initial diagnosis of diabetes.

Risky Behavior and Possible Consequences

RISKY BEHAVIOR	POSSIBLE CONSEQUENCES
Amber-tinted glasses worn at night	Reduction in ability to see
Looking directly at the sun	Permanent vision loss
Not wearing safety glasses while using power tools, including lawn mowers and trimmers	Serious eye damage
Not wearing eye protectors while playing sports like handball and squash	Serious eye damage
Not wearing swim goggles while in chlorinated water	Chemical burns to the cornea
Swimming in non-chlorinated pools or stagnant lakes and ponds	Eye infections
Coming into contact with dog or cat feces	Choroiditis. Becoming infected with toxoplasmosis, which can cause eye inflammation leading to permanent eye damage.

RISKY BEHAVIOR	POSSIBLE CONSEQUENCES
Coming into contact with dog or cat feces (cont.)	Pregnant women can pass the infection to their unborn babies. Children are especially vulnerable.
Contracting German measles during pregnancy	The baby may develop congenital cataracts
The use of certain drugs during pregnancy	The baby may develop congenital cataracts
Exposure to radiation, such as from microwaves, infrared rays, or x-rays	Cataracts
Not treating amblyopia	Impaired vision or functional blindness in one eye
Not wearing sunglasses when appropriate	Cataracts
Borrowing eye makeup	Eye infections, conjunctivitis
Sharing washcloths	Eye infections, conjunctivitis, or towels
Borrowing eye medications	Eye infections, conjunctivitis
Using outdated eye medications	Eye infections
Exposure to the bacteria *Chlamydia*	Trachoma, trachomatous
Smoking	Macular degeneration, cataracts
Unprotected sex (males have the highest risk), especially those with AIDS	Reiter's syndrome

Visit www.healthwatchguide.com for updates on the eyes.

NOTES

The Gallbladder

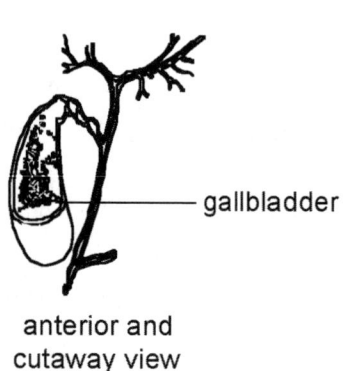

anterior and cutaway view

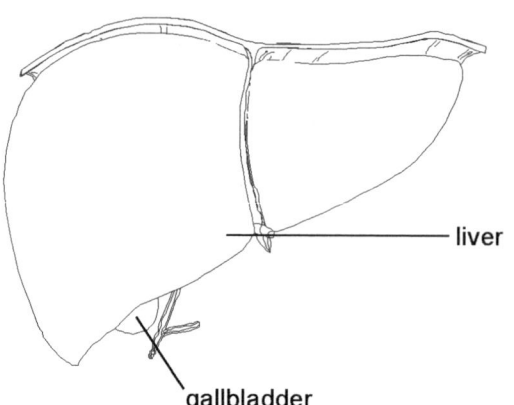

Function

The gallbladder is a small organ located just below the liver. It concentrates and stores bile produced by the liver and releases it as needed for digestion of food passing through the small intestine.

Keeping the Gallbladder Healthy

A certain amount of fat in the diet is necessary to overall health, but too much fat can cause real problems for the gallbladder.

Beneficial Foods and Nutrients

See Part Four, The Importance of Nutrients, for a list of foods containing choline.

Choline

Choline is necessary for proper gallbladder functioning.

What Can Go Wrong

Gallbladder Cancer

Gallbladder cancer is uncommon. Only 7,000 cases are diagnosed annually in the United States. The following factors increase your risk of developing gallbladder cancer.

Age. Usually affects those over age seventy.

Blood types. Type A has a higher risk. Type AB has a moderate-to-high risk. Types B and O have a moderate risk.

Ethnicity/ancestry. In descending order of risk: Hispanics, Native Americans, whites, and blacks.

Gender. Women have three times the risk of men.

What you can do: Know your risk factors. For more information, type GALLBLADDER CANCER into an Internet search engine.

Gallstones (Cholethiasis)

Gallstones usually consist of hardened cholesterol. This condition affects 1 person in 1,000. The following factors increase your risk of developing gallstones.

Age. Most at risk are those over age forty.

Blood types. Types A and AB have a higher risk. Types B and O have a moderate risk.

Ethnicity/ancestry. Native Americans have the highest risk.

Family history. This condition runs in families.

Gender. Women have twice the risk of men.

Medical conditions. These medical conditions are risk factors:
- Cirrhosis of the liver
- Diabetes

Personal history. Long-term IV use (total parenteral nutrition) is a risk factor.

What you can do: Know your risk factors. Maintain a healthy weight. Follow your treatment regimen for diabetes and liver conditions. For more information, type GALLSTONES into an Internet search engine.

Medical Conditions That Can Affect Gallbladder Health

It is important to properly treat any medical condition with which you are diagnosed, because the condition may affect other parts of your body. The body's organs and systems are inextricably connected to one another, so what goes wrong in one part may create problems in another. Conditions that can affect the gallbladder include:

- *Cirrhosis of the liver*
- *Diabetes*
- *Elevated cholesterol levels*

| Risky Behavior and Possible Consequences ||
RISKY BEHAVIOR	POSSIBLE CONSEQUENCES
Obesity	Gallstones

Visit www.healthwatchguide.com for updates on the gallbladder.

NOTES

The Hands

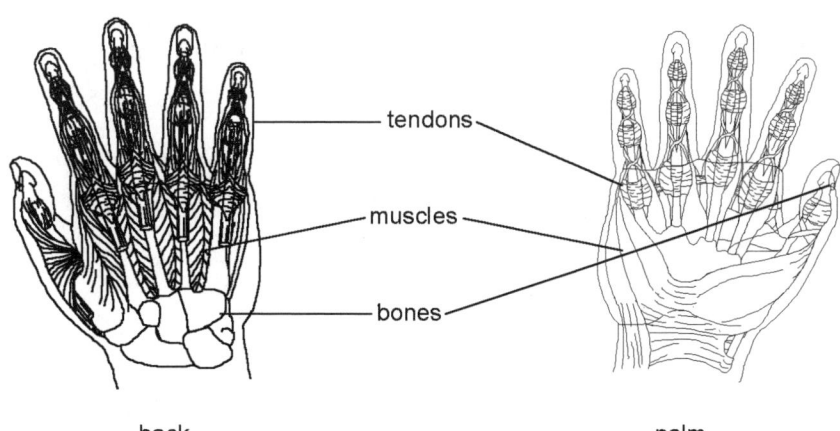

back   palm

Function

There are twenty-seven bones in the hand and wrist, as well as nerves, blood vessels, muscles, and tendons. These components work together to make it possible for us to perform an astounding variety of tasks—grasping, lifting, scratching, twisting, pulling, and pushing, to name just a few.

Keeping the Hands Healthy

- Keep your wrists straight as much as possible—including when you are sleeping, typing, or using tools. Constant flexing and/or extending of the wrists, as well as other repetitive movements, contribute to the risk of carpal tunnel syndrome. If you must flex (bend) your wrists for work or

play, use strengthening and conditioning exercises frequently.
- Use care when holding or carrying heavy objects; avoid straining the tendons and muscles of the hand and wrist.
- Take frequent breaks when typing, sewing, writing, and so forth. Open and close your fists, shake your hands out, wiggle your fingers.
- Avoid leaning on your flexed wrist while sitting or lying down.

What Can Go Wrong

Dupuytren's Contracture

This involves a thickening of the fascia (muscle covering tissue) at the base of the palm. The following factors may increase your risk of developing Dupuytren's contracture.

Age. Usually seen after age forty, though sometimes it appears in teenagers and young children.

Ethnicity/ancestry. Whites of northern European descent have the greatest risk.

Family history. Dupuytren's contracture is a hereditary condition.

Gender. Men have seven times the risk of women.

Medical conditions. These medical conditions are risk factors:
- Epilepsy
- Diabetes
- Pulmonary tuberculosis
- Liver disease

What you can do: Know your risk factors. Minimize your controllable risks. Familiarize yourself with symptoms and seek treatment early. For more information, type DUPUYTREN'S CONTRACTURE into an Internet search engine.

Medical Conditions That Can Affect the Hands

It is important to properly treat any medical condition with which you are diagnosed, because the condition may affect other parts of your body. The body's organs and systems are inextricably connected to one another, so what goes wrong in one part may create problems in another.

- *Diabetes* affects the nerves, making them vulnerable to compression injury, such as carpal tunnel syndrome.
- *Diabetes, rheumatoid arthritis,* and *gout* may lead to trigger-finger problems and tendonitis.

Risky Behavior and Possible Consequences	
RISKY BEHAVIOR	**POSSIBLE CONSEQUENCES**
Repetitive grasping motions with the thumb	De Quervain's disease (inflammation of tendons in the thumb). Women are affected almost ten times more often than men.
Alcoholism	Dupuytren's syndrome

Visit www.healthwatchguide.com for updates on the hands.

NOTES

The Heart

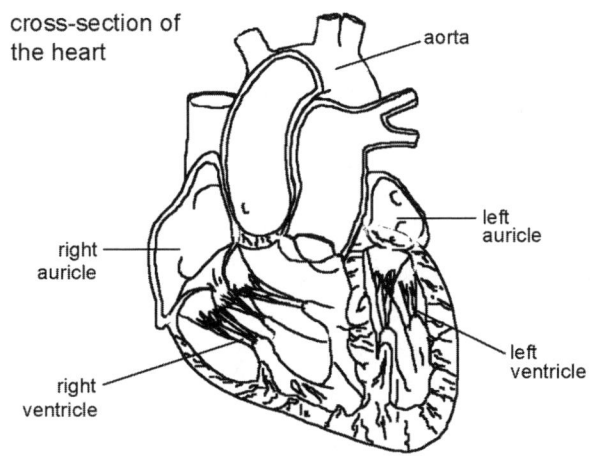

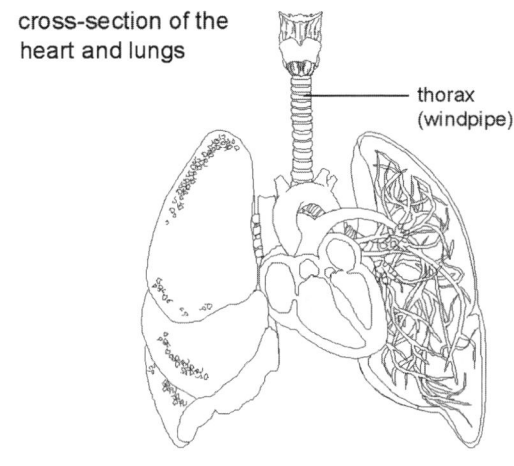

Function

The heart is a muscle about the size of a closed fist, weighing ten ounces on average. Day in and day out it pumps blood throughout the body—about one and a half gallons per minute, 2,000 gallons daily, averaging 100,000 beats every twenty-four hours. Blood is pumped into the lungs to collect oxygen, and out of the lungs to transport the oxygen throughout the body. The fetal heart begins to beat and pump blood at four weeks. The heart will beat approximately 2.5 billion times over a seventy-year lifetime.

Keeping Your Heart Healthy

While there are many things that can go wrong with the heart, most of them can be prevented. A number of heart problems are due to congenital abnormalities over which one has no control, but the rest are the result of lifestyle choices—eating too much, eating the wrong foods, smoking, getting little or no exercise, and allowing cholesterol and blood pressure levels to get dangerously high.

Watch your cholesterol level. Refer to "Cholesterol Screenings" in Part Two for more information on cholesterol numbers and ratios.

Follow these important lifestyle habits for a healthy heart:

- Get the right amount of sleep. Research has shown that eight hours a night is the optimum amount. More or less than that can lead to heart problems, or it can be an indicator of existing trouble.
- Control your blood pressure. Current medical advice is to keep the blood pressure at or below 120/80.
- Get an adequate amount of exercise—this has been shown to reduce the levels of C-reactive protein, especially in men. The inflammation that contributes to heart disease causes C-reactive protein levels to rise. A reduction in the levels of C-reactive protein indicates a similar decline in the inflammation condition.
- Keep your weight under control and fat consumption to no more than 30 percent of daily calories.
- Don't smoke, and avoid breathing in secondhand smoke.
- Keep your life as stress-free as possible, or find good ways to decompress.
- Limit your intake of hydrogenated, partially hydrogenated, and trans-fatty acids.
- If you have early heart disease or a family history of early heart disease, consider testing your levels of homocysteine, C-reactive protein, lipoprotein (a), and apolipoproteins A and B.
    - **DANGER SIGN**: Elevated levels of homocysteine in the blood (normal levels are 5–15 micromoles per liter, with the risk of heart disease rising above levels of 9)
    - **DANGER SIGN**: High levels of C-reactive protein in the liver (safe levels are 0.55–0.99 milligrams per liter)
    - **DANGER SIGN**: Elevated levels of lipoprotein (risks of heart disease increase above 30 mg/dL)

Apolipoproteins carry cholesterol through the bloodstream to dangerous locations in the body. Tests can measure these levels and identify potential problems. Good ranges for apoA-1 are 101–199 mg/dL (milligrams per deciliter) for women and 94–178 mg/dL for men. Good ranges for apoB are 49–103 mg/dL for women and 52–109 mg/dL for men.

What You and Your Doctor Should Know
- Family history of heart disease
- Personal history of heart disease
- Your cholesterol level
- Your blood pressure

Beneficial Foods and Nutrients

See Part Four, The Importance of Nutrients, for a list of foods containing the vitamins, minerals, and trace elements mentioned in this section.

Saffron Flower
Saffron flower is a spice known for its distinctive yellow color. It has a beneficial effect on lipoprotein oxidation in healthy people, when used regularly.

Green Tea
One Japanese study found that people who drank at least two cups of green tea daily reduced the risk of myocardial infarction by 44 percent. Researchers suspect that flavonoids (components that neutralize free radicals) in the tea are responsible. Green tea was not shown to have any effect on the risk of coronary artery disease.

Alcohol
Alcohol in moderation (one drink daily for women, two drinks for men) has been shown to reduce the risk of heart attack. But that doesn't mean that you should start drinking if you have religious or medical reasons for abstaining from alcohol.

Omega-3 Fatty Acids
The omega-3 fatty acids can reduce levels of cholesterol and triglycerides. They are found in salmon, mackerel, herring, and flax seed.

Vitamin B_1
Vitamin B_1 benefits the heart.

Vitamin B_3 (Niacin)
Niacin helps reduce blood cholesterol levels.

Vitamin B_6
Vitamin B_6 helps reduce homocysteine levels.

Vitamin B_{12}
Vitamin B_{12} helps reduce homocysteine levels.

Vitamin C
Vitamin C has antioxidants, which help fight against heart disease.

Folic Acid (Folate)
Folate helps to protect against heart disease by lowering homocysteine levels.

Choline
Choline helps control cholesterol levels.

Pantothenic Acid
Pantothenic acid helps in the synthesis of cholesterol.

Calcium
Calcium helps the heart to maintain a steady beat.

Magnesium
Magnesium is needed for normal heart rhythm.

Phosphorus
Phosphorus helps to regulate the heartbeat.

Potassium
Potassium helps to regulate the heartbeat.

Sodium
Sodium is necessary for optimum cardiac function, but too much salt can be dangerous.

Copper
Copper is necessary for a healthy heart.

Other Tips

- Too much iron may increase your risk of heart attack by stimulating the creation of free radicals. Excess iron also is stored in the liver, the pancreas, the eyes, the brain, and the skin.
- Endocarditis is an inflammation of cardiac valves, often caused by bacterial infection following dental surgery. Make sure your dentist knows about any heart conditions you may have, as protective measures can be taken before the operation.
- Rheumatic fever is a common complication of strep throat and scarlet fever, and it is a major cause of many heart conditions. Strep throat is easily spread, especially among young children, although any age can be infected. Ask your doctor for information on how to identify and treat strep throat.

What Can Go Wrong

Be Aware! African Americans have the highest risk of heart disease of all the ethnic groups.

Myocardial Infarction (Heart Attack)

One out of five deaths are caused by heart attacks, including 250,000 women and even more men, annually. The following factors increase your risk of suffering a heart attack.

Age. Risk increases with age.

Blood types. Types A and AB have a higher risk, and types B and O have a moderate risk. Nonsecretors of all types have a higher risk.

Ethnicity/ancestry. Blacks have the highest risk of heart attack.

Family history. A family history increases the risk.

Gender. Men have the highest risk, but women are catching up, especially postmenopause.

Medical conditions. The following conditions are risk factors:
- Arterial blockages
- Diabetes
- Hemochromatosis
- High blood cholesterol
- High blood pressure
- High levels of C-reactive protein
- High levels of homocysteine

What you can do: Know your risk factors. Minimize your controllable risks. Don't smoke, watch your diet, get some exercise and sleep, control your cholesterol and blood pressure levels. For more information, type HEART ATTACK into an Internet search engine.

Peripartum Cardiomyopathy

Peripartum cardiomyopathy is a weakened heart diagnosed in the mother within a few months of giving birth. Occurs once in every 3,000 to 4,000 deliveries. The following factors increase the risk of developing peripartum cardiomyopathy:

Age. Most common after age thirty.

Ethnicity/ancestry. Blacks have the highest risk.

Personal history. These conditions place one at risk:
- Heart disease
- Malnutrition
- Pregnant with twins, triplets, or more

What you can do: Know your risk factors and make sure to get prenatal care during your pregnancy. Make sure your doctor knows your complete health history, especially any history of heart disease. For more information, type PERIPARTUM CARDIOMYOPATHY into an Internet search engine.

Heart Conditions That Tend to Run in Families

These conditions have no known genetic links:
- Atrial myxoma
- Coronary artery disease
- Early heart attacks
- Mitral valve prolapse

Medical Conditions That Can Affect Heart Health

It is important to properly treat any medical condition with which you are diagnosed, because the condition may affect other parts of your body. The body's organs and systems are inextricably connected to one another, so what goes wrong in one part may create problems in another.

- *Acromegaly* can cause *cardiovascular disease*
- *Atherosclerosis*
- *Chlamydiae pneumoniae*
- *Chronic bronchitis*
- *Degenerative conditions*
- *Diabetes mellitus*
- *Gum disease*, or periodontal disease, has been linked to heart disease. Bacteria from the infected gums can easily get into the bloodstream and infect the heart. Swollen and/or bleeding gums need early treatment.
- *H. pylori* infection
- *Hemochromatosis* is an inherited condition where the body absorbs too much iron and stores it in the heart and other organs.
- *Inflammatory diseases*
- *Kidney failure*
- *Lung diseases*
- *Lupus*
- *Marfan's syndrome*
- *Rheumatic fever* can cause
  - *Aortic insufficiency*
  - *Aortic stenosis*
  - *Chronic mitral regurgitation*
  - *Mitral stenosis*
  - *Pulmonary stenosis*
  - *Tricuspid regurgitation*
- *Scoliosis* can cause
  - *Mitral valve prolapse*

- *Stroke*
- *Syndrome X*, which is related to insulin resistance, may be inherited.
- *Thyroid disorders*

Aortic Insufficiency
Risk factors include:
- Aortic dissection
- Ankylosing spondylitis
- Congenital aortic abnormalities
- Endocarditis
- High blood pressure
- Marfan's syndrome
- Reiter's syndrome
- Rheumatic fever
- Syphilis

Rheumatic Fever
Risk factors include:
- Blood type B has the greatest risk—Strep throat and scarlet fever are the two biggest risk factors for rheumatic fever. People with blood type B have the greatest risk of rheumatic fever, and blood type B newborns with blood type B mothers have twice the risk of neonatal group B streptococci infections, thus also increasing their risk for rheumatic fever.

Beware of Snow Shoveling

Shoveling snow may be one of the most heart-strenuous activities many Americans ever perform. Don't assume you are free of heart disease. You are at risk if you are a man or woman over age forty and have:
- a personal or family history of heart disease
- chest pain
- dizziness or a throbbing heartbeat when you exert yourself
- a smoking habit
- high blood pressure
- elevated blood cholesterol
- a sedentary lifestyle

Get a checkup—don't wait until you are shoveling snow to find out that you have heart disease.

Risky Behavior and Possible Consequences	
RISKY BEHAVIOR	**POSSIBLE CONSEQUENCES**
Snow shoveling	Heart failure
Smoking	Twice the risk of heart disease and arrhythmias, peripartum cardiomyopathy
Sedentary lifestyle	Heart disease
Obesity	Cardiomyopathy, peripartum cardiomyopathy
Excessive use of alcohol	Arrhythmias, alcoholic cardiomyopathy, peripartum cardiomyopathy
Having a total cholesterol level of 240 mg or more	Twice the risk of heart attack of those with a total cholesterol level of 200 mg
Use of oral contraceptives by smokers	Blood clots (thrombosis)
Sudden, overwhelming stress	Heart attack
Excessive use of caffeinated products	Arrhythmias
Cocaine use	Arrhythmias
Amphetamine use	Arrhythmias
Using drugs, alcohol, or retinoic acid while pregnant	Babies born with heart abnormalities
Exposure to rubella while pregnant	Babies born with heart abnormalities

Visit www.healthwatchguide.com for updates on the heart.

The Hormones

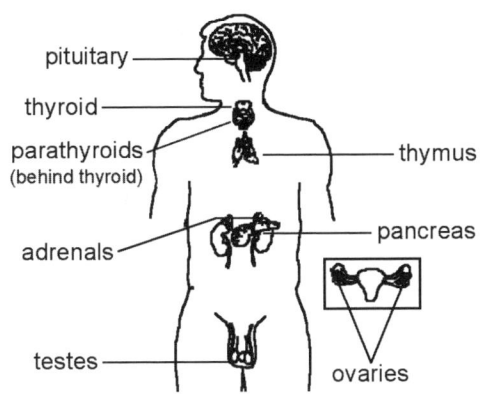 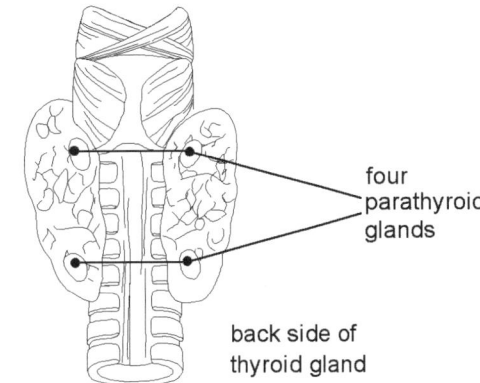

Function

Hormones are specialized substances, such as testosterone, adrenaline, cortisol, and estrogen, produced by the body, many by glands, such as the thyroid and the pituitary. They are designed to regulate cellular activities and are vital to the proper functioning of the whole system.

Beneficial Foods and Nutrients

See Part Four, The Importance of Nutrients, for a list of foods containing pantothenic acid.

Pantothenic Acid

Pantothenic acid helps in the synthesis of hormones.

Other Tips

- Diseases that affect a hormone-producing gland can cause a hormonal deficiency. These diseases might be benign or malignant tumors.
- Inadequate exposure to the sun can result in insufficient production of melatonin by the pineal gland. This can mean sleep difficulties for some people.
- Sometimes the body's chemical processes can malfunction, leading to hormonal imbalances.

What Can Go Wrong

Prolactinoma

A prolactinoma is the most common type of pituitary tumor. It causes high levels of prolactin, which in turn may cause infertility or impotence. It is usually benign. In the United States, 25 percent of the population has small tumors. Significant tumors affect approximately 40,000 people per year. The following factors increase your risk of developing prolactinomas.

Medical conditions. The following conditions are risk factors:

Pituitary Gland

The pituitary is a small gland inside the head, behind the bridge of the nose. It plays a critical role in regulating growth, development, metabolism, and reproduction. The pituitary produces the following hormones:

Prolactin—controls formation of breast milk, influences the pituitary, and affects bone strength.

Growth hormone—regulates body growth, especially during adolescence.

Adrenocorticotropic hormone (ACTH)—stimulates the adrenal glands to produce cortisol.

Thyrotrophic-stimulating hormone (TSH)—stimulates the thyroid to produce thyroid hormone.

Luteinizing hormone (LH)—stimulates the ovaries or testes to produce sex hormones that determine many features of "maleness" or "femaleness".

Follicle-stimulating hormone—regulates fertility in women through ovulation and production of estrogen and progesterone, and in men through sperm formation and the production of testosterone.

- Acromegaly-causing tumors
- Cushing's syndrome tumors
- Hypothyroidism

Medications. Medications used for the following conditions are risk factors:
- Antinausea
- Gastroesophageal reflux disease (GERD)
- Hypertension
- Tranquilizers

What you can do: Prolactinoma is not caused by genetic factors. If you are taking any of the mentioned medications or have any of the listed medical conditions, be sure to follow your doctor's advice. For more information, type PITUITARY GLAND into an Internet search engine.

Cushing's Syndrome

Cushing's syndrome is a hormonal disorder caused by prolonged exposure of the body's tissues to high levels of the hormone cortisol. Relatively rare, it affects some 3,000 Americans annually. The following factors increase your risk of developing Cushing's syndrome.

Age. Those twenty to fifty years of age are most at risk.

Blood type. In blood type A, high levels of cortisol, a stress hormone, linked to heart attacks, lowered immunity, loss of muscle tissue; in blood type B, high cortisol levels are linked to Alzheimer's disease and senile dementia.

Family history. A family history of Cushing's disease is a risk factor for:
- Primary pigmented micronodular adrenal disease
- Multiple endocrine neoplasia (MEN) type I.

Medications. Use of glucocorticoid hormones for conditions such as asthma, rheumatoid arthritis, lupus, and other inflammatory diseases, or for immunosuppression after transplantation are risk factors.

Overproduction of cortisol by the body. This is caused by the following:
- Pituitary adenomas (Cushing's disease)—women have five times the risk for this rare disease. The average age at diagnosis is twenty-five to forty-five.
- Ectopic ACTH syndrome—usually caused by tumors elsewhere in the body, especially lung tumors. Men have three times the risk.
- Adrenal tumors—average age at onset of this rare tumor is forty. Women have four to five times the risk of men.

What you can do: Know your family history. Follow your doctor's advice if you are being treated with glucocorticoid hormones. For more information, type CUSHING'S SYNDROME into an Internet search engine.

Primary Hyperparathyroidism

Primary hyperparathyroidism involves the secretion

Adrenal Glands

The adrenal glands are located at the top of each kidney. They produce the following hormones:

Cortisol—helps to maintain blood pressure and cardiovascular functions; reduces the immune system's inflammatory response; balances the effects of insulin in breaking down sugar for energy; and regulates the metabolism of proteins, carbohydrates, and fats. One of cortisol's most important jobs is to help the body respond to stress. Women in their last trimester of pregnancy and highly trained athletes normally have high levels of cortisol. People suffering from depression, alcoholism, malnutrition, and panic disorders also have increased cortisol levels.

Aldosterone—regulates salt and water levels in the tissues; helps to regulate blood pressure and volume.

Androgens, primarily testosterone—needed for the development of the male reproductive system. They influence male characteristics, such as facial and chest hair, baldness, deepening of the voice, bone growth, and the thickening and strength of muscle fibers. Androgens also affect the kidneys, blood cells, skin pigmentation, and sweat and oil-producing glands.

Parathyroid Glands

The parathyroid glands are located behind the thyroid gland and produce parathyroid hormone (PTH).

Parathyroid hormone—helps to maintain a normal supply of calcium and phosphorus in the blood, bones, and urine. PTH regulates the release of calcium from bone, the absorption of calcium in the intestines, and the excretion of calcium in the urine.

Other Glands

Ovaries—produce estrogen and progesterone (see the section "The Ovaries" for more information).

Pancreas—produces insulin, glucagon, and somatostatin (see the section "The Pancreas" for more information).

Testicles—produce testosterone and androgen (see the section "The Testicles" for more information).

Thyroid—produces thyroid hormone (see "The Thyroid" for more information).

---

of too much parathyroid hormone. This leads to too much calcium in the blood, which in turn causes excess calcium in the urine, and results in kidney stones or kidney damage. Some 100,000 Americans are diagnosed each year. The following factors increase your risk of developing primary hyperparathyroidism:

Age. The risk increases with age. In women sixty or older, 2 in 1,000 will develop the condition.

Family history. Some 5 percent of patients have a family history of hyperparathyroidism. This is a risk factor for:

- Familial endocrine neoplasia type I
- Familial hypercalciuric hypercalcemia
- Multiple endocrine neoplasia type I

Gender. Women have twice the risk of men.

Medical conditions. The following conditions are risk factors:

- Tumor on one of the parathyroid glands
- Two or more enlarged parathyroid glands (hyperplasia)

What you can do: Know your family history and make sure to tell your family doctor or endocrinologist about risk factors. All women should be vigilant about having regular physicals including blood tests. For more information, type PRIMARY HYPERPARATHYROIDISM into an Internet search engine.

Risky Behavior and Possible Consequences	
RISKY BEHAVIOR	**POSSIBLE CONSEQUENCES**
Alcoholism in men	Low testosterone levels

Visit www.healthwatchguide.com for updates on the hormones.

NOTES

The Immune System

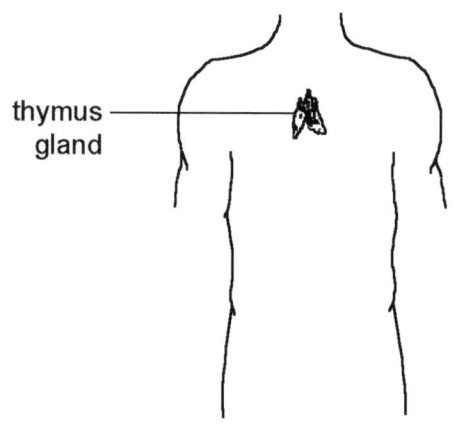
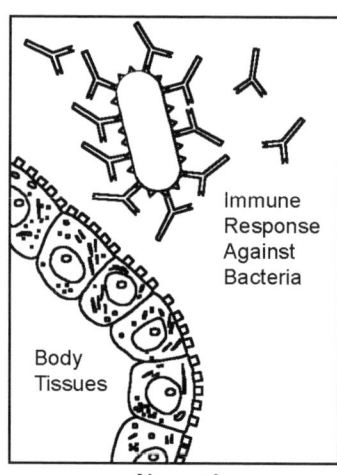
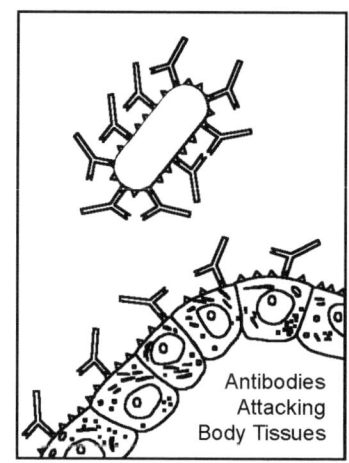

Normal | Autoimmune Disorder

Function

The immune system protects the body against attack by foreign substances (antigens), including bacteria, viruses, and fungi. The body has several innate barriers to try to prevent these antigens from gaining access to vulnerable organs. The skin (with its oils) acts as a very effective barrier, except when it is broken open by cuts, burns, and other wounds. The mucus in your nose and throat is a sticky substance that tries to trap antigens that are being inhaled or swallowed; the body then tries to expel the trapped antigens through sneezing or coughing. Tears protect the eyes. Stomach acid is another way the body tries to destroy antigens. Your tonsils, adenoids, thymus gland, spleen, lymph nodes, appendix, and bone marrow are other vital immune system components.

Specialized white blood cells that surround and kill foreign germs are critical to the immune system. The inflammation around a wound is an attempt of the body to protect itself by isolating germs and keeping them from spreading. Pus forms at the wound site when the white blood cells kill germs and then die themselves.

In addition to the generalized barriers with which we are born, the body occasionally needs to develop immune responses to specific antigens. This is called "acquired immunity," and it can be developed by the body itself through vaccination or after exposure to a particular virus, for instance, chicken pox. The next time you encounter the virus, your body will be able to mobilize these acquired defenses to protect you from infection. (See the immunization schedules in Part Two.)

Many immune system cells are produced by the thymus gland and the spleen and carried by lymph vessels to the lymph glands for storage until needed. (See "The Lymphatic System" for more information.)

Keeping the Immune System Healthy

- Exercise promotes blood circulation and a good supply of oxygen in the body.
- Eat a balanced diet.
- Minimize your exposure to illness, allergens, or other factors that can stress the immune system. Some situations just can't be avoided, but by eating right, getting enough exercise, sleep, and exposure to sunlight, as well as maintaining a sensible weight, you can keep the immune system healthy.
- Pregnant women can stimulate their babies' immune systems by eating yogurt for several days before delivery. The beneficial bacteria in yogurt are transferred to the fetus.

Be Aware! Food allergies are most frequently seen in children younger than three years of age. Most common are allergies to eggs, peanuts, and cow's milk. Adults are more commonly allergic to shellfish, tree nuts, and peanuts.

Beneficial Foods and Nutrients

See Part Four, The Importance of Nutrients, for a list

of foods containing the vitamins, minerals, and trace elements mentioned in this section.

Green Tea
Green tea is a good immune system booster for some people.

Vitamin A
Vitamin A helps to regulate the immune system.

Vitamin B_2 (Riboflavin)
Vitamin B_2 helps with antibody production.

Vitamin B_6
Vitamin B_6 helps strengthen the immune system and fight cancer.

Vitamin C
Vitamin C is an immune system booster.

Vitamin D
Vitamin D is important to the immune system.

Vitamin E
Vitamin E helps with antibody production.

Pantothenic Acid
Pantothenic acid helps with antibody production.

Calcium
Calcium is necessary for immune system health.

Copper
Copper helps destroy free radicals.

Iron
Iron is vital to immune system function.

Selenium
Selenium is necessary for immune system functions.

Zinc
Zinc supports a healthy immune system.

Other Tips
- Stimulate the growth of the thymus gland (which shrinks as we age) by tapping on the middle of your breastbone every morning for five minutes.
- Maintaining an indoor humidity of between 30 and 50 percent keeps your mucous membranes moist and able to act as a barrier against germs.
- Dairy products can increase production of mucus and inhibit breathing, especially in those who suffer from asthma.

What Can Go Wrong
Occasionally the immune system malfunctions and either overresponds or actually begins to attack its own body tissues. Sometimes the immune response is deficient.

Note: Periodontal disease, an inflammation of the gums, is caused by an immune deficiency. See "The Teeth" for more information.

Chronic Fatigue Syndrome
This syndrome may be due to inflammation caused by an inadequate immune system response. The following factors increase your risk of developing chronic fatigue syndrome.

Age. Most affected are individuals ages thirty to fifty.

Blood types. Types B and O have a higher risk; types A and AB have a moderate risk.

Family history. Having relatives who have or have had this condition increases your risk.

Gender. Women are affected more than men.

Medical conditions. Viral infections that depress the immune system are a risk factor.

What you can do: Know your risk factors. Treat viral infections promptly or make sure you get vaccinated against viruses, such as influenza. Keep your immune system healthy with a good diet, exercise, and adequate sleep. For more information, type CHRONIC FATIGUE SYNDROME into an Internet search engine.

AIDS (Acquired Immune Deficiency Syndrome)
AIDS is the fifth leading cause of death among people aged twenty-five to forty-five in the United States. The following factors increase your risk of developing AIDS.

Age. Any age is at risk, but most diagnoses are made in those in their twenties and thirties.

Blood types. All types have a moderate risk. Non-secretors of all types have a higher risk.

Gender. Men, especially homosexual and bisexual, have the greatest risk.

Medical conditions. Stress, which weakens the immune system, is a risk factor.

What you can do: AIDS is an almost completely avoidable disease. Donated blood is carefully screened to minimize the risk from transfusions. The most common risk factors are lifestyle choices (see the list of risky behaviors in the chart at the end of this section). Avoid exposure to the human immunodeficiency virus (HIV). For more information, type AIDS into an Internet search engine.

Autoimmune Diseases

The following is a list of autoimmune diseases, in which the immune system attacks its own organs, tissues, muscles, nervous system, and other body parts. Often, causes of autoimmune disorders are unknown, and much research is being done in this area. Unfortunately, there is not much that can be done to prevent the development of these conditions, except to be aware of risk factors and become familiar with symptoms.

Fibromyalgia

This illness causes generalized pain and tenderness in muscles, joints, and tendons. The following factors increase your risk of developing fibromyalgia.

Age. Most at risk are those ages twenty to fifty.

Blood types. Type O has a moderate risk; types A, B, and AB have a lower risk. Nonsecretors of all types have a higher risk.

Family history. This illness may run in families.

Gender. Women are more affected than men.

What you can do: Fibromyalgia is considered an autoimmune disorder in which, for no apparent reason, the body's immune system begins attacking itself. There is not much you can do to prevent this, but if you know it runs in your family, you can be alert to symptoms and seek treatment as early as possible. For more information, type FIBROMYALGIA into an Internet search engine.

Systemic Lupus Erythematosus

Systemic lupus erythematosus affects one in 2,000 people in America. The following conditions increase your risk of developing lupus.

Age. Lupus usually appears between ages ten and fifty.

Blood types. Type B has a moderate risk; types A, AB, and O have a lower risk. Nonsecretors of all types have a moderate-to-high risk.

Ethnicity/ancestry. Blacks, Asians, Hispanics, and Native Americans have the highest risks.

Family history. Ten percent of lupus patients have a close relative with the disease.

Gender. Women have nine times the risk of men.

Medications. Certain medications may cause drug-induced lupus erythematosus. The condition will end when medication is discontinued.

What you can do: Know your risk factors. Know your family history. For more information, type SYSTEMIC ERYTHEMATOSUS LUPUS into an Internet search engine.

Multiple Sclerosis (MS)

MS is an inflammation of tissue in the central nervous system, including the brain and the spinal cord. It affects 1 in 1,000 people. The following factors increase your risk of developing multiple sclerosis.

Age. Symptoms usually appear between ages fifteen and sixty.

Blood types. Types B and AB have a moderate-to-high risk; types A and O have a lower risk. Nonsecretors have a moderate-to-high risk. Rh-positive individuals have a moderate risk.

Ethnicity/ancestry. Whites have twice the risk of any other group. Ashkenazi Jews have a high risk.

Family history. This disease may have a genetic connection.

Gender. Women have twice the risk of men.

Geographic location. People living in northern Europe, northern United States, southern Australia, and New Zealand have a risk factor. Very high risk is associated with certain islands in Scotland.

What you can do: Know your family history. If the condition runs in your family or you live in one of the high-risk regions, become familiar with symptoms so that you can seek treatment as early as possible. For more information, type MULTIPLE SCLEROSIS into an Internet search engine.

Myasthenia Gravis

This neuromuscular disorder affects 3 in 10,000 people. The following factors increase your risk of developing myasthenia gravis.

Age. Two groups are at risk: teenagers and young people, and those over age forty.

Blood types. Type B has a moderate risk; types A, AB, and O have a lower risk. Nonsecretors have a moderate-to-high risk. Rh-negative individuals have a moderate risk.

Gender. Women have the highest risk at younger ages. Men have the higher risk at older ages.

Medical conditions. A tumor of the thymus gland places one at risk.

Rheumatoid Arthritis

Rheumatoid arthritis is a chronic inflammatory disease that most often affects the joints, but other parts of the body can be involved as well. It affects some 2 million Americans. The following conditions increase your risk of developing rheumatoid arthritis.

Age. The usual onset of the disease is between the ages of twenty-five and fifty-five, but it can occur at any age.

Gender. Women have two and a half times the risk of men.

Blood types. Type O has a moderate risk; types A, B, and AB have a lower risk. Nonsecretors of all types have a moderate-to-high risk.

Family history. Rheumatoid arthritis often runs in families.

What you can do: Know your risk factors. There is not much you can do to prevent this disease, but becoming familiar with the signs and symptoms can enable you to seek early treatment. For more information, type RHEUMATOID ARTHRITIS into an Internet search engine.

Sarcoidosis

This inflammation can affect various parts of the body. The cause is unknown. The following factors increase your risk of developing sarcoidosis:

Age. Most at risk are people aged thirty to fifty.

Blood types. Type A has a moderate-to-high risk for the most severe form of the disease. Types B, AB, and O have a low-to-moderate risk. Nonsecretors are moderate-to-high risk.

Ethnicity/ancestry. African, northern European, Japanese, and Irish are most at risk.

Family history. This condition may run in families.

Gender. Women have the greatest risk.

What you can do: Know your risk factors. If sarcoidosis runs in your family, be sure to tell your doctor. For more information, type SARCOIDOSIS into an Internet search engine.

Sjögren's Syndrome

This is a chronic condition characterized by insufficient moisture production. It affects 1 million Americans. The following conditions increase your risk of developing Sjögren's syndrome.

Age. Postmenopausal women are most at risk.

Blood types. Types A, B, AB, and O have a lower risk. Nonsecretors of any blood type have a moderate-to-high risk.

Gender. Ninety percent of those affected are women.

Medical conditions. The following conditions are risk factors:

- Lupus
- Rheumatoid arthritis
- Scleroderma
- Thyroid disease
- Vasculitis

What you can do: Know your risk factors. For more information, type SJÖGREN'S SYNDROME into an Internet search engine.

Immune System Disorders That Tend to Run in Families

These conditions have no known genetic links:

- Fibromyalgia
- Graves' disease (see "The Thyroid")
- Hashimoto's disease (see "The Thyroid")
- Multiple sclerosis
- Pernicious anemia (see "The Blood Supply")
- Rheumatoid arthritis
- Sarcoidosis
- Systemic lupus erythematosus

Medical Conditions That May Affect Immune System Health

It is important to properly treat any medical condition with which you are diagnosed, because the condition may affect other parts of your body. The body's organs and systems are inextricably connected to one another, so what goes wrong in one part may create problems in another. These conditions can affect immune health:

- *Diseases affecting the white blood cells*
- *Blood type A*—high cortisol levels are linked to lowered immunity.

- *Blood types B and O* are susceptible to slow-moving viruses and are at risk for problems with the immune system.
- *Nonsecretors of all blood types* are at greater risk of autoimmune diseases, including ankylosing spondylitis, reactive arthritis, Sjögren's syndrome, multiple sclerosis, Graves' disease, and fibromyalgia.
- *Family history of allergies*
- *Free radicals* (unstable oxygen molecules) in the body can damage immune system cells and render them useless.
- *Poor diet*
- *Stress*
- *Toxins in food and the environment*

Risky Behavior and Possible Consequences

RISKY BEHAVIOR	POSSIBLE CONSEQUENCES
Unprotected sex	AIDS
Anal sex	AIDS
Sex with someone known or suspected of having AIDS	AIDS
Sex with multiple partners	AIDS
Sex with someone who has multiple partners	AIDS
Sex with someone who injects drugs	AIDS
Sharing a needle with an infected person	AIDS
Contact with the blood of an infected person	AIDS
Becoming pregnant while HIV-positive	Having a baby born with AIDS
Breastfeeding while HIV-positive	Transmitting AIDS to the baby
Poor nutrition	Contributes to the number of free radicals
X-rays (have them when needed, but no more than necessary)	Contributes to the number of free radicals
Smoking	Contributes to the number of free radicals
Pollutants	Contributes to the number of free radicals

Visit www.healthwatchguide.com for updates on the immune system.

NOTES

The Intestines

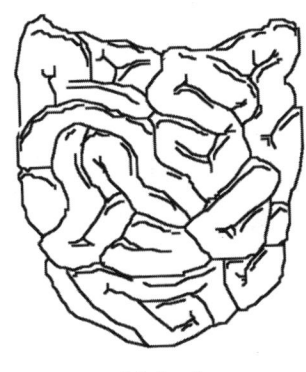

small intestine

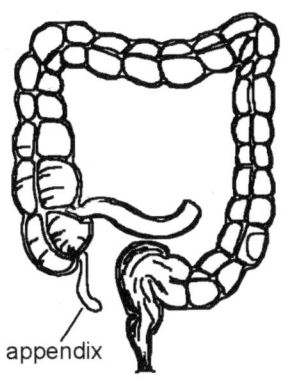

large intestine (colon)

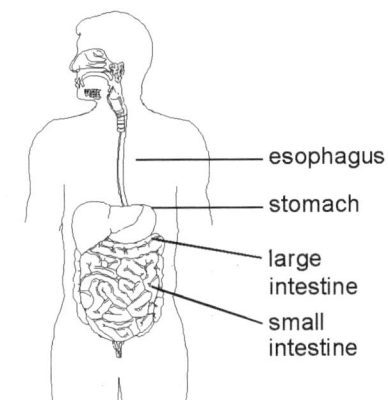

Function

The intestines comprise one part of the digestive tract, which handles the digestion of food. The digestive tract begins with the alimentary canal, which food enters via the mouth. Food passes from the alimentary canal into the stomach, and from there into the intestines, where muscular contractions propel it along. Digestive juices convert the food into materials that can be absorbed for the body to use, or into fecal matter for excretion.

Keeping the Intestines Healthy

- Drink plenty of water in addition to other fluids. Caffeine and alcohol tend to dry out your system.
- Eat foods high in fiber. Fiber is not absorbed by the intestines, which push it out along with other unwanted material in the intestines. Water keeps this material soft, so elimination is not uncomfortable.
- Exercise regularly—even light walking helps with regularity.
- Never ignore the need to have a bowel movement; try to schedule a regular time of day and give yourself enough time.

What You and Your Doctor Should Know

- Family or personal history of polyps, colon cancer, celiac disease (sprue), Crohn's disease, ulcers, and ulcerative colitis

Recommended Tests

For everyone over age fifty:

- Annually—fecal occult blood test, if recommended by your doctor
- Every ten years—colonoscopy for people of average risk *or* air-contrast barium enema with flexible sigmoidoscopy, if recommended by your doctor.

Note: This schedule should be modified for people at high risk of colorectal cancer. Make sure your doctor knows your risk factors.

Beneficial Foods and Nutrients

See Part Four, The Importance of Nutrients, for a list of foods containing the vitamins, minerals, and trace minerals mentioned in this section.

Green Tea

Green tea contains polyphenols, which may help to reduce the risk of colon cancer.

High-Fiber Foods

High-fiber foods should be a part of a healthy diet. They include acorn squash, apples, black-eyed peas, broccoli (raw), Brussels sprouts, cabbage, carrots (raw), cauliflower (raw), fava beans, kidney beans, lima beans, mushrooms, oat bran, peaches, raspberries, spinach, tangerines, wheat bran, and zucchini.

Peppermint

Peppermint oil (found in candies and mints) and peppermint tea help the digestive process and are used to reduce intestinal spasms and pain, but too much can contribute to GERD.

Other Food Supplements

- Hamburger cooked with one and a quarter teaspoon of garlic powder per pound has 90 percent

fewer pathogens than ground meat cooked without the spice. One tablespoon of prune puree per pound of ground meat will work almost as well, without changing the taste.
- A teaspoon of cinnamon stirred into a gallon of unpasteurized apple juice will kill almost 100 percent of any *E. coli* present.

Vitamin A
Vitamin A contributes to the health of intestinal mucous membranes that serve to fight off bacterial infection.

Vitamin B_1 (Thiamine)
Thiamine aids digestion.

Vitamin B_3 (Niacin)
Niacin is necessary for a healthy digestive system.

Zinc
Zinc assists with digestion.

Folic Acid (Folate)
Folic acid appears to be useful in lowering the risk of colon cancer (but may be harmful if taken by people who have advanced cancer, have pernicious anemia, or are taking medications for epilepsy).

Other Tips
- Take precautions when traveling to avoid developing diarrhea.
- Babies who are breastfed are less likely to suffer from diarrhea.
- Blood type O is at the greatest risk of contracting severe cases of cholera.
- Some studies have shown that a daily low-dose aspirin tablet may help to reduce the risk of colorectal cancer in susceptible individuals. See your doctor before taking any medications, however, because aspirin can irritate your stomach, cause ulcers, or thin your blood, which may not be good for you.
- There may be a connection between working at night and an increased risk of colorectal cancer in women. Bright light in dark hours disrupts melatonin production and increases estrogen levels, which appears to influence the risk.

When You Cook
- Thoroughly wash fruits and vegetables to remove bacteria, fertilizers, and pesticides.
- Rinse meat and poultry with cold water to remove surface contaminants.
- Cook meats, poultry, and fish thoroughly to kill any internal bacteria or parasites, such as tapeworms.
- Use meat thermometers.
- Use separate cutting boards and knives for fruits/vegetables and meat/poultry. Never let juices from uncooked meat, poultry, or fish come into contact with fruits and vegetables, or cooked meats, fish, and poultry. This includes preparations in which meats have been marinating.
- Don't put cooked foods on the same platter you used for the raw foods.
- When cleaning up after a meal, wipe cutting boards and countertops with a diluted bleach solution to kill germs.
- Take care not to let raw meat juices spill onto shelves or food in the refrigerator.
- Keep cold foods cold and hot foods hot—bacteria grow rapidly in a very short amount of time. Put the leftovers away first if you like to linger at the table and talk. Don't eat anything (for instance, at a picnic) that has been sitting at room temperature—potato chips excepted! Mayonnaise is a prime breeding ground for bacteria. Store-bought mayonnaise is more acidic than homemade, however, and *slightly* less risky for salmonella.
- Divide large amounts of hot foods into small storage containers and refrigerate. They will cool faster, and then you can safely freeze them.
- Thaw frozen food in a microwave oven, in the refrigerator, or under cold running water, NOT on the counter.

What Can Go Wrong

Celiac Disease (Sprue)
Sprue is thought to be an immune system response to certain proteins, such as glutens, that causes damage to the lining of the intestine. It may affect as many as 1 in 150 people. Celiac disease predisposes patients to the eventual development of lymphoma (see "The Lymphatic System"). The following factors increase your risk of developing celiac disease.

Age. Sprue usually appears in babies shortly after wheat products are introduced into the diet.

Blood types. Types A, B, AB, and O have a moderate risk. Nonsecretors of all types have a higher risk.

Ethnicity/ancestry. Whites of northern and southern European ancestry have the highest risk. It is very common in Italy, where all children are screened for celiac disease by age six.

Family history. Sprue runs in families.

Gender. Women account for some 70 percent of cases.

What you can do: Know your family history. Treatment can make a big difference. If you are expecting a baby and the condition runs in your family, talk to your doctor about signs and symptoms. For more information, type CELIAC DISEASE into an Internet search engine.

Colon Cancer

Colon cancer is the second leading cause of cancer deaths in the United States. Some 150,000 new cases are diagnosed annually in the United States. The following factors increase your risk of developing colorectal cancer.

Age. Colon cancer is most common in people over the age of fifty but can occur at any age.

Blood types. Types A and AB have a higher risk. Type A individuals with a history of thyroid cancer may have a very high risk of developing colon cancer. Types B and O have a moderate risk.

Cancer history. Women who have had ovarian or uterine cancer are at greater risk of developing colorectal cancer. Also, those who have had colorectal cancer once can develop it a second time.

Ethnicity/ancestry. In descending order of risk: Alaska Natives, Japanese, blacks, non-Hispanic whites, Chinese, Hawaiians, white Hispanics, Filipinos, Koreans, Vietnamese, and Native Americans. Some 6 percent of Ashkenazi Jews have a genetic alteration doubling their risk.

Family history. Your risk increases if you have:
- Family members with juvenile polyposis
- Family members with hyperplastic polyposis
- Parents, siblings, or children who have had colorectal cancer

Medical conditions. These conditions increase risk:
- Colon adenomas
- Crohn's disease
- Gardner's syndrome (familial adenomatous polyposis)
- Polyps—some types increase the chances of developing cancer
- Ulcerative colitis.

What you can do: Know your family history! Make sure your doctor knows your family history! Your doctor may recommend early intervention treatments if you are at high risk. Have regular colon screenings appropriate for your age and risk factors. For instance, have a colonoscopy every five years if a first-degree relative (parent or sibling) has or had colon cancer. Begin to screen at an age ten years younger that the age of the relative when their cancer was diagnosed. Don't let squeamishness prevent you from doing this; the tests are not that uncomfortable and may save your life. (See "Colon Cancer Screenings" in Part Two) Minimize or eliminate your controllable risk factors. For more information type COLON CANCER into an Internet search engine.

Colon Polyps

Colon polyps are growths that jut out from the wall of the colon. They are often benign, but those larger than one centimeter have an increased risk of malignancy. The following factors increase your risk of developing polyps in the colon.

Age. The risk increases with age.

Family history. Having a parent or sibling with:
- Colon cancer (greatly increases your risk of polyps)
- Inflammatory bowel disease (increases your risk of polyps)
- Polyps (puts you at risk of polyps)

Blood types. Types A and AB have a higher risk; types B and O have a moderate risk.

Genetic links. These conditions are risk factors:
- Gardner's syndrome (familial adenomatous polyposis)
- Juvenile polyposis
- Peutz-Jeghers syndrome

Medical conditions. Acromegaly increases the risk of malignancy.

Environment. Living in industrialized societies increases risk. This is perhaps connected with less exercise and high-fat, low-fiber diets.

What you can do: Know your risk factors and

your family history. Have the necessary screenings, perhaps at an earlier age. Early detection can give your doctor a chance to remove the polyps before they become malignant. Eat a diet low in fat and high in fiber. Minimize your controllable risks. For more information, type COLON POLYPS into an Internet search engine.

Crohn's Disease

Crohn's disease, a chronic inflammation anywhere along the digestive tract, affects about 1 person in 15,000. The following factors increase your risk of developing Crohn's disease.

Age. This is most common in young adults.

Blood types. Type O has a higher risk. Types A, B, and AB have a moderate risk, but often develop inflammatory bowel conditions when under stress.

Ethnicity/ancestry. Being Jewish increases the risk.

Family history. About 20 percent of patients have a close relative with some form of inflammatory bowel disease. If both parents have an inflammatory bowel disease, you have a 50 percent chance of developing Crohn's disease or colitis.

Geography. This disease is most common in people living in northern climates.

What you can do: Know your family history. Treatment is available. For more information, type CROHN'S DISEASE into an Internet search engine.

Duodenal Ulcer

A duodenal ulcer is an erosion in the lining of the duodenum, the part of the small intestine that connects to the stomach. The following factors increase your risk of developing duodenal ulcers.

Gender. Men have the greater risk.

Blood types. Types A, B, and AB have a moderate risk; type O has a higher risk. Nonsecretors of all types have a higher risk.

Family history. Duodenal ulcers tend to run in the family.

Medical conditions. Poor nutrition and *H. pylori* infections are risk factors.

Medications. Excessive use of NSAIDs (nonsteroidal anti-inflammatory drugs) and aspirin increase risk.

Professions. Nurses and gastroenterologists are at high risk of *H. pylori* infection.

What you can do: If you have risk factors, minimize your use of NSAIDs and aspirin. Don't smoke. Treat any *H. pylori* infection you may have. For more information, type DUODENAL ULCER into an Internet search engine.

Ulcerative Colitis

Ulcerative colitis is an inflammation of the lining of the large intestine (colon) and rectum. It affects about 1 person in 10,000. The following factors increase your risk of developing ulcerative colitis.

Age. Most patients are between the ages of fifteen and thirty, or between fifty and seventy.

Blood types. Type O has a high risk of colitis and for the form that includes bleeding with elimination. Types A, B, and AB are moderate risk and develop more of a mucous colitis, which is not as bloody.

Ethnicity/ancestry. Jews of European descent are five times more likely to develop colitis or Crohn's disease.

Environmental factors. This disease occurs most often in people living in cities and industrial nations.

Family history. About 15 to 20 percent of patients have a close relative with the disease.

What you can do: Know your risk factors. Ulcerative colitis increases the risk of colon cancer, so make sure to get prompt treatment for the condition. For more information, type ULCERATIVE COLITIS into an Internet search engine.

Intestinal Conditions That Tend to Run in Families

There are no known genetic links for:
- Celiac disease (sprue)
- Colorectal cancer
- Colorectal polyps
- Crohn's disease
- Lactose intolerance
- Ulcerative colitis

PART FIVE • DISEASE PREVENTION GUIDE

Risky Behavior and Possible Consequences

RISKY BEHAVIOR	POSSIBLE CONSEQUENCES
Careless food handling	Food poisoning (salmonella infection)
Diets high in fat and calories, low in fiber	Colorectal cancer, polyps
Inadequate fiber and fluid intake	Constipation Diverticulosis (pouches on the intestinal lining)
Sedentary lifestyle	Constipation
Laxative overuse	Laxative dependency and damage to the intestines
Eating contaminated food	Diarrhea, cholera, shigella, typhoid fever, amebiasis
Drinking contaminated water	Diarrhea, cholera, shigella, typhoid fever, amebiasis
Persistent or intense pressure on the abdomen	Hiatal hernia

RISKY BEHAVIOR	POSSIBLE CONSEQUENCES
High-stress lifestyle	Irritable bowel syndrome
Smoking	Colorectal polyps
Alcohol use	Increases the risk of developing polyps
Rectal intercourse with a man infected with *E. hystolica* (an amoebic parasite)	Amebiasis (a parasitic disease)
Direct contact with soil containing human feces	Hookworm
Failure to wash hands after using the toilet or changing diapers, especially in day care centers	Parasitic infection

Visit www.healthwatchguide.com for updates on the intestines.

NOTES

The Joints

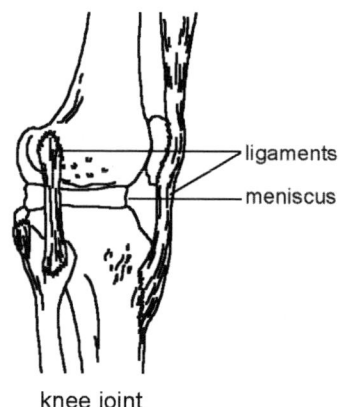
knee joint

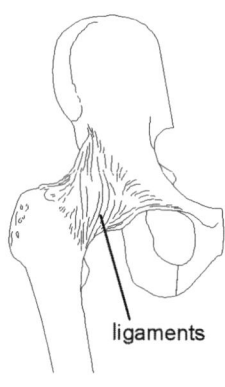
hip joint

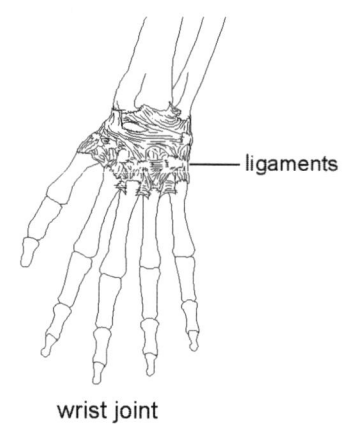
wrist joint

Function

Joints are the points of contact between two parts of the skeleton. Tendons, ligaments, or membranes may connect the bones. Joint flexibility is important for ease of movement in places such as the knee, shoulder, elbow, and wrist.

Keeping the Joints Healthy

- Maintain a healthful weight. Obesity puts additional strain on the spine and knees and increases the risk of developing osteoarthritis, as well as other joint diseases.
- Exercise strengthens the joints.
- Avoid tennis elbow by minimizing repetitive arm, elbow, and wrist movements.

What You and Your Doctor Should Know

- Family or personal history of arthritis

Beneficial Foods and Nutrients

See Part Four, The Importance of Nutrients, for a list of foods containing zinc.

Citrus Fruits

Citrus fruits, such as grapefruit, lemons, limes, oranges, and tangerines, may help to reduce the risk of rheumatoid arthritis.

Zinc

Zinc may help to reduce the risk of rheumatoid arthritis.

What Can Go Wrong

Benign Hypermobility Joint Syndrome (BHJS)

BHJS is joint looseness often associated with day or nighttime pain, or discomfort after exercising. The following factors increase your risk of developing BHJS.

Age. Children and young adults are at risk.

Ethnicity/ancestry. Asians are the most affected, followed by whites.

Family history. A family history of BHJS places one at risk.

Gender. Girls are more at risk than boys.

Personal history. These conditions place one at risk:
- Congenital hip dislocations
- Frequent sprains of the wrist or ankle
- Scoliosis (curvature of the spine)
- Shoulder, elbow, or kneecap dislocations

Medical conditions. The following conditions place one at risk:
- Cleidocranial dysostosis
- Down syndrome
- Ehlers-Danlos syndrome
- Marfan's syndrome
- Morquio's syndrome

What you can do: Know your family history. There is an increased risk of joint dislocation with this condition, so precautions may be necessary. For more information, type HYPERMOBILE JOINTS into an Internet search engine.

Gout

Gout is caused by uric acid deposits in the joints, causing painful arthritis. It is found in 1 in 200 people and usually affects the legs and feet. The following factors increase your risk of developing gout.

Age. Any age can be affected.

Family history. Gout often runs in families.

Gender. Men are primarily affected. Women are at risk primarily postmenopause.

Medical conditions. The following conditions place one at risk:
- Diabetes
- Hypertension
- Kidney disease
- Sickle-cell anemia

Personal history. Recurrent attacks are common.

What you can do: Know your risk factors and tell your doctor if the condition runs in your family, especially if you have any of the medical conditions listed above. For more information, type GOUT into an Internet search engine.

Osteoarthritis

Osteoarthritis is a degenerative joint disease that usually affects hips, knees, spine, the joints of the fingers, the base of the thumb, and the base of the big toe. Some 70 million Americans have a form of arthritis. The following factors increase your risk of developing osteoarthritis.

Age. Most humans show some signs of arthritis in their joints by age forty.

Blood types. Types A and AB have a moderate-to-high risk; types B and O have a low-to-moderate risk.

Ethnicity/ancestry. In descending order of risk: blacks, whites, Hispanics, Asians, and Pacific Islanders.

Family history. Heredity is a factor in osteoarthritis.

Gender. Risks are equal before age fifty-five. Women have a greater risk than men after age fifty-five.

Medical conditions. The following conditions place one at risk:
- Being double-jointed
- Scoliosis (curvature of the spine)

Personal history. Joint injury and overuse places one at risk.

What you can do: Know your risk factors. Exercise regularly to maintain joint flexibility; use stretches. Keep your weight down—the more you weigh, the more pressure you put on your joints, especially the knees. For more information, type OSTEOARTHRITIS into an Internet search engine.

Psoriatic Arthritis (PA)

This form of arthritis develops in association with psoriasis. The following factors increase your risk of developing psoriatic arthritis.

Age. Most at risk are those ages thirty to fifty.

Family history. About 40 percent of sufferers have a family history of skin or joint disease. Having a parent with PA increases your risk.

Gender. Men and women are equally affected.

Medical conditions. Approximately 5 percent of psoriasis patients will develop psoriatic arthritis.

What you can do: If you have psoriasis, be aware of the risk of developing arthritis. Become familiar with the symptoms and seek treatment promptly. For more information, type PSORIATIC ARTHRITIS into an Internet search engine.

Rheumatoid Arthritis

Rheumatoid arthritis is a chronic inflammatory disease that most often affects the joints, but other parts of the body can be involved as well. This disease affects some 2 million Americans. The following factors increase your risk of developing rheumatoid arthritis.

Age. The usual onset of the disease is between ages twenty-five and fifty-five, but it can occur at any age.

Blood types. Type O has a moderate risk; types A, B, and AB have a lower risk. Nonsecretors of all types have a moderate-to-high risk.

Family history. Rheumatoid arthritis often runs in families.

Gender. Women have two and a half times the risk of men.

What you can do: Know your risk factors. There is not much you can do to prevent this disease, but becoming familiar with the signs and symptoms can enable you to seek early treatment. For more information, type RHEUMATOID ARTHRITIS into an Internet search engine.

Joint Conditions That Tend to Run in Families

There are no known genetic links for these conditions:

- Arthritis
- Benign hypermobility joint syndrome
- Juvenile rheumatoid arthritis
- Osteoarthritis
- Psoriatic arthritis
- Rheumatoid arthritis

Medical Conditions That Can Affect the Joints

It is important to properly treat any medical condition with which you are diagnosed, because the condition may affect other parts of your body. The body's organs and systems are inextricably connected to one another, so what goes wrong in one part may create problems in another. Conditions that can affect the joints are:

- *Inflammations of the digestive system*
- *Osteoarthritis, kidney disease, and thyroid conditions,* which increase the risk of pseudogout, an inflammation of the knee or wrist.

Risky Behavior and Possible Consequences

RISKY BEHAVIOR	POSSIBLE CONSEQUENCES
Obesity	Osteoarthritis, gout
Popping or cracking fingers	May aggravate BHJS or lead to arthritis
Excessive use of alcohol	Gout
A diet high in fat	Rheumatoid arthritis

Visit www.healthwatchguide.com for updates on the joints.

NOTES

The Kidneys

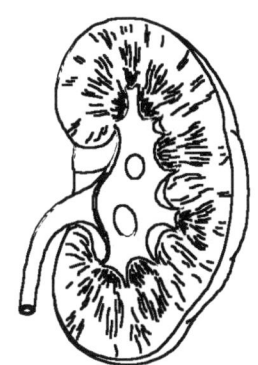
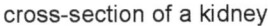
cross-section of a kidney

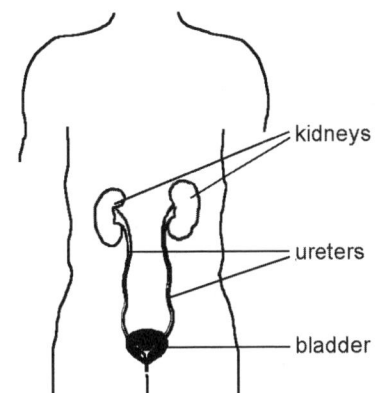

Function

Kidneys are vital to the optimum functioning of the body. Almost everyone is born with two, but amazingly enough, the work they do—filtering the blood, regulating blood pressure, maintaining the body's normal chemical levels, balancing the body's water supply, and excreting wastes, excess salt, and fluids—can all be handled by only one kidney if necessary. Kidneys filter some 500 gallons of blood per day, generating approximately one to two quarts of urine. Ridding the body of harmful metabolic products is crucial to good health. The kidneys also help to regulate blood pressure. When the kidneys fail to work properly, poisons begin to accumulate in the bloodstream.

Keeping Your Kidneys Healthy

- Drink six to eight 8-ounce glasses of water daily (in addition to any other beverages you consume). This keeps your kidneys flushed out and prevents toxins from building up.
- Urinate when you feel the urge. Holding back can encourage bacteria buildup.

Beneficial Foods and Nutrients

See Part Four, The Importance of Nutrients, for a list of foods containing the vitamins and minerals mentioned in this section.

Diuretic Foods

Diuretic foods are those that encourage water loss, such as asparagus, watercress, cranberries, peaches, nectarines, potatoes, celery, and cucumbers.

Cranberry Juice

Cranberry juice helps keep the kidneys healthy.

Vitamin D

Vitamin D is vital for kidney health.

Choline

Choline is necessary for properly functioning kidneys.

Phosphorus

Phosphorus helps with kidney function.

Other Tips

Exercise to encourage calcium absorption in the bones, instead of in the kidneys.

What Can Go Wrong

Atheroembolic Renal Disease

Atheroembolic renal disease causes blood clots that form in the kidney artery and/or narrowing of kidney blood vessels. It affects 1 person in 2,500 annually. The following factors increase your risk of developing atheroembolic renal disease.

Age. At risk are those age sixty and up.

Family and/or personal history. The following conditions are risk factors:

- Cerebrovascular disease
- Coronary artery disease
- Diabetes mellitus
- Heart disease
- High blood pressure
- Peripheral vascular disease

Gender. Men have the greater risk.

Medical conditions. Having the following conditions or procedures increases your risk:
- Aortic surgery
- Aortography
- Arteriography
- Blood clots elsewhere in the body
- Treatment for blood clots

What you can do: Minimize your controllable risk factors, such as smoking, obesity, high blood pressure, high cholesterol levels. Follow your treatment program for diabetes and heart disease. For more information, type ATHEROEMBOLIC RENAL DISEASE into an Internet search engine.

Kidney Cancer (Renal Cell Carcinoma)

About 31,000 cases of kidney cancer are diagnosed annually in the United States. The following factors increase your risk of developing kidney cancer.

Age. People aged fifty to seventy are at risk.

Ethnicity/ancestry. In descending order of risk: blacks, Hispanics, and whites.

Family history. These conditions are risk factors:
- Hereditary papillary renal cell carcinoma
- Hereditary renal oncocytoma
- Von Hippel-Lindau disease—an inherited condition

Gender. Men have twice the risk of women.

Medical conditions. The following conditions are risk factors:
- Chronic kidney failure that requires long-term use of dialysis
- Wilms' tumor

Personal history. The following place one at risk:
- Extended use of the painkiller phenacetin
- Radiation therapy for uterine disorders

Workplace. These conditions increase risk:
- Working with coke ovens in steel plants
- Exposure to asbestos

What you can do: Know your personal risks. Minimize your controllable risks, especially smoking and diet. For information on symptoms, type KIDNEY CANCER into an Internet search engine.

Kidney Stones (Nephrolithiasis)

Kidney stones are hardened formations of urine/calcium in the kidneys. Some 600,000 cases are diagnosed annually. The following factors increase your risk of developing kidney stones.

Age. Kidney stones are most likely between the ages of twenty and forty.

Blood types. Types A, B, and AB have a higher risk. Type O has a moderate risk.

Ethnicity/ancestry. Whites have a greater risk than blacks for kidney stones.

Family history. The risk of kidney stones is inherited.

Gender. Men are at greater risk of kidney stones, but the number of women getting kidney stones is increasing.

Medical conditions. The following conditions are risk factors:
- Chronic inflammation of the bowel
- Cystic kidney disease
- Cystinuria—an inherited disease
- Excess vitamin D
- Gout
- Hypercalciuria—an inherited disease
- Hyperoxaluria—an inherited disease
- Hyperparathyroidism
- Hyperuricosuria
- Renal tubular acidosis—an inherited disease
- Urinary tract blockage
- Urinary tract infections

Medications. The use of indinavir is a risk factor.

Personal history. The following place one at risk:
- Ostomy surgery
- Previous kidney stone

What you can do: Know your personal risks. Minimize your controllable risks. Maximize the amount of fluids you drink each day. Be aware of the amount of calcium you take in the form of supplements. For more information, type KIDNEY STONES into an Internet search engine.

Membranous Nephropathy

This inflammation of the inner structure of the kidney affects 1 in 5,000 people annually. In 70 to 90 percent of patients, some form of irreversible kidney damage develops within two to twenty years. The following factors increase your risk of developing membranous nephropathy.

Age. This disease usually affects people who are over age forty.

Environment. Exposure to the mineral mercury increases risk.

Gender. Both men and women are at risk.

Medical conditions. The following conditions are risk factors:
- Malaria
- Malignant "solid" tumors
- Non-Hodgkin's lymphoma
- Systemic lupus erythematosus

Medications. Use of the following medications increases risk:
- Penicillamine
- Trimethadione

What you can do: Avoid exposure to diseases and substances that can lead to this condition. If you develop a medical condition that increases your risk, be sure to follow your doctor's treatment advice. For more information, type MEMBRANOUS NEPHROPATHY into an Internet search engine.

Kidney Conditions That Tend to Run in Families

There are no known genetic links for these conditions:
- Berger's disease
- Goodpasture's syndrome
- Lupus nephritis
- Nephrolithiasis (kidney stones)
- Wilms' tumor

Medical Conditions That Can Affect Kidney Health

It is important to properly treat any medical condition with which you are diagnosed, because the condition may affect other parts of your body. The body's organs and systems are inextricably connected to one another, so what goes wrong in one part may create problems in another.

Kidney Failure

Risk factors are:
- *Chronic kidney infections*
- *Chronic kidney stones*
- *Churg-Strauss vasculitis*
- *Diabetes,* both type I and type II
- *E. Coli infection*
- *High blood pressure*—blacks ages twenty-five to forty-nine are twenty times more likely than whites to develop hypertension-related kidney failure.
- Others at risk for this condition are Native Americans, Hispanics, Pacific Islanders, older people, and those with a family history of hypertension-related kidney failure.
- *Polycystic kidney disease*—an inherited condition
- *Sickle-cell disease*
- *Scleroderma*
- *Use of medications that cause kidney toxicity*

Note: Pregnant women with a history of kidney disease have an increased risk of preeclampsia.

Risky Behavior and Possible Consequences	
RISKY BEHAVIOR	**POSSIBLE CONSEQUENCES**
Sedentary lifestyle	Kidney stones
High-fat, low-fiber diet	Kidney stones, atheroembolic renal disease
Using antacids with calcium	Kidney stones (Note: calcium-rich foods are okay, but too many calcium supplements cause calcium to accumulate in the kidneys)
Smoking	Kidney cancer, atheroembolic renal disease (smokers have twice the risk of nonsmokers)
Obesity	Kidney cancer, atheroembolic renal disease, kidney failure
Hypertension	Kidney cancer, atheroembolic renal disease
Diets high in oxalates (nuts, tea, chocolate, beets, rhubarb, strawberries, wheat bran, coffee, cola, spinach)	Kidney stones
Excessive consumption of phosphate-based soft drinks	Kidney stones
High cholesterol levels	Atheroembolic renal disease
Infection with syphilis	Membranous nephropathy
Infection with hepatitis B	Membranous nephropathy
Heavy use (more than 3 pills daily) of acetaminophen for prolonged periods of time	Kidney damage

Visit www.healthwatchguide.com for updates on the kidneys.

NOTES

The Liver

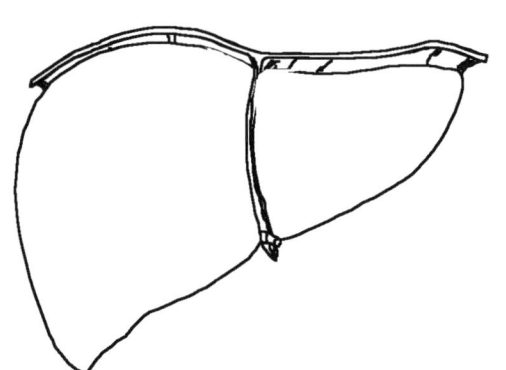
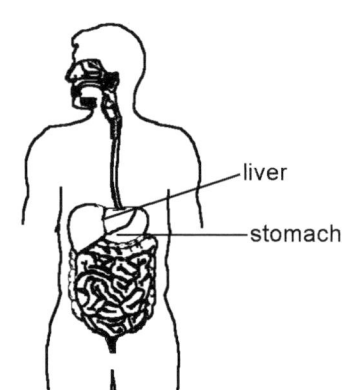

Function

The liver is the body's largest gland, weighing about three pounds. It is located in the upper side of the abdomen, mostly under the lower ribs. The liver converts food into energy, filters toxins and alcohol from the blood and converts them into substances that can be excreted from the body, processes medications and drugs so that the body can effectively use them, and manufactures vital chemicals needed by the body. It produces clotting factors, bile, and blood proteins, metabolizes cholesterol, maintains normal blood sugar concentrations, regulates several hormones, and produces more than a thousand enzymes. The liver is still being studied and researchers don't know all of its functions yet, but clearly the liver is one of the body's most important organs.

Keeping the Liver Healthy

- Limit alcohol consumption to no more than two drinks per day.
- Avoid taking unnecessary medications, especially acetaminophens
- Exercise caution when mixing alcohol and medication
- Avoid exposure to industrial chemicals
- Get vaccinated against hepatitis B (see the immunization schedule in Part Two).
- Tapeworms found in foxes and coyotes can infect

the liver. Dogs and cats that catch and eat rodents can also be infected by the tapeworm, which can then be transmitted to their human owners. This tapeworm is found worldwide. The transmission rate is low, but safeguard yourself and your family by taking the following steps:

- Never eat fruits and vegetables picked directly from the ground (where they may have come into contact with feces). Always wash foods thoroughly before eating.
- Don't touch any wild animals with your bare hands.
- Try to keep your pets from catching or eating rodents, especially in areas where there are fox and coyote populations. Talk to your veterinarian about treatments for suspected infections.
- Always wash your hands after petting or playing with your pets.

Beneficial Foods and Nutrients

See Part Four, The Importance of Nutrients, for a list of foods containing the vitamins, minerals, and trace elements mentioned in this section.

Artichokes
Artichokes help the liver process chemicals and hormones more efficiently, and they can help the liver regenerate cells and repair itself.

Radishes
Radishes stimulate the secretion of liver bile, aiding the digestive process.

Vitamin B_2
Vitamin B_2 promotes the metabolism of lipids, tryptophan, proteins, fats, and carbohydrates.

Vitamin C
Vitamin C activates liver detoxification systems.

Vitamin E
Vitamin E can help stop neurological problems associated with liver disease early in their progression.

Choline
Choline helps transport fats from the liver.

Pantothenic Acid
Pantothenic acid synthesizes fat and cholesterol.

Chromium
Chromium is important for cholesterol synthesis.

Manganese
Manganese assists with liver functions.

Copper
Copper helps with cholesterol metabolism.

Other Tips

- Pregnant women should be sure they are vaccinated against hepatitis B and C.
- The Food and Drug Administration has advised of a possible link between kava kava use and liver failure.

What Can Go Wrong

Hepatitis

Hepatitis is a viral inflammation of the liver. There are several forms of the hepatitis virus, the most infectious of which are A, B, and C. Hepatitis D is a defective viral form that affects only those infected with hepatitis B. These are dangerous, but largely preventable, infections. Autoimmune hepatitis is sometimes seen with other autoimmune disorders. Drug-induced hepatitis may occur when people who drink alcohol take medications containing acetaminophen (such as Tylenol).

The following factors increase your risk of developing hepatitis A.

Environment. These environments increase risk:
- Nursing homes
- Day-care centers

Exposure. Exposure factors include:
- Exposure to a family member with hepatitis A
- Travel and immigration to or from certain at-risk countries

What you can do: Hepatitis A is such a preventable disease, but 100,000 cases are diagnosed annually. The virus is primarily spread through the feces, but blood and other bodily fluids also carry the virus. A vaccination is available for those at risk of infection, but normal precautions with food and hygiene also offer effective safeguards. Men who have sex with men and people who inject drugs have a high risk of infection, as do travelers to certain countries in Asia and South and Central America. Fortunately, hepatitis A is rarely fatal although there is no specific treatment. For more information, type HEPATITIS A into an Internet search engine.

The following factors increase your risk of developing hepatitis B.

Blood types. Type AB has a higher risk, type B has a moderate-to-high risk, and types A and O have a moderate risk.

Exposure. Exposure to a family member with hepatitis B is a risk factor.

Workplace. Any occupation that exposes you to blood, such as healthcare worker or athletic trainer, is a risk factor.

What you can do: See the list of risky behaviors in the chart at the end of this section for the best ways to avoid exposure to the hepatitis B virus. Infants now are routinely vaccinated against hepatitis B because infection by the virus leads to such dire consequences—90 percent of newborns infected with the virus develop chronic hepatitis B, as do 50 percent of children. For more information, type HEPATITIS B into an Internet search engine.

The following factors increase your risk of developing hepatitis C.

Workplace. Any occupation, such as in healthcare, that exposes workers to blood or blood products is a risk factor.

Medical treatment. These medical treatments increase risk:
- Long-term kidney dialysis
- Blood transfusion before 1992. Donated blood now is routinely screened for hepatitis.

Blood types. Type AB has a higher risk, type B has a moderate-to-high risk, types A and O have a moderate risk.

What you can do: Hepatitis C is a huge problem in the United States—approximately 1 in 70 to 100 people are infected. However, it is largely preventable. Take sensible precautions to avoid exposure to blood. See the list of risky behaviors in the chart at the end of this section for controllable lifestyle risks. Hepatitis C is one of the leading causes of chronic liver disease and is the number-one reason for liver transplants in the United States. For more information, type HEPATITIS C into an Internet search engine.

Liver Cancer (Hepatocellular Carcinoma)

Liver cancer occurs in 1 person in 2,500. The following factors increase the risk of developing liver cancer.

Age. The usual age at diagnosis is between fifty and sixty.

Blood types. Types A and AB have a higher risk; types B and O have a moderate risk.

Ethnicity/ancestry. The risk appears to be affected more by geography than ethnicity. Liver cancer is found more often in Africa and Asia than in the Americas and Europe.

Gender. Men have a greater risk than women.

Medical conditions. The following conditions place one at risk:
- Hemochromatosis
- Liver disease
- Viral hepatitis, particularly hepatitis B and C

What you can do: Many cases of liver cancer are preventable through the use of vaccinations against hepatitis B and by avoiding exposure to other forms of hepatitis. Never share needles, avoid using steroids, don't drink water contaminated by arsenic, and practice safe sex. For more information, type LIVER CANCER into an Internet search engine.

Sarcoidosis

Sarcoidosis is an inflammation that can affect the liver. The cause of this illness is unknown. The following factors increase your risk of developing sarcoidosis.

Age. Those between thirty and fifty years old are most at risk.

Blood types. Type A has a moderate-to-high risk for the most severe form of the disease. Types B, AB, and O have a low to moderate risk. Nonsecretors have a moderate-to-high risk.

Ethnicity/ancestry. Most at risk are those of African, northern European, Japanese, and Irish decent.

Family history. This illness may run in families.

Gender. Women have the greatest risk.

What you can do: Know your risk factors. If sarcoidosis runs in your family, be sure to tell your doctor. For more information, type SARCOIDOSIS into an Internet search engine.

Sclerosing Cholangitis

This is an autoimmune disease of the bile ducts. The following factors increase the risk of developing sclerosing cholangitis.

Age. Onset is usually between the ages of thirty-five and forty.

Blood types. Types A, B, and AB have a moderate-to-high risk; type O has a low-to-moderate risk. Nonsecretors of all types have a moderate-to-high risk.

Family history. This disease may have a genetic link.

Gender. Sclerosing cholangitis is more common in men.

Medical conditions. These conditions place one at risk:
- Inflammatory bowel disease
- An infection of the bile ducts

Bile Duct Cancer (Cholangiocarcinoma)

Risk factors for this rare cancer include:
- Choledochal cysts
- Chronic biliary irritation
- Being over age sixty-five
- Primary sclerosing cholangitis

Primary Biliary Cirrhosis

Risk factors for this rare disease include:
- Chronic bile obstruction
- Hypothyroidism
- Being a middle-aged woman
- Raynaud's syndrome

Medical Conditions That Can Affect Liver Health

It is important to properly treat any medical condition with which you are diagnosed, because the condition may affect other parts of your body. The body's organs and systems are inextricably connected to one another, so what goes wrong in one part may create problems in another.

- *Hereditary hemochromatosis* is a genetic disease that affects approximately 1 in 200 Americans of northern European descent, especially those of Scandinavian, English, Irish, Scottish, and Welsh ancestry. People with this disease absorb iron too efficiently and can rapidly build up too much iron in various organs, which leads to cirrhosis of the liver or heart failure. A simple blood test can tell if you are at risk of hemochromatosis.

- *Sub-Saharan African hemochromatosis* appears to result from a high iron intake along with an as-yet-unidentified genetic factor. Although it is seen primarily in South Africa where iron cooking pots are used, African Americans who are diagnosed with iron overload may have inherited the genetic mutation.

- *Wilson's disease* is a rare hereditary condition in which too much copper is stored in the liver.

Risky Behavior and Possible Consequences	
RISKY BEHAVIOR	**POSSIBLE CONSEQUENCES**
Consuming food or water contaminated with human excrement	Hepatitis A
Anal sex	Hepatitis A
Injecting drugs by needle	Hepatitis A
Injecting drugs by needle while infected with hepatitis B	Hepatitis D
Excessive consumption of alcohol	Cirrhosis of the liver
Becoming pregnant while infected with hepatitis B	Passing the infection to the unborn baby Baby is born with neonatal hepatitis
Exposure to the Indian Ocean	Contracting the virus that causes hepatitis E
Traveling to infected areas without being vaccinated	Hepatitis A
Obesity	Fatty liver
Chronic hepatitis B	Cirrhosis of the liver, liver cancer
IV drug use	Hepatitis B and C
Unprotected and/or promiscuous sex	Hepatitis B and C
Chronic hepatitis B and C infections	Cancer of the liver
Exposure to infected bodily fluids	Hepatitis B
Using unsterile needles for tattoos or piercings	Hepatitis B
Sharing razors, toothbrushes, or pierced earrings	Hepatitis B and C
Contracting rubella (German measles) while pregnant	Baby develops neonatal hepatitis

RISKY BEHAVIOR	POSSIBLE CONSEQUENCES
Giving aspirin (and medications containing aspirin) to a child with chicken pox	Child develops Reye's syndrome (liver damage)
Infection with hepatitis B	Liver cancer
Infection with hepatitis C	Liver cancer
Use of anabolic steroids	Liver cancer
Consuming arsenic in drinking water	Liver cancer
Smoking	Liver cancer
Developing cirrhosis of the liver	Liver cancer
Being born to a mother with hepatitis C	Hepatitis C as a newborn
Heavy use (more than 3 pills daily) of acetaminophen for prolonged periods of time	Liver damage

Visit www.healthwatchguide.com for updates on the liver.

NOTES

The Lungs

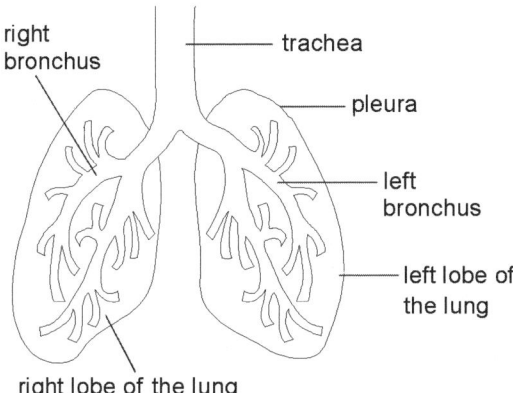
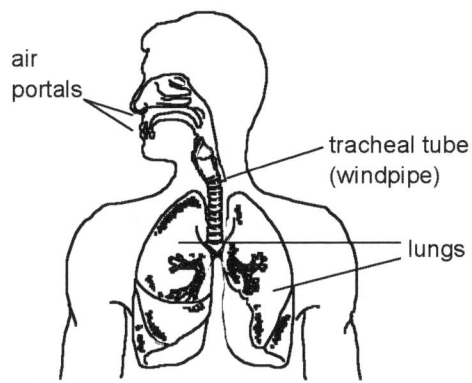

Function

The lungs are spongy, cone-shaped organs located on both sides of the upper chest cavity. When you inhale, bronchial tubes in the lungs take in oxygen and send it to the rest of the body via the blood circulatory system. Veins collect the waste product carbon dioxide and return it to the lungs for removal when you exhale. Over a twenty-four-hour period you will use approximately 3,000 gallons of air.

Keeping the Lungs Healthy

- Drink lots of liquids to keep the respiratory tract from becoming clogged with mucus.
- Stop smoking. Better yet, don't ever start. The bronchial tubes of the lungs are coated with millions of tiny hairs called "cilia" (Latin for hair). These cilia constantly sweep germs, dust, and other contaminants out of the lungs so that they can be exhaled before getting into the rest of your body. Tobacco smoke deadens these cilia, so that they can't do their job. As a result, smokers are defenseless against many airborne diseases.
- Observe pneumonia and influenza vaccination schedules (see "Immunizations" in Part Two) and get boosters against diphtheria when necessary.
- Some forms of pneumonia-causing bacteria, including those responsible for Legionnaire's disease, live in residential water heaters where temperatures of 90 to 120 degrees provide perfect breeding grounds. Bacteria can be accidentally inhaled or swallowed during showers, cleaning, and other similar activities. Researchers suggest that you can kill these bacteria by raising the temperature of your house's water heater to 140 degrees and letting the water run from the hot-water faucets for half an hour. Then return the water to its usual (lower) temperature. Do this every three to four months.

What You and Your Doctor Should Know

- Personal history of allergies
- Personal and family history of asthma
- Personal history of smoking

Beneficial Foods and Nutrients

See Part Four, The Importance of Nutrients, for a list of foods containing the vitamins and minerals mentioned in this section.

Vitamin A

Vitamin A contributes to the health of mucous membranes, which fight off bacterial infection.

Vitamin C

Vitamin C helps ward off colds and helps to protect asthmatic children from the effects of pollution.

Vitamin E

Vitamin E also helps to protect asthmatic children from the effects of pollution.

Iron

Iron is vital to the respiration process.

What Can Go Wrong

Asthma

Asthma affects about 3 percent of the general population. There are two types of asthma: *Intrinsic asthma* usually is caused by infection, cold air, emotional trauma, physical exertion, or inhalation of an irritating substance. *Extrinsic asthma* usually is caused by allergens (animal dander, foods, molds, pollens, dust, cockroaches, dust mites). The following factors increase your risk of developing asthma.

Age. Asthma is most common in those under age ten and before age thirty.

Blood types. Type B has a higher risk, type O has a moderate risk, and types A and AB have a lower risk. Nonsecretors of all types have a moderate-to-high risk.

Family history. A family history increases the risk but is not always a factor.

Gender. Women have a higher risk than men.

Medical conditions. The following conditions place one at risk:
- Allergies
- Eczema

Occupation/workplace. Working in the following workplaces or industries puts you at risk: bakeries, detergent manufacturing, farming, grain elevators, laboratories, metalworking, milling, pharmaceuticals, plastics, and woodworking. The risk also increases with exposure to diesel fumes.

What you can do: If you know that asthma runs in your family, be very aware of environmental factors that might trigger attacks in young children, especially tobacco smoke. Sometimes asthma appears without warning. For instance, asthma may develop in response to cold weather. If your occupation puts you at risk, be alert to any breathing problems. For more information, type ASTHMA into an Internet search engine.

Chronic Bronchitis (Chronic Obstructive Pulmonary Disease, COPD)

Chronic bronchitis is a long-term or frequent inflammation of the airways in the lungs. The following factors increase your risk of developing chronic bronchitis.

Blood types. Type A has a higher risk of severity; types B, AB, and O have a moderate risk. Nonsecretors of all types have a higher risk of susceptibility. Type A children with type A fathers and type O mothers may have an increased risk of fatal bronchopneumonia in infancy and young childhood.

Environment. Exposure to secondhand tobacco smoke and pollution are risk factors.

Family history. This condition may have a genetic link.

Medical conditions. Allergies are a risk factor for bronchitis.

What you can do: If you smoke, stop. If you have risk factors for chronic bronchitis, be sure to take care of any cold or respiratory illness. Never ignore a cough that lasts for six weeks or more. Together with emphysema and asthma, chronic bronchitis is the fourth leading cause of death in the United States. For more information, type CHRONIC BRONCHITIS into an Internet search engine.

Lung Cancer

Lung cancer is the second most common cancer and the leading cause of cancer deaths in the United States. Cigarette smoking accounts for 90 percent of lung cancers. The following factors increase your risk of developing lung cancer.

Age. Lung cancer is rare before age forty. The average age at diagnosis is sixty.

Blood types. Type A has a higher risk, especially in patients under age fifty. Type B has a higher risk of bronchial lung cancer. Type AB has a higher risk, and type O has a moderate risk.

Environment. Exposure to the following increases risk:
- Air pollutants—studies are ongoing
- Radon in the home
- Secondhand smoke

Ethnicity/ancestry. In descending order of risk: blacks, whites, Asians/Pacific Islanders, Hispanics, Native Americans, and Alaska Natives.

Gender. Men have a slightly higher risk.

Medical conditions. Tuberculosis is a risk factor.

Personal history. These conditions place one at risk:
- Having once had lung cancer, which increases your chances of developing a second lung cancer
- Women with a history of breast cancer

Workplace. These workplace conditions are risk factors:
- Asbestos exposure from shipbuilding, asbestos mining and manufacturing, insulation work, and brake repair
- Mining (possible exposure to radon)

What you can do: First of all, obviously, DON'T SMOKE! If you do smoke, quit. Your risk will begin to decrease the instant you stop smoking. Next, minimize your other controllable risks. For more information, type LUNG CANCER into an Internet search engine.

Sarcoidosis

Sarcoidosis is an inflammation that can affect the lungs. It is one of a group of conditions called "interstitial lung disease." The cause of sarcoidosis is unknown. The following factors increase your risk of developing the disease:

Age. Sarcoidosis is most likely to affect those who are thirty to fifty years of age.

Blood types. Type A has a moderate-to-high risk for the most severe form of the disease. Types B, AB, and O have a low-to-moderate risk. Nonsecretors have a moderate-to-high risk.

Ethnicity/ancestry. Most at risk are those of African, northern European, Japanese, and Irish decent.

Family history. This condition may run in families.

Gender. Women have the greatest risk.

What you can do: Know your risk factors. If you have this condition in your family, make sure to tell your doctor. Minimize your controllable risks for lung damage. For more information, type SARCOIDOSIS into an Internet search engine. Also check out DIFFUSE INTERSTITIAL PULMONARY FIBROSIS, a lung disease often caused by sarcoidosis.

Pneumonia

The following conditions increase your risk of developing pneumonia:

- Aspiration of foreign matter into the lungs
- Blood type B, which is the most susceptible—type B children of type B mothers have twice the risk of other babies of developing neonatal streptococcal infection.
- Bone marrow transplants
- Bronchitis
- Cancer treatments
- Coma
- Early childhood exposure to respiratory infections
- Emphysema
- Excessive buildup of tooth plaque
- Exposure
- Extended bed rest or immobility
- Hospitalization
- HIV infection
- Infections of the upper respiratory system
- Leukemia
- Organ transplants
- Periodontal disease

Note: Pneumonia can result from infection due to bacteria, viruses, and fungi. There are several vaccines available to help fight off pneumonia agents. See the immunization schedule in Part Two for the recommended vaccines.

Tuberculosis (TB)

The following factors increase your risk of developing tuberculosis.

Blood types. Type O has a moderate risk, with Europeans having a greater susceptibility than other type O people; type B has a higher risk, especially Asians; type AB has a moderate risk; type A is at low risk; Rh-negative of all types have a higher risk, with Europeans having the worst prognosis.

Environment. Exposure to crowded environments, such as:

- Airplanes (lengthy flights)
- Cities
- Homeless shelters
- Migrant work camps
- Prisons
- Nursing homes
- Hospitals

Age. Extreme youth or old age puts one at risk.

Medical conditions. People with immunocompromised systems, such as from chemotherapy or bone marrow transplants, are at risk.

Note: Once a feared killer, tuberculosis was all but wiped out in the United States when, to the dismay of the medical profession, it began to claim new victims at a growing rate. Much of this is due to AIDS, which compromises the immune system and increases vulnerability to TB and other infections. Drug-resistant strains of TB are appearing, often due to patients failing to take medications as prescribed. As a result, the general population is becoming more at risk for the disease.

Lung Conditions That Tend to Run in Families

The following conditions have no known genetic links:

- Allergies

- Asthma
- Familial Mediterranean fever
- Sarcoidosis

Medical Conditions That Can Affect Lung Health

It is important to properly treat any medical condition with which you are diagnosed, because the condition may affect other parts of your body. The body's organs and systems are inextricably connected to one another, so what goes wrong in one part may create problems in another. Conditions that can affect the lungs include the following:

- *Allergies*
- *Ankylosing spondylitis* may cause pain during breathing or reduce the ability to breathe deeply.
- *Chronic conditions*
- *Rheumatoid arthritis, scleroderma, and lupus* may contribute to interstitial lung disease.
- *Stress*
- *Viral influenza* may lead to pneumonia, especially in young children, hospitalized patients, IV drug users, and those with debilitated immune systems.

Risky Behavior and Possible Consequences

RISKY BEHAVIOR	POSSIBLE CONSEQUENCES
Smoking (cigarettes, cigars, pipes)—***the primary risk factor***	Bronchial cancer, lung cancer, chronic bronchitis, emphysema, interstitial lung disease
Not observing precautions with food and beverages while traveling	Diphtheria
Alcoholism	Pneumonia
Traveling in Third World countries	Tuberculosis exposure, typhoid fever

Visit www.healthwatchguide.com for updates on the lungs.

NOTES

The Lymphatic System

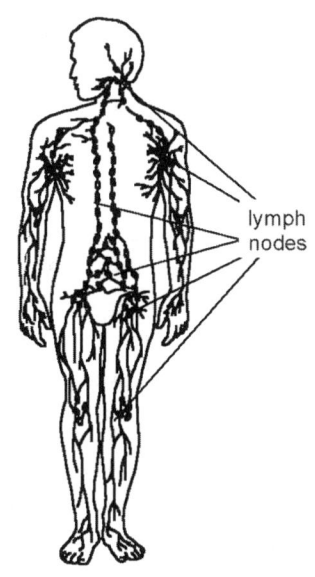

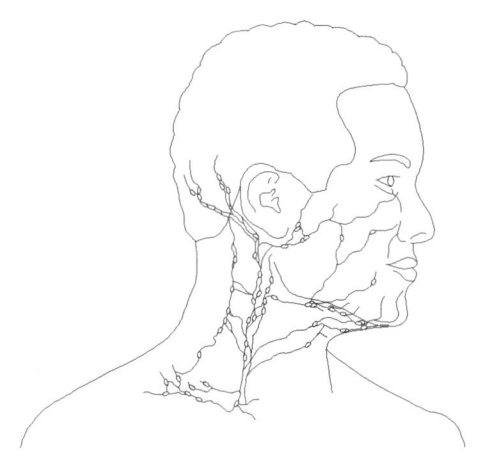

lymph nodes of the head and neck

Function

The lymphatic system is part of the body's immune system. Clusters of lymph nodes at various parts of the body—the neck, the armpits, the groin, the chest, and the abdomen—form lymph fluid containing lymphocytes, which help to defend the body against infection. Other parts of the lymphatic system are the spleen, tonsils, adenoids, and thymus. The lymph nodes are usually located at places where the arms and legs join the trunk of the body and where the head joins the trunk. These positions help the lymph nodes serve as gatekeepers. As germs try to invade the body through the mouth and nose, for instance, they are stopped by the tonsils, which swell up with defender cells and dead germs. Medical practice used to dictate removal of tonsils in response to frequent infections. Now physicians realize that a tonsillectomy removed a major barrier to infection and left the patient more vulnerable. Today tonsils are removed only as a last resort. The lymphatic system is connected by a series of thin tubes that extend throughout the body.

Beneficial Foods and Nutrients

See Part Four, The Importance of Nutrients, for a list of foods containing vitamin B_6.

Vitamin B_6

Vitamin B_6 helps the body maintain the health of the lymphatic system.

What Can Go Wrong

Hodgkin's Lymphoma

Hodgkin's lymphoma is a rare cancer of the lymphatic system. The following factors increase your risk of developing Hodgkin's lymphoma.

Age. The ages of fifteen to thirty-four and over fifty-five are most at risk.

Family history. Having a brother or sister with Hodgkin's lymphoma increases your risk.

Gender. This disease is more common in men than in women.

What you can do: It is difficult to take preventive measures since this is such a rare cancer, with so few known risk factors. Be sure to let your doctor know if the condition has afflicted any family members.

Non-Hodgkin's Lymphoma (NHL, Cancer of the Lymph System)

This is the fifth most common cancer in the United States, affecting 3 in 10,000 people. The following factors increase your risk of developing non-Hodgkin's lymphoma.

Age. The average age at diagnosis is forty. The risk increases with age.

Blood types. Types B and AB have a higher risk, type A has a moderate risk, and type O has a lower risk.

Environment. Recent studies have shown a link between NHL and nitrates in drinking water.

Ethnicity/ancestry. In descending order of risk: *men*—whites, Vietnamese, Hispanics, blacks, Filipinos, Hawaiian, Chinese, Japanese; *women*—whites, Hispanics, Filipinos, Japanese, blacks, Chinese.

Gender. Men have a higher risk than women.

Medical conditions. The following medical conditions are risk factors:
- Autoimmune disorders
- HIV/AIDS
- Inherited immune deficiencies

Medical treatments. Use of immunosuppressant drugs following organ transplants is a risk factor.

Personal history. The following conditions may place one at risk:
- Epstein-Barr virus (possible connection)
- Human T-lymphotropic virus type -1

Workplace. Exposure to solvents, fertilizers, and pesticides is a risk factor.

What you can do: Know your personal history. If you have risk factors, minimize your controllable risks. For more information, type NON-HODGKIN'S LYMPHOMA into an Internet search engine.

Mononucleosis

Mononucleosis, often called "mono," is a viral infection linked to the herpes viruses. The following factors increase your risk of being infected with mononucleosis.

Age. This illness is common between ages seven and thirty-five, and most common between ages fifteen and twenty-four.

Blood types. Types A, AB, and O have a low-to-moderate risk; type B has a moderate-to-high risk. Rh-negative of all types have a higher risk.

Exposure. This disease is usually transmitted through exposure to the saliva of an infected person.

Medical conditions. The following infections place one at risk:
- Epstein-Barr virus
- Cytomegalovirus

Note: The African form of Burkitt's lymphoma is closely associated with Epstein-Barr infection in childhood. Tell your doctor if you were born in Africa and had mononucleosis there as a young child.

What you can do: Mononucleosis is not life threatening, although serious complications arise occasionally. However, treatment requires four to six weeks of rest, as well as abstention from sports because of the risk to the swollen spleen. It is better to avoid becoming ill in the first place. The good news is that infection generally confers future immunity from the illness. For more information, type MONONUCLEOSIS into an Internet search engine.

Sarcoidosis

Sarcoidosis is an inflammation that can affect the lymph glands. The cause is unknown. The following factors increase your risk of developing sarcoidosis.

Age. Individuals aged thirty to fifty are most likely to contract sarcoidosis.

Blood types. Type A has a moderate-to-high risk for the most severe form of the disease. Types B, AB, and O have a low-to-moderate risk. Nonsecretors have a moderate-to-high risk.

Ethnicity/ancestry. Those with African, northern European, Japanese, and Irish ancestry are most at risk.

Family history. This illness may run in families.

Gender. Women have the greatest risk.

What you can do: Know your risk factors. Be sure to tell your doctor if this condition runs in your family. For more information, type SARCOIDOSIS into an Internet search engine.

Lymphatic System Conditions That Tend to Run in Families

There are no known genetic links for this condition:
- Sarcoidosis

Medical Conditions That Can Affect Lymphatic Tissue Health

It is important to properly treat any medical condition with which you are diagnosed, because the condition may affect other parts of your body. The body's organs and systems are inextricably connected to one another, so what goes wrong in one part may create problems in another.

Any bacteria or virus that tries to gain entry to your body is going to stimulate a response from your immune system. Serious problems arise when the immune system is compromised (weakened) in any way. For instance, AIDS (acquired immune deficiency syndrome) is a devastating disease because the virus attacks the immune system and leaves the patient vulnerable to innumerable infections and cancers.

PART FIVE • Disease Prevention Guide

Risky Behavior and Possible Consequences	
RISKY BEHAVIOR	POSSIBLE CONSEQUENCES
Contracting AIDS	AIDS-related lymphoma (cancer of the lymphatic system)

Visit www.healthwatchguide.com for updates on the lymphatic system.

NOTES

The Mouth

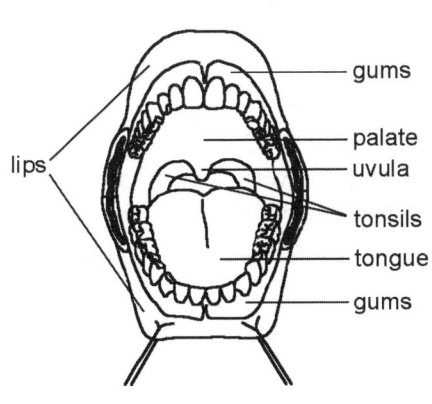

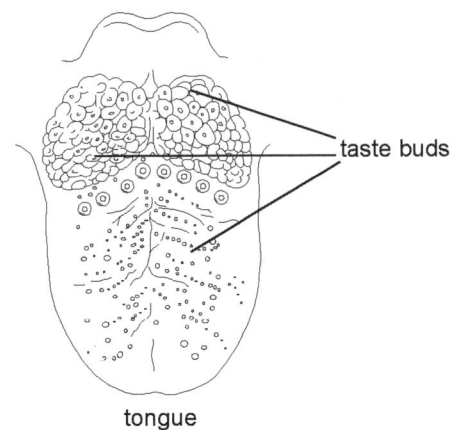

Function

The mouth is an important gateway to the internal organs. Food, fluids, air, and bacteria all pass through the mouth on a constant basis. Contained within the mouth is the tongue, which is important for the function of speech and central to the sense of taste. The taste buds, located on the tongue, are necessary for distinguishing between salty, sour, sweet, and bitter. Salivary glands within the mouth initiate the process of digestion. The mouth also is home to the teeth (see "The Teeth" for more information). The mouth is a central point that facilitates communication between the ears, the nose, and throat.

Keeping the Mouth Healthy

- Regular dental checkups will help to catch problems early.
- Avoid the use of tobacco products—they cause the vast majority of oral cancers.

Beneficial Foods and Nutrients

See Part Four, The Importance of Nutrients, for a list of foods containing the vitamins and trace elements mentioned in this section.

Vitamin A
Vitamin A contributes to the health of the mucous membranes in the mouth.

Vitamin B_3
Vitamin B_3 contributes to the health of the tongue.

Vitamin C
Vitamin C contributes to the health of the gums.

Zinc
Zinc helps to maintain the sense of taste.

Other Tips

- Ill-fitting dentures increase the risk of cancer of the oropharynx.
- Pregnant women with advanced gum disease have an increased risk of delivering underweight babies.

What Can Go Wrong

Oral Cancer

Oral cancer can affect the lips, tongue, cheeks, and gums. The following factors increase your risk of developing oral cancer:

Age. People aged forty and older are more at risk.

Blood types. Types A and AB have a higher risk, and types B and O have a moderate risk. Nonsecretors of all types have a higher risk.

Gender. Men have a greater risk than women.

Medical conditions. The following conditions place one at risk:

- Cancers of the lungs, esophagus, or larynx
- Constant irritation from teeth, fillings, or dentures
- Infection with HPV (human papillomavirus)
- Mouth ulcers

What you can do: The use of tobacco products is associated with 70 to 80 percent of oral cancers. If you smoke or use chewing tobacco, stop, especially if you have any of the other risk factors. See your dentist regularly. Leukoplakia (whitish patches) and erythroplakia (red patches) are often found in the mouths of people who subsequently develop oral cancers. Your dentist checks for signs of these conditions at your regular checkups. For more information, type ORAL CANCER into an Internet search engine.

Mouth Conditions That Tend to Run in Families

There are no known genetic links for this condition:

- cleft lip or palate

Risky Behavior and Possible Consequences	
RISKY BEHAVIOR	**POSSIBLE CONSEQUENCES**
Smoking	Cancers of the lip, tongue, gums, and cheeks
Chewing tobacco	Cancers of the lip, tongue, gums, and cheeks
Heavy alcohol use	Cancers of the lip, tongue, gums, and cheeks
Overexposure to the sun	Cancer of the lip
Poor oral hygiene	Cancer of the oropharynx
Use of mouthwash with a high alcohol content	Cancer of the oropharynx
Chewing betel nuts	Oral cancer

Visit www.healthwatchguide.com for updates on the mouth.

The Muscles

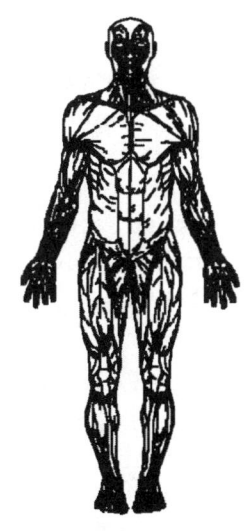
front view of the muscles

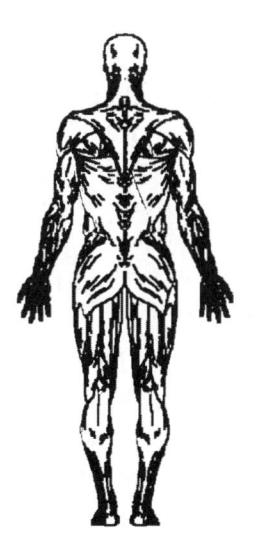
back view of the muscles

Function

The muscles are responsible for moving every part of the body. The muscles are tissues made of specialized cells that contract when stimulated. These contractions produce movement. Voluntary muscles work on command, such as when you take a step. Smooth muscles (such as those in the intestines) function without needing input from you. Muscles require energy from fats, sugars, and oxygen.

Keeping the Muscles Healthy

Exercise regularly. The more muscles are used, the more smoothly and efficiently they function. For instance, the heart is a muscle whose contractions push blood through the body. The more the heart muscle is stimulated through exercise, the more blood it can pump with fewer contractions (heartbeats). The same is true for all of the body's muscles. Regular exercise will keep the muscles from becoming flabby, and your body will be a more efficient machine.

What You and Your Doctor Should Know

- Family history of amyotrophic lateral sclerosis, fibromyalgia, and/or muscular dystrophy

Beneficial Foods and Nutrients

See Part Four, The Importance of Nutrients, for a list of foods containing the vitamins and minerals mentioned in this section.

Vitamin B_1 (Thiamine)

Thiamine benefits the muscles.

Vitamin D

Vitamin D is important for muscle function.

Calcium

Calcium is vital to the ability of the muscles to contract.

Magnesium

Magnesium is needed for normal muscle function.

Phosphorus

Phosphorus is needed for muscle contraction.

Potassium

Potassium helps with muscle contraction.

Sodium

Sodium is needed for muscle contraction.

What Can Go Wrong

Amyotrophic Lateral Sclerosis (ALS, Lou Gehrig's Disease)

This is a disease of the motor nerves that control the voluntary muscles. One in 100,000 people are affected annually. The following factors increase your risk of developing ALS.

Age. Symptoms usually develop after age fifty.

Blood types. Type B has a moderate-to-high risk; types A, AB, and O have a low-to-moderate risk. Nonsecretors of all types have a moderate risk.

Ethnicity/ancestry. Ashkenazi Jews have the highest ethnic incidence.

Family history. About 10 percent of cases are caused by an inherited genetic defect. In other cases there is no known cause.

What you can do: Be aware if ALS runs in your family. For more information, type AMYOTROPHIC LATERAL SCLEROSIS into an Internet search engine.

Fibromyalgia

Fibromyalgia is a generalized pain and tenderness in muscles, joints, and tendons. The following factors increase your risk of developing fibromyalgia.

Age. This disease is commonly diagnosed between the ages of twenty and fifty.

Blood types. Type O has a moderate risk, while types A, B, and AB have a lower risk. Nonsecretors of all types have a higher risk.

Family history. This illness may run in families.

Gender. Women are more affected than men.

What you can do: Fibromyalgia is considered an autoimmune disorder in which, for no apparent reason, the body's immune system begins attacking itself. There is not much you can do to prevent this, but if you know it runs in your family, you can be alert to symptoms and seek treatment as early as possible. For more information, type FIBROMYALGIA into an Internet search engine.

Myasthenia Gravis

This autoimmune neuromuscular disorder affects 3 in 10,000 people. The following conditions increase your risk of developing myasthenia gravis.

Age. Myasthenia gravis affects two age groups: teenagers and younger adults, and people over age forty.

Blood types. Type B has a moderate risk; types A, AB, and O have a lower risk. Nonsecretors have a moderate-to-high risk. Rh-negative has a moderate risk.

Gender. Women have the higher risk at younger ages. Men have the higher risk at older ages.

Medical conditions. Tumor of the thymus gland is a risk factor.

What you can do: Myasthenia gravis is considered an autoimmune disorder in which, for no apparent reason, the body's immune system begins attacking itself. Myasthenia gravis is characterized by severe weakness of voluntary muscles (those you can control). It is not the same as fibromyalgia, which is characterized by diffuse pain in muscles, joints, and tendons. There is not much you can do to prevent this disorder, but if you have any other autoimmune disorders or trouble with the thymus gland, you can be alert to symptoms and seek treatment as early as possible. For more information, type MYASTHENIA GRAVIS into an Internet search engine.

Muscular Dystrophy

Muscular dystrophy refers to a group of inherited disorders in which the muscles grow progressively weaker and muscle tissue is lost. These are inherited autosomal conditions, and your risk depends on whether or not you inherit the defective gene. See the section "Hereditary Conditions" in Part One for more information.

| Risky Behavior and Possible Consequences ||
RISKY BEHAVIOR	POSSIBLE CONSEQUENCES
Overstressing muscles	Muscle strain
Cold drafts	Muscle aches and pains

Visit www.healthwatchguide.com for updates on the muscles.

NOTES

The Nervous System

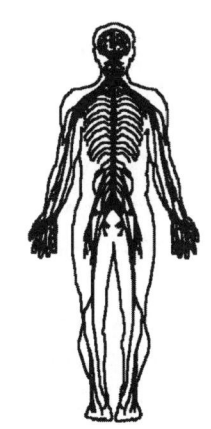

major nerves of the body

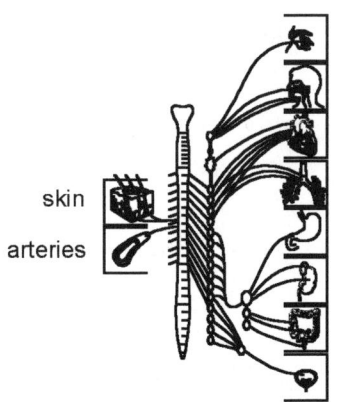

sympathetic nervous system and the spinal nerves

Function

The nervous system is an amazing network of transmitters that send messages to the brain and the spinal cord, which interpret the impulses and relay instructions to the various organs. The nerves can send a message about a cut in the skin to the brain in a fraction of a second. Before you have time to say "ouch" the brain has received and sent thousands of messages along the nerve pathways, sending signals to the body's defense and repair systems.

Keeping the Nervous System Healthy

- Damage to nerves or a nerve path often occurs as a result of trauma to the nerve or compression. Avoid activities or behaviors that put prolonged pressure on body parts. For instance, the use of crutches can compress the nerves of the arm and the shoulder. Rotate your arm, shrug your shoulders, and otherwise try to minimize the pressure from the top of the crutch.

- Habitual leg crossing and wearing high, tight boots can compress the nerves of the legs.
- Being extremely thin reduces the padding that protects the nerves and can cause problems.
- Carpal tunnel syndrome is a common problem resulting from constant repetitive wrist motions, such as keyboard typing, and tennis and golf swings. Using wrist boards while typing and taking frequent breaks to flex the wrists and hands can help.

Beneficial Foods and Nutrients

See Part Four, The Importance of Nutrients, for a list of foods containing the vitamins, minerals, and trace elements mentioned in this section.

Vitamin B_1 (Thiamine)
Thiamine benefits the nervous system.

Vitamin B_3 (Niacin)
Niacin benefits the nervous system.

Vitamin B_6
Vitamin B_6 helps to strengthen the nerves.

Vitamin B_{12}
Vitamin B_{12} helps to maintain healthy nerve cells.

Vitamin C
Vitamin C is necessary for a healthy nervous system.

Choline
Choline contributes to a properly functioning nervous system.

Pantothenic Acid
Pantothenic acid contributes to the health of the central nervous system.

Calcium
Calcium helps to ensure that the nervous system is able to transmit signals to and from the brain.

Magnesium
Magnesium is needed for normal nerve function.

Phosphorus
Phosphorus is necessary for nerve conduction.

Potassium
Potassium is needed for nerve conduction.

Sodium
Sodium is needed for nerve impulse transmission.

Copper
Copper is needed for healthy nerves.

What Can Go Wrong

Amyotrophic Lateral Sclerosis (ALS, Lou Gehrig's Disease)

This is a disease of the motor nerves that control the voluntary muscles. It affects 1 in 100,000 people annually. The following factors increase your risk of developing ALS.

Age. Symptoms usually develop after age fifty.

Blood types. Type B has a moderate-to-high risk; types A, AB, and O have a low-to-moderate risk. Nonsecretors of all types have a moderate risk.

Ethnicity/ancestry. Ashkenazi Jews have the highest ethnic incidence.

Family history. About 10 percent of cases are caused by an inherited genetic defect. In other cases there is no known cause.

What you can do: Be aware if ALS runs in your family. For more information, type AMYOTROPHIC LATERAL SCLEROSIS into an Internet search engine.

Multiple Sclerosis (MS)

MS is an inflammation of tissue in the central nervous system, including the brain and the spinal cord. It affects 1 in 1,000 people. The following factors increase your risk of developing multiple sclerosis.

Age. Symptoms usually appear between ages fifteen and sixty.

Blood types. Types B and AB have a moderate-to-high risk; types A and O have a lower risk. Nonsecretors have a moderate-to-high risk. Rh-positive has a moderate risk.

Ethnicity/ancestry. Whites have twice the risk of any other group. Ashkenazi Jews have a high risk.

Family history. There may be a genetic connection for this disease.

Gender. Women have twice the risk of men.

Geographic location. Risk is associated with northern Europe, northern United States, southern Australia, and New Zealand. Very high risk exists in certain islands in Scotland.

What you can do: Know your family history. If the condition runs in your family and you live in one of the high-risk regions, become familiar with symptoms so that you can seek treatment as early as possible. For more information, type MULTIPLE SCLEROSIS into an Internet search engine.

Neurosarcoidosis

Neurosarcoidosis is an inflammation that can affect the nervous system. The cause is unknown. The following factors increase your risk of developing neurosarcoidosis.

Age. Most at risk are people aged thirty to fifty.

Blood types. Type A has a moderate-to-high risk for the most severe form of the disease. Types B, AB, and O have a low-to-moderate risk. Nonsecretors have a moderate-to-high risk.

Ethnicity/ancestry. At risk are people of African, northern European, Japanese, and Irish decent.

Family history. This disease may run in families.

Gender. Women have the greatest risk.

What you can do: Know your risk factors. If this runs in your family, be sure to tell your doctor. For more information, type NEUROSARCOIDOSIS into an Internet search engine.

Neuralgia

Neuralgias are pains that occur along specific nerve paths. Risk factors include:
- Chemicals
- Chronic renal insufficiency
- Compression
- Diabetes
- Infections
- Inflammation
- Lyme disease
- Multiple sclerosis
- Porphyria, an inherited condition (a number of medications can aggravate porphyria and trigger nerve pain)
- Shingles
- Syphilis
- Trauma to the nerve

Nervous System Conditions That Tend to Run in Families

There are no known genetic links for these conditions:
- Enuresis (bed-wetting)
- Essential tremor
- Febrile seizure
- Multiple sclerosis
- Neurosarcoidosis
- Stuttering

Medical Conditions That Can Affect Nervous System Health

It is important to properly treat any medical condition with which you are diagnosed, because the condition may affect other parts of your body. The body's organs and systems are inextricably connected to one another, so what goes wrong in one part may create problems in another. Conditions that can affect the nervous system include:

- *Diabetes mellitus*—50 percent of diabetics will eventually develop temporary or permanent nerve damage.

Risky Behavior and Possible Consequences	
RISKY BEHAVIOR	**POSSIBLE CONSEQUENCES**
Heavy metal exposure	Stress
Constant exposure to white noise	Stress
Lack of adequate sleep	Stress
All work and no play	Stress
Sedentary lifestyle	Stress
Heavy use of alcohol	Alcoholic neuropathy
Infection with syphilis	Neurosyphilis (infection of the brain or spinal cord)

Visit www.healthwatchguide.com for updates on the nervous system.

NOTES

The Nose

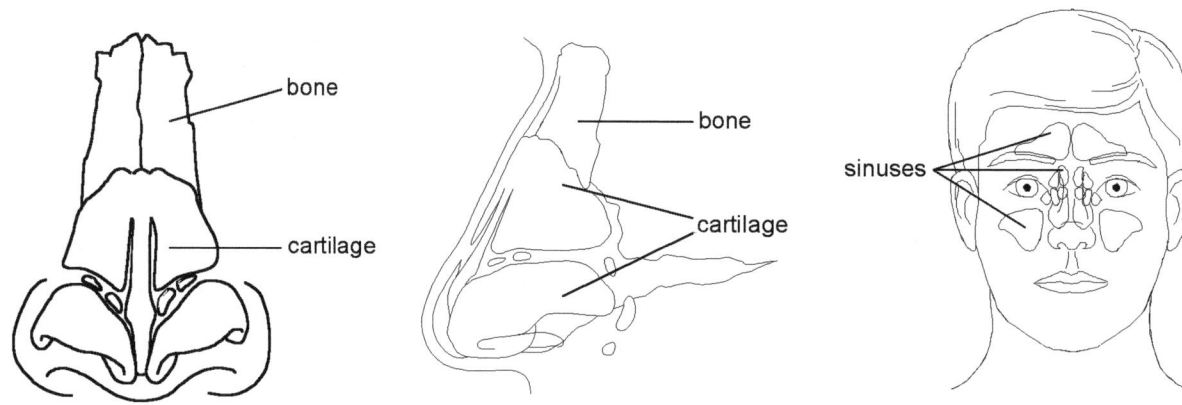

Function

The nose is a remarkable part of the body. Although the outward appearance is variable and depends on genes for its size and shape, the functions it performs are universal. Air enters the body through the nostrils, the two halves of the nose, and is cleaned, warmed, filtered, and moistened before it reaches the lungs. Large hairs, microscopic hairs called cilia, and mucus help to trap dust, bacteria, soot, and other unwanted material. The nose contains olfactory cells that support the sense of smell. The cartilage that makes up the rigid part of the nose is both flexible enough to give when necessary, but strong enough to keep the nose from collapsing during inhalation.

Keeping the Nose Healthy

- Nasal congestion often is caused by allergic responses. Mucus is one of the body's defense

mechanisms—the sticky mucus traps germs, dust, pollen, and fur, and then sneezes and coughs expel the trapped matter from your nose and mouth. Reduce congestion by minimizing exposure to allergens whenever possible. Chronic congestion can interfere with speech, hearing, and breathing, so it should be treated. Mucus also forms when something to which the body is allergic is eaten.
- Don't suppress sneezes. The pressure created in your nose and throat by suppression can push infection into your sinuses and ears.

Beneficial Foods and Nutrients

See Part Four, The Importance of Nutrients, for a list of foods containing vitamin C and zinc.

Vitamin C
Vitamin C helps to ward off colds.

Zinc
Zinc helps to maintain the sense of smell.

What Can Go Wrong

Cancers of the Nasal Cavity and Sinuses

The following factors increase your risk of developing these cancers.

Ethnicity/ancestry. Asians, especially Chinese, are particularly at risk of cancer of the nasopharynx. They are followed by Filipinos, blacks, Hispanics, and non-Hispanic whites.

Workplace. Wood and nickel dust inhalation are risk factors.

What you can do: These cancers are rare in the United States, but if you were born in China or Taiwan and emigrated to America, you may want to become familiar with the symptoms in order to start treatment as early as possible. For more information type NASOPHARYNGEAL CANCER into an Internet search engine.

Sinusitis

Sinusitis is a chronic or acute inflammation of the sinuses. This affects some 31 million Americans annually. The following factors increase your risk of developing sinusitis.

Blood types. Types B and O have the greatest risk of sinusitis due to allergies; types A and AB have moderate risk.

Medical conditions. The following conditions are risk factors:

- Allergies
- *Aspergillus* fungal allergies
- Asthma
- Cancer
- Colds
- Cystic fibrosis
- Dental work
- Deviated septum
- Frequent swimming or diving
- Immotile cilia syndrome
- Kartagener's syndrome
- Nasal polyps
- Nasal bone spurs
- Tooth abscesses
- Tumors of the nose or face

Medical Treatments. Medical treatments that create risk include:

- Chemotherapy
- Immunosuppressants for organ or bone marrow transplants

What you can do: Treat colds promptly. Keep the mucus thin and flowing well with humidifiers and by drinking plenty of fluids. Avoid temperature extremes. For more information, type SINUSITIS into an Internet search engine.

Nasal Conditions That Tend to Run in Families

There are no known genetic links for this condition:
- Allergies

Risky Behavior and Possible Consequences	
RISKY BEHAVIOR	POSSIBLE CONSEQUENCES
Smoking	Cancers of the nose and sinuses, sinusitis
Excessive consumption of alcohol	Cancers of the nose and sinuses
Excessive consumption of Cantonese salted fish	Cancer of the nasopharynx
Excessive use of decongestants	Sinusitis
Becoming infected with HIV	Sinusitis

Visit www.healthwatchguide.com for updates on the nose.

NOTES

The Ovaries

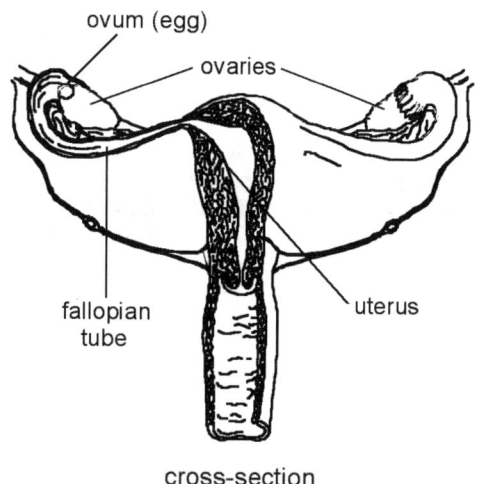

cross-section

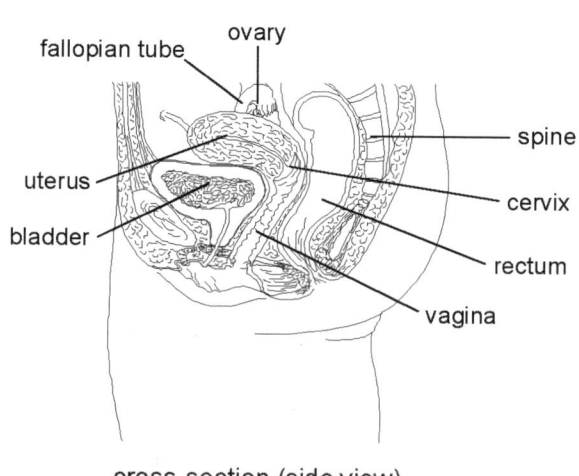

cross-section (side view)

Function

The ovaries are the reproductive organs in women, which produce ova (eggs) and the hormones estrogen and progesterone. Girls have between 150,000 and 500,000 immature ova at birth. By the time they begin to menstruate, the number has diminished to some 34,000 ova, and as women age the number decreases steadily until menopause, when the last eggs vanish.

Once a month, during the reproductive years, one of the eggs matures and is released into one of the two fallopian tubes for possible fertilization. If fertilization doesn't occur, the egg is washed out of the body during menstruation. Of the 34,000 immature follicles present at adolescence, only about 400 ever reach maturity. Once ovulation (the monthly maturation and release of an egg) stops, estrogen and progesterone production declines considerably but never ceases altogether. These hormones are vital to the reproduction process, and estrogen is also a major requirement for bone health.

Keeping the Ovaries Healthy

Avoiding diabetes may reduce your risk of developing polycystic ovary disease, a condition whose symptoms include infertility, hirsutism (excess facial and body hair), and irregular or missing periods.

What You and Your Doctor Should Know

- Family and personal history of breast, uterine, ovarian, and gastrointestinal cancers
- Personal history of having the breast cancer gene mutations BRCA1 or BRCA2

What Can Go Wrong

Hypogonadism

Hypogonadism is the inability of the ovaries to produce hormones. The following factors increase your risk of hypogonadism.

Age. This condition can occur at any age. One in 2,500 to 10,000 girls is born with hypogonadism.

Medical conditions. The following conditions increase risk:

- Autoimmune disorders
- Brain tumors
- Chemotherapy
- Hemochromatosis
- Infection
- Kidney disease
- Liver disease
- Nutritional deficiencies
- Pituitary tumors
- Premature menopause
- Surgery
- Radiation therapy
- Trauma
- Turner's syndrome

What you can do: Minimize your controllable risks. Treat any medical conditions that are considered to be risk factors. For more information, type HYPOGONADISM into an Internet search engine.

Ovarian Cancer

Ovarian cancer is the fifth leading cause of cancer death in women. American women have a one in fifty chance of developing ovarian cancer in their lifetime. The following factors increase your risk of developing ovarian cancer.

Age. One-fourth of deaths occur in women aged thirty-five to fifty-four, and half in women aged fifty-five to seventy-four. Most women are diagnosed postmenopause.

Blood types. Types A and AB have a higher risk; types B and O have a moderate risk. Rh-positive in all types have a high risk.

Family history. A family history of ovarian cancer is a risk factor.

- A woman's risk is 5 percent if she has a mother or sister with ovarian cancer.
- The risk is 7 percent with two or more relatives.
- If a woman's mother and grandmother or great-grandmother had the disease, the risk increases to 40 to 50 percent.
- The risk increases with a family history of uterine or colon cancer.

Genetic factors. Having the breast cancer gene mutations BRCA1 or BRCA2 is a risk factor.

Geographic location. Risk increases for those in industrialized nations, except Japan.

Personal history. Your risk increases with the following conditions:

- Breast cancer
- Older age (thirty or above) at the first pregnancy

What you can do: One reason that the death rate is so high for ovarian cancer is because this disease has no specific symptoms, and many cases are misdiagnosed as other conditions. Research has shown that the risk is reduced by oral contraceptive use, early pregnancy, breastfeeding, and the more children you have. These behaviors all reduce the number of times you ovulate during your life, which seems to be a major factor in the development of the cancer. However, oral contraceptive use may be risky for other reasons. Discuss your situation with your doctor, and do what seems right to you. Knowing your family history is crucial. Talk to your doctor about genetic screening if breast, ovarian, uterine, or gastrointestinal cancers run in your family. For more information, type OVARIAN CANCER into an Internet search engine.

Ovarian Conditions That Tend to Run in Families

These conditions have no known genetic links:
- Ovarian cancer
- Stein-Leventhal syndrome

Medical Conditions That Can Affect the Ovaries

It is important to properly treat any medical condition with which you are diagnosed, because the condition may affect other parts of your body. The body's organs and systems are inextricably connected to one another, so what goes wrong in one part may create problems in another. Conditions that may affect the ovaries include:

- *Insulin-resistant diabetes*
- *Stein-Leventhal syndrome* (polycystic ovary disease)

Risky Behavior and Possible Consequences	
RISKY BEHAVIOR	POSSIBLE CONSEQUENCES
Having or having had an infection from chlamydial trachomatis	Ovarian cancer
Being significantly overweight	Ovarian cancer
Estrogen-only hormone replacement therapy (not enough data yet on the risks, if any, of estrogen-progestin therapy)	Ovarian cancer

Visit www.healthwatchguide.com for updates on the ovaries.

NOTES

The Pancreas

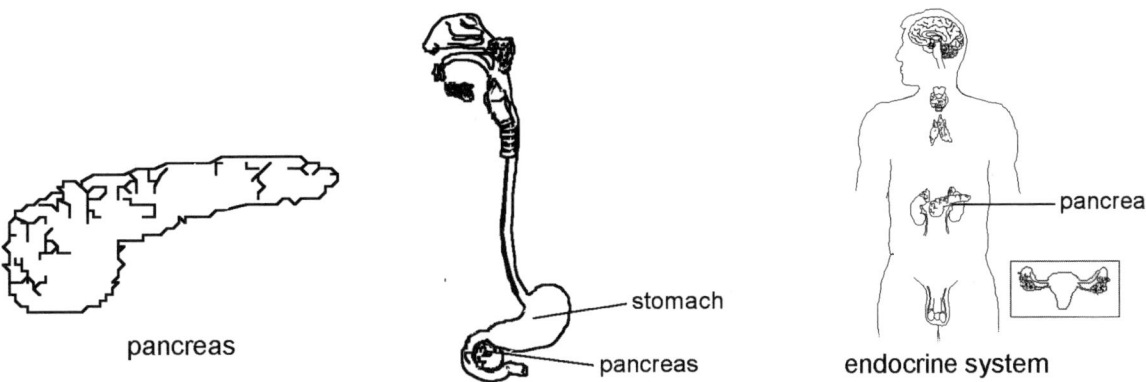

Function

The pancreas is located behind the stomach, surrounded by the small intestine, spleen, and liver. It produces a number of hormones, including insulin and glucagon, which regulate blood sugar levels in healthy people by controlling the body's absorption of glucose into muscles, fat, and liver cells. Insulin lowers blood sugar levels and glucagon raises them. The cells use the glucose as energy, or if there's too much glucose, store it as fat. When the body fails to produce insulin, excess glucose builds up in the bloodstream, causing the kidneys to work overtime trying to excrete it through the urine.

Normal fasting blood glucose levels are between 70 and 115 mg/dL (milligrams per deciliter) for people without diabetes.

Beneficial Foods and Nutrients

See Part Four, The Importance of Nutrients, for a list of foods containing the vitamins and trace elements mentioned in this section.

Green Tea
Green tea contains polyphenols, which may help to reduce the risk of pancreatic cancer.

Wine and Beer
Studies show that men who have a daily glass of wine or beer have a 36 percent lower risk of developing type II diabetes, compared with men who don't drink or who drink smaller amounts.

Note: This does not mean you should start drinking if you have medical or religious objections to alcohol consumption.

Vitamin B_6
Vitamin B_6 helps to maintain normal ranges of blood glucose.

Vitamin D
Vitamin D is important to insulin secretion.

Chromium
Chromium helps to regulate blood sugar.

Manganese
Manganese assists with glucose production.

Zinc
Zinc is needed for the body's effective use of insulin.

Other Tips

- Regular exercise can help to keep weight at a safe level.
- Eat foods low in fat and high in fiber.

Note: Type II diabetes historically has occurred in people over the age of fifty. But children who eat high-fat diets and get little or no exercise are developing type II diabetes at an alarming rate.

What Can Go Wrong

There are two major risks to the pancreas—diabetes and cancer.

Type I (Juvenile) Diabetes

Type I diabetes accounts for 3 percent of all new diabetes cases in the United States. The following factors increase your risk of type I diabetes.

Age. Most at risk are those in infancy or young childhood. Most cases are diagnosed under age thirty.

Blood types. Types A and O have a higher risk; types B and AB have a moderate risk. The risk for type A increases over type O with age. The risk of a child developing type I (juvenile) diabetes is greater when the mother is type O and the child is type A. Nonsecretors of all types have a higher risk.

Ethnicity/ancestry. Juvenile diabetes is more common in whites than in non-whites.

Family history. Having a mother with diabetes greatly increases the risk for the child.

What you can do: The exact cause of type I diabetes is still unknown. Know your blood type and that of your mother (or child). While these are not guaranteed predictors, they may give you a better awareness of symptoms for early diagnosis or treatment. For more information, type TYPE I DIABETES into an Internet search engine.

Diabetes Mellitus, Type II (Adult-Onset) Diabetes

Type II diabetes is the most common form of diabetes. There are some 17 million cases in the United States. The following factors increase your risk of type II (adult-onset) diabetes.

Age. There is risk especially after age forty-five, but the age is dropping as more young people become obese. Older diabetics are at risk of limb amputation due to circulation problems from restricted blood flow.

Blood types. Types A and O have a higher risk; types B and AB have a moderate risk. Nonsecretors of all types have a higher risk.

Certain medications. Medications that increase risk are:
- Blood pressure medicine
- Hydantoin medicines
- Medications for transplant recipients
- Steroids

Ethnicity/ancestry. In order of risk: blacks, Hispanics, Native Americans, Asians, Pacific Islanders, non-Hispanic whites.

Family history. Having a parents or siblings with diabetes is a risk factor.

Gender. The risk is the same for both men and women, but men who consume processed meats, such as hot dogs, bologna, sausage, bacon, and salami more than five times per week are forty-six times more likely to develop type II diabetes than men who consume lesser amounts.

Medical conditions. These conditions are risk factors:
- Abnormal cholesterol levels—HDL under 35 or triglyceride level over 250
- Acromegaly
- Addison's disease
- Glucose intolerance
- Hypertension
- Multiple endocrine neoplasia
- Pancreatic tumors

Medical History. The following factors increase risk for women:
- A history of gestational diabetes
- Early menstruation
- Giving birth to one or more babies weighing more than nine pounds

Note: Coronary artery disease is the leading cause of death for diabetics.

What you can do: Adult-onset diabetes is a very preventable disease. Obviously, some factors are uncontrollable, but by avoiding obesity, staying fit, and controlling blood pressure, the chance of becoming diabetic can be tremendously reduced. This disease is particularly troublesome given the many children who are developing diabetes. Children are meant to be active, and the exercise they get provides lifelong health benefits. For more information, type DIABETES MELLITUS into an Internet search engine.

Diabetes Insipidus

This is a rare condition resulting from the kidneys' inability to hold on to water. Risk factors include:
- Certain medications
- Damage to the hypothalamus or pituitary gland from trauma, surgery, infection, tumor
- Polycystic kidney disease
- X-linked hereditary disorder, affecting boys

Complications of Diabetes
- Atheroembolic renal disease
- Atherosclerosis
- Bladder infections
- Blindness
- Cataracts
- Endometrial cancer
- Foot amputation
- Gallstones
- Gout
- Heart attack
- Hypertension
- Kidney failure

- Malignant ear infections
- Nerve damage
- Neurogenic bladder
- Open-angle glaucoma
- Pancreatic cancer
- Periodontal disease
- Preeclampsia (for pregnant women)
- Retinal detachment
- Stroke
- Urinary tract infections
- Uterine cancer
- Vaginal yeast infections

Pancreatic Cancer

This is the fourth leading cause of cancer in the United States, with 29,000 cases diagnosed annually. The following conditions increase your risk of pancreatic cancer.

Age. Most at risk are those between ages thirty-five and seventy, with most cases diagnosed around age sixty.

Blood types. Types A and B have a higher risk, type B has a moderate risk, and type O is at low risk.

Ethnicity/ancestry. In descending order of risk: blacks, Native Hawaiians, whites, Asians, and Hispanics. Ashkenazi Jews also have a high risk.

Family history. The risk triples if a parent or sibling has or had pancreatic cancer. Other risk factors are:
- Hereditary non-polyposis colorectal cancer
- Inflammatory pancreatic problems (chronic pancreatitis)
- Multiple endocrine neoplasia
- Ovarian cancer
- Peutz-Jeghers syndrome

Gender. Men have three to four times the risk of women.

Medical conditions. Diabetes mellitus is a risk factor, especially for women.

What you can do: Know your family history. If you smoke, STOP. Smoking accounts for one-third of pancreatic cancers. Postmenopausal women may reduce their risk by taking aspirin. Talk to your doctor. For more information, type PANCREATIC CANCER into an Internet search engine.

Pancreatic Conditions That Tend to Run in Families

These conditions have no known genetic links:
- Diabetes
- Multiple endocrine neoplasia (MEN) type 1
- Pancreatic cancer

Medical Conditions That Can Affect Pancreatic Health

It is important to properly treat any medical condition with which you are diagnosed, because the condition may affect other parts of your body. The body's organs and systems are inextricably connected to one another, and what goes wrong in one part may create problems in another.

- *Chronic periodontal disease* aggravates diabetes and interferes with diabetes control.
- *Gallbladder disease*
- *Polycystic ovary disease* is connected with insulin resistance.
- *Viral infections*

Risky Behavior and Possible Consequences	
RISKY BEHAVIOR	POSSIBLE CONSEQUENCES
Obesity	Type II diabetes, pancreatic cancer
Alcohol abuse/overuse	Type II diabetes, pancreatic cancer, pancreatitis
Smoking	Type II diabetes, pancreatic cancer
Exposure to certain petroleum products, dry-cleaning agents, and other chemicals	Pancreatic cancer
Diets low in fiber	Pancreatic cancer
Diets high in fat (Western diet)	Pancreatic cancer, type II diabetes
Diets high in white bread, potatoes, and rice, especially in combination with obesity and lack of exercise	Pancreatic cancer

Visit www.healthwatchguide.com for updates on the pancreas.

The Penis

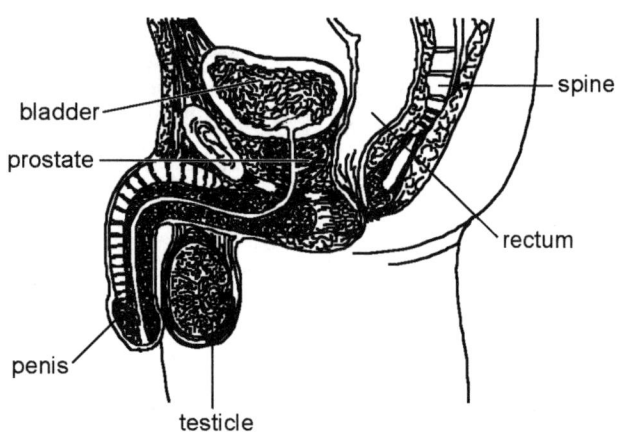

Function

The penis is a male organ that serves two functions: the excretion of urine and the transfer of semen into the female reproductive tract.

Keeping the Penis Healthy

- Practice good hygiene. If you are uncircumcised, be sure to retract and wash beneath the foreskin daily, or more often as needed.
- Unprotected sex can be dangerous. Why take chances? *Be Aware!* Genital warts are caused by infection with the human papilloma virus (HPV), the primary cause of cervical cancer in women. HPV infection does not always manifest with warts; you may have HPV infection with no symptoms for years, but you can still infect someone else.

Beneficial Foods and Nutrients

See Part Four, The Importance of Nutrients, for a list of foods containing vitamin E.

Vitamin E

Vitamin E is thought to be helpful in preventing Peyronie's disease (see below).

Other Tips

- Use protective devices, such as athletic cups, as recommended for specific sports.
- Narrow, unpadded bicycle seats can restrict penile blood flow, which may eventually contribute to erectile dysfunction problems.

What Can Go Wrong

Cancer of the Penis

Cancer of the penis is not a common disease in the United States; only 1,000 cases are diagnosed annually. However, cancer of the penis accounts for 20 to 30 percent of all male cancers diagnosed in Asia, Africa, and South America. The following factors increase your risk of developing penile cancer.

Age. This cancer is more common in older men, with sixty being the average age at diagnosis.

Personal history. Anyone who has had penile cancer is at risk of redeveloping the disease. Circumcision as an infant dramatically reduces the risk of squamous cell (skin) cancer of the penis. Circumcision in adolescence or adulthood does not reduce the risk.

What you can do: Know your personal risks and minimize your controllable risks. Practice good hygiene, especially if you are uncircumcised. For more information on symptoms and treatment, type PENILE CANCER into an Internet search engine.

Peyronie's Disease

This curvature of the penis is often associated with a hard, benign lump that forms on the penis. It occurs in about 1 percent of men. The following factors increase your risk of developing Peyronie's disease.

Age. This disease occurs mostly in middle age.

Family history. A family history of Peyronie's disease may increase the risk.

Medical conditions. Dupuytren's contracture of the hand may increase risk.

Personal history. Peyronie's disease may result from even minor trauma to the penis.

What you can do: Know your personal risks. See your doctor if you feel a lump. For more information, type PEYRONIE'S DISEASE into an Internet search engine.

Congenital Conditions

- Ambiguous genitalia—very rare
- Hypospadias—the urethral opening is in the wrong place on the penis; this condition tends to run in families
- Micropenis—very rare

Medical Conditions That Can Affect Penile Health

It is important to properly treat any medical condition with which you are diagnosed, because the condition may affect other parts of your body. The body's organs and systems are inextricably connected to one another, and what goes wrong in one part may create problems in another.

- *AIDS* and *chlamydial infections* can lead to *Reiter's syndrome*, a form of arthritis affecting the urethra.

Risky Behavior and Possible Consequences	
RISKY BEHAVIOR	POSSIBLE CONSEQUENCES
Smoking	Cancer of the penis
Unprotected sex	Sexually transmitted diseases, such as gonorrhea
Infection from genital herpes and human papillomavirus	Cancer of the penis
Poor hygiene in uncircumcised men	Cancer of the penis

Visit www.healthwatchguide.com for updates on the penis.

NOTES

The Prostate

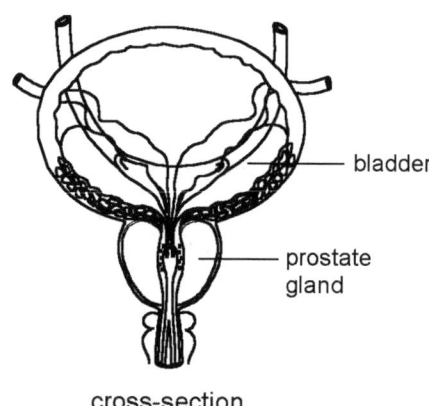

cross-section

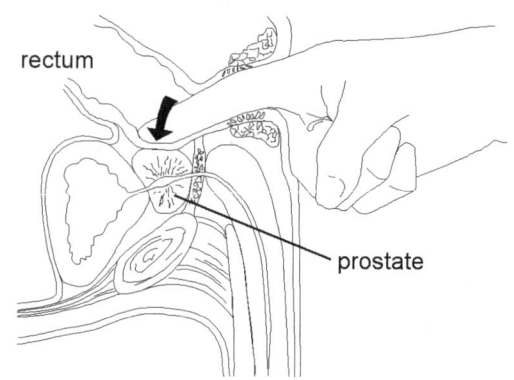

digital prostate exam

Function

The prostate gland is located below the bladder, in front of the rectum, and is about the size of a walnut. It produces and stores seminal fluid, a milky liquid that nourishes sperm.

Keeping the Prostate Healthy

What You and Your Doctor Should Know

- Family history of prostate cancer
- Your last PSA (prostate-specific antigen) reading
- Your current PSA reading

Beneficial Foods and Nutrients

See Part Four, The Importance of Nutrients, for a list of foods containing the vitamins and trace elements mentioned in this section.

Allium Foods

Chives, onions, scallions, leeks, and garlic may help to reduce the risk of prostate cancer.

Green Tea

Green tea contains polyphenols, which may help to reduce the risk of prostate cancer.

Cruciferous Vegetables

Broccoli, kale, cauliflower, and Brussels sprouts contain compounds called indoles that help to reduce the risk of prostate cancer.

Vitamin E

Vitamin E assists with prostate function.

Selenium

Selenium helps lower the risk of prostate cancer.

Lycopene

Lycopene may help to reduce the risk of prostate cancer. Foods containing lycopene include tomatoes, apricots, guava, pink grapefruit, papaya, and watermelon.

Other Tips

- Have a PSA (prostate-specific antigen) blood test and a digital exam annually if you are a man age fifty or older, or beginning at age forty for men of African ancestry or with a family history of prostate cancer. Keep track of your visits and record the results in "Tests for Men" in Part Two. Note each PSA reading and take steps if you see an increase in the numbers.
- Research has shown that the more ejaculations a man has, the lower his lifetime risk of prostate cancer.

What Can Go Wrong

Prostate Cancer

This is the most common cancer in men, other than skin cancer, and the second leading cause of cancer death in men, after lung cancer. Close to 200,000 new cases are diagnosed each year in the United States. Fortunately, this is a very slow-growing cancer with an excellent prognosis if caught in time. The following factors increase the risk of developing prostate cancer.

Age. Risk increases after age forty. Average age at diagnosis is seventy-two.

Blood types. Types A and AB have a higher risk; types B and O have a moderate risk. Secretors have a higher risk.

Ethnicity/ancestry. In descending order of risk: blacks, whites, Asians, Native Americans.

Family history. Your risk of developing prostate cancer is much higher if your father, son, or brother had (has) it. Research is being done to see if there is a genetic link in prostate cancer cases, particularly where men under age fifty-five have been diagnosed with the disease.

Height. Risk increases by 23 to 43 percent for men over the age of fifty who are 5'11" or taller.

Occupations. The following occupations are at risk:
- Cadmium mining
- Farming
- Painting
- Tire manufacturing

Personal history. Having high testosterone levels may increase your risk.

What you can do: Know your personal risks. Minimize your controllable risks, especially concerning a high-fat diet. Be sure to have the appropriate digital and PSA exams. Prostate cancer is highly treatable when caught early, so don't allow a little squeamishness about the checkup keep you from going to the doctor each year. For more information, type PROSTATE CANCER into an Internet search engine.

Benign Prostatic Hyperplasia (BPH)

Approximately 80 percent of men will probably experience this enlargement of the prostate. There is no known connection between BPH and prostate cancer. The following factors increase your risk of developing BPH.

Age. Risk increases over the age of fifty.

Blood types. Types A and AB have a moderate-to-high risk; types B and O have a moderate risk. Secretors have a moderate-to-high risk.

Medical conditions. Prostatitis places one at risk.

What you can do: Know your personal risk factors, the most significant of which is being male. The only sure way to prevent the development of BPH, is castration before puberty, which is pretty drastic—few men would opt for it. Luckily, there are other treatment options. If you begin to experience symptoms of an enlarged prostate, talk to your doctor. For more information, type BENIGN PROSTATIC HYPERPLASIA into an Internet search engine.

Prostatitis

Prostatitis is an inflammation of the prostate gland. There are several different forms, some of which are caused by bacterial infections. Most cases are diagnosed between ages thirty and seventy.

Acute prostatitis. This form is more common in younger men. Its causes include bladder outlet obstruction, infection from *E. coli,* or prolonged catheterization.

Chronic bacterial prostatitis. This form is a recurrent urinary tract infection. It is the most common urologic concern for men over age fifty.

Risky Behavior and Possible Consequences

RISKY BEHAVIOR	POSSIBLE CONSEQUENCES
Diets high in fat	Prostate cancer
Excess consumption of alcohol	Prostate cancer, chronic prostatitis
Infection from chlamydia and gonorrhea	Acute prostatitis
Rectal intercourse without a condom	Chronic and acute prostatitis
Being significantly overweight	Prostate cancer
Multiple sexual partners	Acute prostatitis

Visit www.healthwatchguide.com for updates on the prostate.

The Rectum

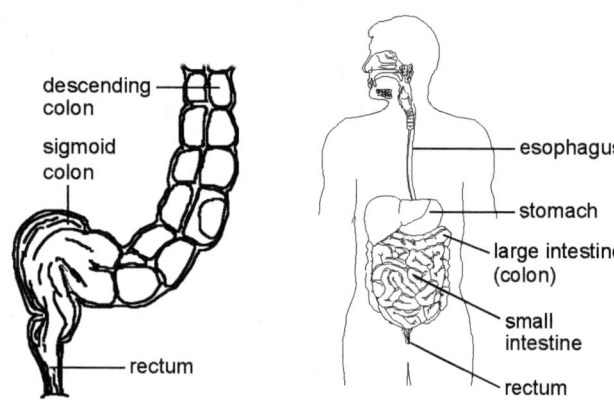

Function

The rectum is located at the end of the large intestine and terminates at the anal canal, which opens at the anus. Fecal matter waiting to be eliminated accumulates in the rectum. Muscular contractions of the rectum push the feces out of the body.

Keeping the Rectum Healthy

Defecation is a natural process in the body's routine handling of food and waste, but many factors can affect it, including a rise in the body's temperature and neurological or psychological factors, such as pain or fear. To get into a normal routine for elimination, try the following:

- Drink plenty of water in addition to other fluids. Caffeine and alcohol tend to dry out your system.
- Eat foods high in fiber. Fiber is not absorbed by the intestines, which push it out along with other unwanted material present. Water keeps this material soft, so elimination is not uncomfortable.
- Exercise regularly—even light walking helps regularity.
- Never ignore the need to have a bowel movement. Try to schedule a regular time of day and give yourself enough time for the process.

Beneficial Foods and Nutrients

See Part Four, The Importance of Nutrients, for a list of foods containing the vitamins, minerals, and trace elements mentioned in this section.

Green Tea

Green tea can reduce a woman's risk of rectal cancer by 60 percent.

Calcium

Calcium appears to be helpful in preventing polyp formation.

Folic Acid (Folate)

Folic acid appears to be useful in lowering the risk of polyps and colon cancer, but it may be harmful if taken by people who have advanced cancer, have pernicious anemia, or are taking medications for epilepsy. See the section "Folic Acid" in Part Four for more information.

Selenium
Selenium may help prevent polyp formation.

Low-Dose Aspirin
Aspirin appears to be helpful in reducing the risk of colorectal polyps. If you are at risk, talk to your doctor about taking one low-dose aspirin daily. Aspirin can cause bleeding problems in some people.

What Can Go Wrong

Colorectal Cancer
Colorectal cancer is the second leading cause of cancer deaths in the United States, with some 150,000 new cases are diagnosed annually. The following factors increase your risk of developing colorectal cancer.

Age. While most common in people over the age of fifty, this disease can occur at any age.

Blood types. Types A and AB have a higher risk. Types B and O have a moderate risk. Type A individuals with a history of thyroid cancer may have a very high risk of developing colon cancer.

Cancer history. Women who have had ovarian or uterine cancer are at greater risk of developing colorectal cancer. Also, those who have had colorectal cancer once can develop it a second time.

Ethnicity/ancestry. In descending order of risk: Alaska Natives, Japanese, blacks, non-Hispanic whites, Chinese, Hawaiians, white Hispanics, Filipinos, Koreans, Vietnamese, and Native Americans. Some 6 percent of Ashkenazi Jews have a genetic alteration that increases their risk by two-fold.

Family history. Your risk increases if you have:
- Family members with hyperplastic polyposis
- Family members with juvenile polyposis
- Parents, siblings, or children who have had colorectal cancer

Medical conditions. The following conditions place one at risk:
- Colon adenomas
- Gardner's syndrome (familial adenomatous polyposis)
- Polyps—some types increase the chances of developing cancer
- Ulcerative colitis—increases the risk of colorectal cancer

What you can do: Know your family history! Make sure your doctor knows your family history! Your doctor may recommend early intervention treatments if you are at high risk. Have regular colon screenings appropriate for your age and risk factors. Don't let squeamishness prevent you from doing this. The tests are not that uncomfortable and may save your life. (See "Colon Cancer Screenings" in Part Two for the recommended screening schedules.) Minimize or eliminate your controllable risk factors. For more information, type COLORECTAL CANCER into an Internet search engine.

Colorectal Polyps
Polyps are growths that jut out from the wall of the rectum. They are often benign, but those larger than one centimeter have an increased risk of malignancy. Not all polyps are cancerous, but most colorectal cancers start as polyps. The following conditions increase your risk of developing polyps in the rectum.

Age. The risk increases with age.

Blood types. Types A and AB have a higher risk; types B and O have a moderate risk.

Environment. Living in industrialized societies increases risk. This may be connected with the tendency for less exercise and high-fat, low-fiber diets common in these environments.

Family history. You are at risk of polyps if you have a parent or sibling with:
- Colon cancer—greatly increases risk
- Inflammatory bowel disease—increases risk
- Polyps—increases risk

Genetic links. There are links between polyps and:
- Gardner's syndrome (familial adenomatous polyposis)
- Juvenile polyposis
- Peutz-Jeghers syndrome

Medical conditions. Acromegaly increases risk of polyps.

What you can do: Know your risk factors and your family history. Have the necessary screenings, perhaps at an earlier age if your family has a history of polyps. Early detection can give your doctor a chance to remove the polyps before they become malignant. Eat a diet low in fat and high in fiber. Minimize your controllable risks. For more information, type COLORECTAL POLYPS into an Internet search engine.

Ulcerative Colitis

Ulcerative colitis is an inflammation of the lining of the large intestine (colon) and rectum. It affects some 1 in 10,000 people. The following conditions increase your risk of developing ulcerative colitis.

Age. Most patients are between ages fifteen and thirty or ages fifty and seventy.

Blood types. Type O has a higher risk for colitis and for the form that includes bleeding with elimination. Types A, B, and AB have a moderate risk and develop more of a mucous colitis, which is not as bloody.

Environment. Ulcerative colitis occurs most often in people living in cities and industrial nations.

Ethnicity/ancestry. Jews of European descent are five times more likely to develop colitis or Crohn's disease.

Family history. 15 to 20 percent of patients have a close relative with the disease.

What you can do: Know your risk factors. Ulcerative colitis increases the risk of colorectal cancer, so make sure to get prompt treatment for the condition. For more information, type ULCERATIVE COLITIS into an Internet search engine.

Hemorrhoids

Risk factors include:
- Childbirth
- Constipation
- Pregnancy

Rectal Conditions That Tend to Run in Families

There are no known genetic links for these conditions:
- Colorectal cancer
- Colorectal polyps
- Ulcerative colitis

Risky Behavior and Possible Consequences	
RISKY BEHAVIOR	**POSSIBLE CONSEQUENCES**
Obesity	Hemorrhoids
Smoking	Colorectal polyps
Diets high in fat	Colorectal cancer
Diets low in fiber	Colorectal cancer
Rectal intercourse	Anal cancer, proctitis (rectal inflammation)
Infection with human papillomavirus (HPV)	Anal cancer
Prolonged sitting during bowel movements	Hemorrhoids

Visit www.healthwatchguide.com for updates on the rectum.

NOTES

The Skin

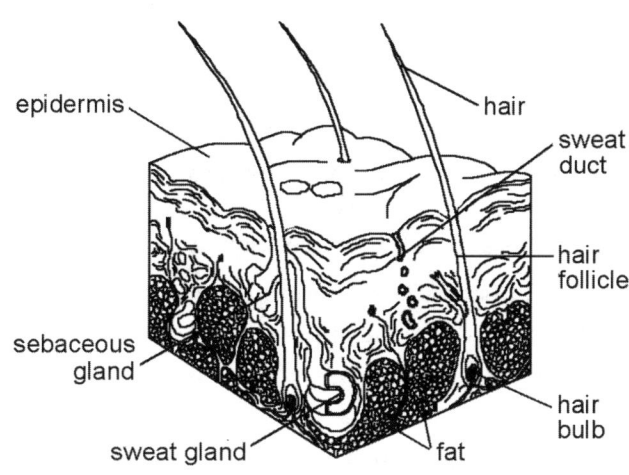

Function

The skin covers the entire body, except for the eyeballs, and it is the body's largest organ. It is designed to protect the inner organs from harm due to heat, injury, infection, and sunlight. The skin stores water and fat, helps regulate body temperature, and produces vitamin D.

Keeping the Skin Healthy

- Never go outside—even in the winter, or on cloudy days—without wearing sunscreen, a hat, a long-sleeved shirt, and long pants. Use sunscreen on your lips, too. The Australians have a saying: "Slip (on a shirt), slap (on a hat), slop (on sunscreen)." However, ten to fifteen minutes of unprotected exposure to the sun each day is important for melatonin and vitamin D production.
- Make sure your hat protects your ears and the back of your neck as well as your face.
- Eat a balanced diet.
- Children are very vulnerable to sunburn and are not immune to melanomas. Monitor their time in the sun and make sure they are well covered with clothes or sunscreen and sunglasses.
- Avoid being out in the midday sun (from 10:00 A.M.–3:00 P.M.).
- Perform a regular monthly skin self-exam. Become familiar with all of your moles, birthmarks, and blemishes so you are able to recognize changes if they occur. The best time to do this is right after a bath or shower, in the nude. Use a hand mirror to examine your back and any other hard-to-see places. Remember to look on your scalp, between your toes, in your genital area, and between your buttocks. Don't be shy about this—it's your body, and no one should know it as well as you. Catching a problem early is the best way to deal with it.

What You and Your Doctor Should Know

- Your family history of melanoma
- Your personal history of melanoma

Beneficial Foods and Nutrients

See Part Four, The Importance of Nutrients, for a list of foods containing the vitamins and trace elements mentioned in this section.

Vitamin A
Vitamin A is necessary for healthy skin.

Vitamin B_2 (Riboflavin)
Riboflavin is necessary for healthy skin.

Vitamin B_3 (Niacin)
Niacin is necessary for healthy skin tissue.

Vitamin B_6
Vitamin B_6 helps prevent acne.

Vitamin C
Vitamin C promotes wound healing.

Vitamin E
Vitamin E helps to heal burns.

Definitions of Terms

SPF (sun protection factor)—A sunscreen with SPF 20 will give you twenty times more protection from the sun than no sunscreen at all. The lighter your skin, the higher the SPF you need.

Moles—also called **nevi** (one nevus, two nevi). These benign growths are very common; most people have between ten and forty. They can be flat or raised, and flesh-colored, pink, tan, or dark. They can be present at birth or appear later, usually before age forty. As you age they may fade away. Moles can be surgically removed and usually do not come back.

Copper
Copper is necessary for skin pigmentation.

Manganese
Manganese assists with wound healing.

Zinc
Zinc assists with wound healing.

Other Tips

- Treat even minor cuts and scrapes promptly with an antibacterial ointment. Note that Mercurochrome and Merthiolate contain mercury and are not good choices for putting on wounds. Use rubbing alcohol for sterilizing needles or tweezers, not for cleaning or treating wounds. Hydrogen peroxide and iodine damage the skin, and iodine also slows the healing process, so use soap and water instead to cleanse wounds.
- Breastfed infants are less likely to develop eczema. The risk of eczema is further reduced if the nursing mother avoids drinking cow's milk. Eggs, fish, peanuts, and soy in the mother's diet may also be culprits.
- Apply insect repellents containing DEET to clothing, not skin.
- Use extra sunscreen and reapply it more frequently than usual if you also are using DEET products on your skin, as the DEET reduces the sunscreen's effectiveness.

What Can Go Wrong

Melanoma (Skin Cancer)

Melanoma is cancer of the melanocytes (pigment-carrying cells). This is the most frequently diagnosed cancer for whites between the ages of twenty-five and twenty-nine. The following factors increase your risk of developing melanoma.

Age. Half of all cases are between ages twenty and forty.

Blood types. Type O has a higher risk; types A, B, and AB have a moderate risk.

Family history. A family history increases risk.
- Familial dysplastic nevus syndrome is an inherited condition. The risk of melanoma is 100 percent if someone inherits this condition and has a family member with melanoma.
- Having two or more members of a family with melanoma increases the risk for other relatives.

Gender. The risk is equal for men and women.

Medical conditions. These conditions increase risk:
- Weakened immune system from certain cancers or from immunosuppressant drugs following organ transplants
- AIDS

Occupation. Three or more years in an outdoor summer job as a teenager or excessive exposure to strong sunlight as an adult increases risk.

Personal history. These conditions increase risk:
- Having had one melanoma
- Three or more sunburns that blister before age twenty
- Having more than fifty moles—the greater the number of moles, the greater the risk of one becoming cancerous
- Having a number of atypical birthmarks
- Significant freckling on the upper back

Pigmentation. People of all skin colors are at risk of melanoma, but the risk doubles if you have the following:
- Blonde or red hair
- Blue eyes
- Fair complexion
- Freckling

Note: Melanoma is rare in dark-skinned people but can occur, usually under fingernails and toenails or on the palms of the hand or the soles of the feet.

What you can do: Know your personal and family history. If you are at high risk, learn the symptoms of melanoma and enlist the support of a good dermatologist. Minimize your controllable risks. For more information, type SKIN CANCER or MELANOMA into an Internet search engine.

Basal Cell or Squamous Cell Carcinoma

Approximately 1 million people are diagnosed with basal cell or squamous cell carcinoma each year in the United States. Basal cell and squamous cell carcinomas are tumors that result from changes in normal skin cells. They often first appear as a change in a mole, wart, or birthmark. The predominant cause is overexposure to sunlight. The following factors increase your risk of developing nonmelanoma skin cancer.

Age. Diagnosis usually occurs after age fifty, but the damage is done at a much earlier age.

Chemical exposure. Exposure to arsenic, possibly in herbicides, is a risk factor.

Ethnicity/ancestry. People with fair complexions have a greater risk than those with dark skin. Freckles, blue or green eyes, and red or blonde hair are all risk factors.

Gender. Slightly more men than women have been diagnosed, possibly because of outdoor occupations and sports activities, but women are at an equal risk.

Habitat. Areas with high amounts of UV radiation, such as deserts, mountains, and areas close to the equator, increase risk.

Radiation. Overexposure to x-rays is a risk factor.

What you can do: Know your skin. Know your risk factors and minimize your controllable risks. Don't take chances with the sun. Conduct regular skin examinations and report anything unusual to your doctor or dermatologist. For more information on symptoms and treatment, type SKIN CANCER into an Internet search engine.

Sarcoidosis

Sarcoidosis is an inflammation that can affect the skin. The cause is unknown. The following factors increase your risk of developing sarcoidosis.

Age. Most at risk are people thirty to fifty years old.

Blood types. Type A has a moderate-to-high risk for the most severe form of the disease. Types B, AB, and O have a low-to-moderate risk. Nonsecretors have a moderate-to-high risk.

Ethnicity/ancestry. In order of risk: African, northern European, Japanese, and Irish.

Family history. This disease may run in families.

Gender. Women have the greatest risk.

What you can do: Know your risk factors. If this disease runs in your family, be sure to tell your doctor. For more information, type SARCOIDOSIS into an Internet search engine.

Skin Conditions That Tend to Run in Families

There are no known genetic links for these conditions:

- Allergies. Common ones are:
    - Drug allergies—penicillin, sulfa, aspirin
    - Food allergies—shellfish, eggs, nuts, strawberries, tomatoes
- Eczema
- Ichthyosis vulgaris
- Lamellar ichthyosis
- Melanoma
- Psoriasis
- Sarcoidosis
- Seborrheic dermatitis
- Vitiligo

Medical Conditions That Can Affect the Skin

It is important to properly treat any medical condition with which you are diagnosed, because the condition may affect other parts of your body. The body's organs and systems are inextricably connected to one another, and what goes wrong in one part may create problems in another. Conditions that can affect the skin include:

- *Gilbert's syndrome*
- *Hepatitis*
- *Hypothyroidism*

Risky Behavior and Possible Consequences	
RISKY BEHAVIOR	**POSSIBLE CONSEQUENCES**
Regular, prolonged sunbathing, frequent sun burns, use of tanning beds	Premature aging of the skin, skin cancer, sun allergy
Exposure to chemicals	Rashes
Sunburns that blister badly before age twenty	Doubles the risk of skin cancer
Stress	Hives, eczema

Visit www.healthwatchguide.com for updates on the skin.

NOTES

The Spine

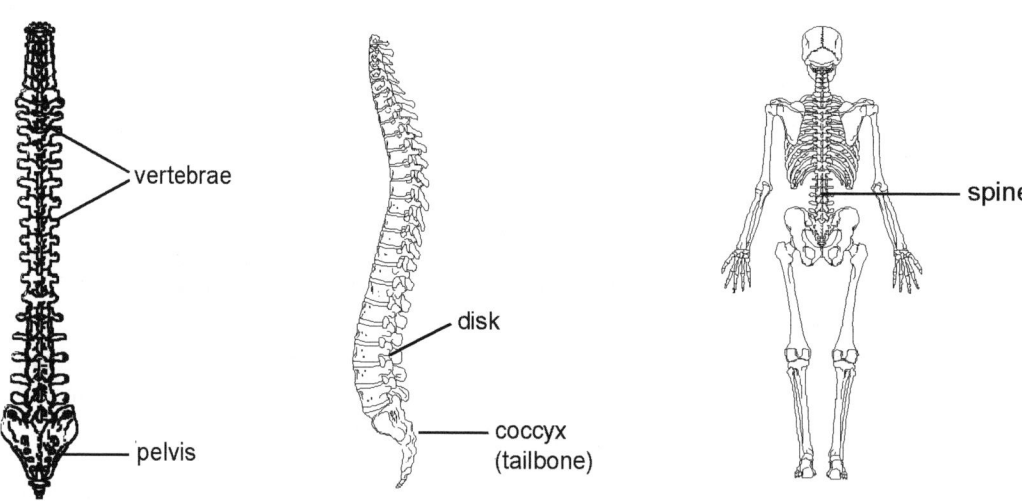

Function

The spine is a flexible column of bones called vertebrae, which stack one on top of the other from the neck to the tailbone. The spine's primary function is to protect the spinal cord, the major nerve that transmits messages between the brain and every part of the nervous system. If a vertebra is misaligned, it can negatively affect the nerve that extends from it to a specific body part. Vertebrae are separated by disks—shock-absorbing materials made of cartilage. Many of the body's muscles are attached to the spinal column.

Keeping the Spine Healthy

- Maintain a proper weight—excess pounds put enormous pressure on your back.
- Lift loads with your legs, not your back.
- Sit up straight (grandmother was right)
- Stretch before strenuous activity
- Sit with your feet flat on the floor or raised on a

footstool—crossing your legs throws your back out of alignment.

Beneficial Foods and Nutrients

See Part Four, The Importance of Nutrients, for a list of foods containing folic acid.

Folic Acid (Folate)

Folic acid (folate) is used to prevent spina bifida. The dosage is 400 micrograms, or 0.4 milligrams daily. Women need to have enough folic acid in their systems before they become pregnant in order to protect their babies. Folic acid supplements should be taken daily as soon as girls become teenagers. Some studies suggest that men also need to have an adequate supply of folate in their systems before they father children. Most multivitamins contain the recommended daily allowance of folic acid.

Other Tips

The birth process puts a lot of stress on the baby's spine, flexible though it is. A chiropractic or osteopathic examination of your infant can identify misalignments affecting other parts of the body.

What Can Go Wrong

Ankylosing Spondylitis (AS)

This condition is a chronic inflammatory arthritis affecting the joints between the vertebrae. Some 20 percent of Americans over age twenty have ankylosing spondylitis. The following factors increase your risk of developing ankylosing spondylitis.

Age. AS usually appears between the ages of twenty and forty.

Blood types. There is equal risk in all types, but nonsecretors have the greatest risk.

Ethnicity/ancestry. Eskimo populations have a high incidence, followed by Japanese and blacks.

Family history. This condition is ten to twenty times more likely in close relatives of AS patients than in the general population.

Gender. Men have three times the risk of women.

What you can do: Because family history is a big predictor of the condition, it is important to be aware if it runs in your family. If it does, learn the symptoms in order to be able to seek early treatment. Affected people may test positive for the HCS-B27 antigen. For more information, type ANKYLOSING SPONDYLITIS into an Internet search engine.

Scoliosis

Scoliosis is a sideways curvature of the spine. It affects 2 to 3 percent of all teenagers. The following factors increase the risk of developing scoliosis.

Age. This condition is commonly diagnosed between ages ten and sixteen.

Family history. Idiopathic scoliosis, the most common form, has a strong hereditary link.

Gender. Girls are affected three times as often as boys.

Medical conditions. The following conditions are risk factors:
- Cerebral palsy
- Congenital deformity
- Muscular dystrophy
- Osteoporosis
- Polio
- Spina bifida

What you can do: Most children are routinely screened for scoliosis during middle school. Treatments are available, and some cases resolve without intervention. Be aware if scoliosis runs in your family, because you may want to have your child screened at an earlier age. For more information, type SCOLIOSIS into an Internet search engine.

Spina Bifida

This condition affects 1 in 2,000 babies. It is a congenital condition in which the bones of the spine fail to form completely, and the top of the bones are open, exposing some or all of the spinal cord. In spina bifida manifesta, a rare but severe form of this condition, the skin over the spine also does not cover the spinal cord. In spina bifida occulta (SBO), the mildest form, the skin forms properly and the defect is hidden (occulta). Some 10 to 24 percent of the population probably has SBO, unbeknownst to them. The following factors increase the risk of having spina bifida.

Blood types. Research suggests that blood type incompatibility, for instance, between a type O mother and a type A father, may be a risk factor for spina bifida. Mother and fetus incompatibility may also be a factor.

Conditions during Early Pregnancy. Excessive heat

exposure, for instance, from a sauna or high fever, is a factor.

Ethnicity/ancestry. British ancestry carries the greatest risk.

Family history. This condition runs in families. Having one child with spina bifida increases the risk for future babies.

Medical conditions. The following conditions are risk factors for having a baby with spina bifida:
- Diabetes
- Medications for treating acne or epilepsy

What you can do: Spina bifida runs in families, so knowing your family history is important. Even more important is making sure that both the prospective mother and father are getting an adequate supply of folic acid in their diets before pregnancy. The spine is formed in the first six weeks of pregnancy and malformations are irreversible, although there have been some successful attempts at spinal repair in utero. If you are thinking of becoming pregnant, ask your doctor to test your serum folate levels. For more information, type SPINA BIFIDA into an Internet search engine.

Spine Conditions That Tend to Run in Families

There are no known genetic links for these conditions:
- Ankylosing spondylitis
- Scoliosis
- Spina bifida

Risky Behavior and Possible Consequences	
RISKY BEHAVIOR	POSSIBLE CONSEQUENCES
Bad posture	Excess pressure on spinal disks can lead to herniated disks
Improper lifting techniques	Disk problems
Bad mattress	Disk problems
Obesity	Excess weight puts a lot of pressure on disks and increases the risk of having a baby with spina bifida
Excessive use of alcohol	Having a baby with spina bifida

Visit www.healthwatchguide.com for updates on the spine.

NOTES

The Stomach

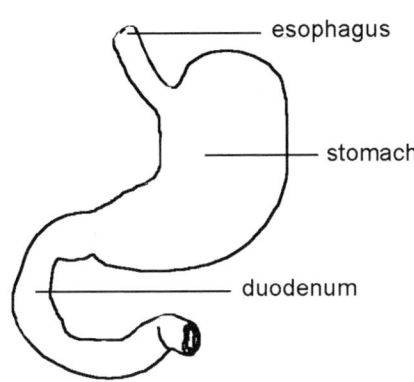

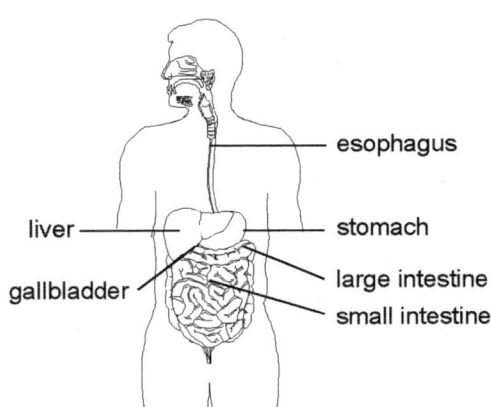

Function

The stomach continues the process of digestion, which begins in the mouth. Saliva starts to digest food when you take a bite and chew it, and hydrochloric acid and pepsin produced by the stomach break the particles down further. Intrinsic factor is produced to help the stomach absorb vitamin B_{12}. Hydrochloric acid is so strong it could blister your bare skin, but the lining of the stomach is protected from damage by an overlapping layer of mucus particles, which also help to lubricate food. Rhythmic contractions of the stomach muscles push digested food toward the intestines, where nutrients and waste are separated. It takes the stomach anywhere from one to seven hours to digest a meal, depending on what you have eaten.

Keeping the Stomach Healthy

- Avoid eating large quantities of foods that are salted, smoked, or pickled. Stomach cancer is very common in countries whose diets feature many such foods, including Latin America, parts of eastern Europe, Japan, and Korea. Eat fresh foods as often as possible.
- Exercising immediately after eating slows down the digestive process and may cause you to feel nauseated.
- Young children in households where iguanas are kept as pets have an increased risk of salmonella poisoning from a coating on the reptile's skin.
- Avoid eating charred meat, which can contain carcinogenic chemicals created during cooking.

Beneficial Foods and Nutrients

See Part Four, The Importance of Nutrients, for a list of foods containing the vitamins and minerals mentioned in this section.

Garlic
Hamburger cooked with one and a quarter teaspoon of garlic powder per pound has 90 percent fewer pathogens than ground meat cooked without the spice.

Prunes
One tablespoon of prune puree per pound of ground meat will work almost as well as garlic, without changing the taste.

Cinnamon
A teaspoon of cinnamon stirred into a gallon of unpasteurized apple juice will kill almost 100 percent of any *E. coli* present.

Peppermint
Peppermint oil (found in candies and mints) and peppermint tea help the digestive process and can help to reduce intestinal spasms and pain, but too much can contribute to GERD.

Green Tea
Green tea has been shown to kill harmful bacteria in the stomach and reduces by half the risk of chronic gastritis.

Vitamin A
Vitamin A contributes to the health of mucous membranes, which fight off bacterial infection.

Vitamin B_1 (Thiamine)
Thiamine aids digestion.

Vitamin B₃ (Niacin)
Niacin is necessary for a healthy digestive system.

Zinc
Zinc assists with digestion.

Other Tips

When you cook:
- Thoroughly wash fruits and vegetables to remove bacteria, fertilizers, and pesticides.
- Rinse meat and poultry with cold water to remove surface contaminants.
- Cook meats, poultry, and fish thoroughly to kill any internal bacteria or parasites, such as tapeworms.
- Use meat thermometers.
- Use separate cutting boards and knives for fruits/vegetables and meat/poultry. Never let juices from uncooked meat, poultry, or fish come into contact with fruits, vegetables, or cooked meats, fish, and poultry. This includes preparations in which meats have been marinating.
- Don't put cooked foods on the same platter you used for the raw foods.
- When cleaning up after a meal, wipe cutting boards and counter tops with a diluted bleach solution to kill germs.
- Take care not to let raw meat juices spill onto shelves or food in the refrigerator.
- Keep cold foods cold and hot foods hot—bacteria grow rapidly in a very short amount of time. Put the leftovers away first if you like to linger at the table and talk. Don't eat anything (for instance, at a picnic) that has been sitting at room temperature—potato chips excepted! Mayonnaise is a prime breeding ground for bacteria. Store-bought mayonnaise is more acidic than homemade, however, and *slightly* less risky for salmonella.
- Divide large amounts of hot foods into small storage containers and refrigerate. They will cool faster, and then you can safely freeze them.
- Thaw frozen food in a microwave oven, in the refrigerator, or under cold running water, NOT on the counter.

What Can Go Wrong

Stomach (Gastric) Cancer
There are 24,000 cases of stomach cancer diagnosed annually in the United States. The following factors increase your risk of stomach cancer.

Age. This cancer is found most often in people over age forty.

Blood types. Types A and AB have a higher risk; types B and O have a moderate risk.

Ethnicity/ancestry. In descending order of risk: Koreans, Vietnamese, Japanese, Alaska Natives, Hawaiians, white Hispanics, Chinese, blacks, Filipinos, and white non-Hispanics.

Note: Rates of stomach cancer are much higher in the native countries than when populations emigrate to the West. Eating a Western diet confers a Western (lower) risk. Countries with the highest risk are Japan, Chile, and Iceland.

Family history. The following increase risk:
- Chromosome 9q34 (an inherited feature) is tied to the stomach's ability to turn cancerous.
- Having a parent or sibling who has or had stomach cancer increases your risk of this cancer.

Gender. Men have twice the risk of women.

Medical conditions. These conditions increase risk:
- Achlorhydria
- Atrophic gastritis (Ménétrier's disease)
- Chronic gastritis
- Familial polyposis
- Gastric atrophy
- Gastric polyps
- *H. Pylori* infection
- Intestinal metaplasia
- Pernicious anemia

Personal history. Having had stomach surgery increases risk.

What you can do: Know your risk factors, and reduce your controllable risks. The most important of these are smoking and the overconsumption of smoked, salted, and/or cured foods. For more information, type GASTRIC CANCER into an Internet search engine.

Gastritis
Gastritis is a chronic inflammation of the stomach lining, affecting 1 in 5,000 people. The following factors increase your risk of developing gastritis.

Age. Most sufferers are over age sixty.

Blood types. Types A and AB have a higher risk; types B and O have a low-to-moderate risk.

Medical conditions. These conditions increase risk:
- Bile reflux
- Blood or lymph system disorders
- *H. Pylori* infection
- Pancreatic enzyme reflux
- Pernicious anemia
- Staph infections
- Stress
- Viral infections

Medications. The following increase risk:
- Prolonged use of NSAIDs (nonsteroidal anti-inflammatory drugs)
- Prolonged use of aspirin

What you can do: Know your risk factors. Chronic gastritis symptoms are similar to those of many other conditions, so you should make sure your doctor knows your health history, especially of pernicious anemia. For more information, type GASTRITIS into an Internet search engine.

Peptic or Gastric Ulcers

Ulcers are acid erosions of the lining of the stomach. The following factors increase your risk of developing stomach ulcers.

Age. Ulcers are most common over age fifty.

Blood types. Types A, B, and AB have a moderate risk, and type O has a higher risk. Nonsecretors of all types have a higher risk.

Gender. Men and women are equally affected.

Medical conditions. These conditions are risk factors:
- Abnormal types of bacterial flora
- Gastritis, which often occurs alongside benign peptic ulcers
- *H. Pylori* bacteria—cause of most gastric ulcers

Medications. The following increase risk:
- Prolonged use of NSAIDs
- Prolonged use of aspirin

Workplace. Nurses and gastroenterologists are at high risk for *H. pylori* infections, a risk factor for ulcers.

What you can do: Treat any ulcers caused by *H. pylori* and avoid aspirin or NSAID use if you have problems with gastritis. For more information, type GASTRIC ULCER into an Internet search engine.

Stomach Conditions That Tend to Run in Families

There are no known genetic links for this condition:
- Gastric cancer

Medical Conditions That Can Affect Stomach Health

It is important to properly treat any medical condition with which you are diagnosed, because the condition may affect other parts of your body. The body's organs and systems are inextricably connected to one another, so what goes wrong in one part may create problems in another. Medical conditions that can affect the stomach include:

- *Bacteria*
- *Mental stress*
- *Tumors*
- *Vertebral misalignment*
- *Viruses*
- *Worms*

Risky Behavior and Possible Consequences

RISKY BEHAVIOR	POSSIBLE CONSEQUENCES
Smoking	Stomach cancer, ulcers
Poor diet	Stomach cancer
Excessive consumption of smoked, salted foods	Stomach cancer
Careless food handling	Food poisoning (salmonella infection), cholera, diphtheria, shigella, typhoid fever
Excessive consumption of alcohol	Gastritis, ulcers
Excessive use of NSAIDs (nonsteroidal anti-inflammatory drugs)	Gastritis, ulcers
Exposure to radiation	Gastritis
Inadequate amounts of vitamins and minerals	Ulcers
Aspirin abuse	Ulcers
Excessive consumption of coffee	Ulcers
Being overweight, especially men	Stomach cancer
Chronic vomiting	Gastritis

Visit www.healthwatchguide.com for updates on the stomach.

NOTES

The Teeth

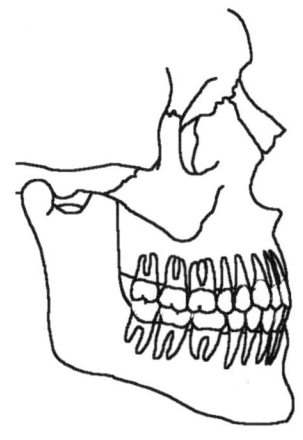
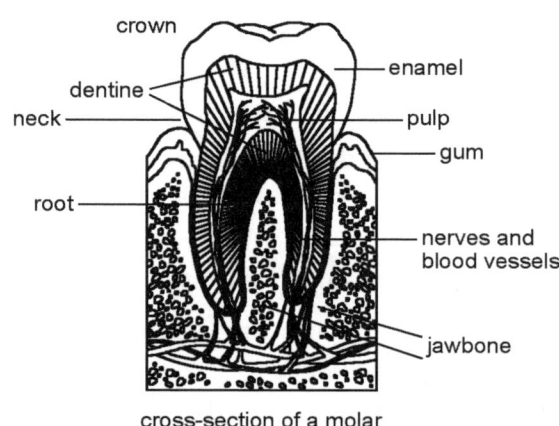

cross-section of a molar

Function

Teeth are the hardest structures in the body and serve several important functions. We use teeth to bite and chew our food, starting the process of digestion. And, along with the tongue, teeth help us form certain sounds necessary for speech.

Keeping the Teeth Healthy

Dental care begins at birth. When the baby is a few days old you can begin to wipe the gums gently with a soft, damp washcloth or piece of gauze. When teeth begin to emerge you can clean them with a tiny bit of toothpaste on one section of a very soft child's toothbrush. Begin to teach your children to brush at age two or three. A parent should begin to floss the child's teeth at this time. At around age eight the child can floss with adult supervision. Children should begin to visit the dentist by their second birthday.

- Brush after every meal.
- Never share your toothbrush.
- Using tap water, rinse the toothbrush thoroughly after each use.
- Let the toothbrush air-dry between uses, prefer-

ably in an upright position. *Note: storing the toothbrush in a closed holder allows the growth of bacteria.*
- Brush for at least two minutes—a lot of people use an egg timer.
- Replace the toothbrush when the bristles are worn or spread.
- It isn't necessary to disinfect toothbrushes, and putting them in the microwave or dishwasher can damage them.
- Floss to clean food and plaque from the spaces between teeth.
- See the dentist at least every six months.
- Avoid eating snacks that are sugary or sticky (even raisins). Incorporate sweets (when appropriate) into a meal, and brush soon after. Try to limit snacks to crisp vegetables, fruits, or popcorn.
- If you can't brush right after eating, chew sugarless gum for about fifteen minutes. This stimulates the production of saliva and reduces the risk of cavities.
- Rinsing with tea after brushing kills germs that cause bad breath and tooth decay.
- Baby bottle tooth decay is a serious problem for children under age three. It is caused by prolonged exposure to sugary substances. To prevent baby bottle tooth decay, take the following precautions:
  - Never put a baby to bed with a bottle of milk, formula, juice, or other liquid containing sugar. The liquids stay in the sleeping baby's mouth and coat the teeth.
  - Never put a sweet or sugary substance on a pacifier.
  - Don't let your child walk around sucking on a bottle.
  - Give your child a bottle of water if he or she needs to drink between feedings.
  - Replace the bottle with a cup by the first birthday.
- A mother with cavities and gum disease can pass oral microbes and bacteria through the placenta to the mouth of the unborn baby.

Beneficial Foods and Nutrients

Eat foods that encourage chewing. Chewing raw fruits and vegetables stimulates the gums and cleans away plaque. See Part Four, The Importance of Nutrients, for a list of foods containing the vitamins, minerals, and trace elements mentioned in this section.

Tea
One cup of green tea a day provides fluoride protection and kills bacteria that cause tooth decay. Black tea also kills germs that cause plaque to form and reduces the acids that lead to tooth decay.

Vitamin A
Vitamin A helps to maintain healthy teeth.

Vitamin B_6
Vitamin B_6 helps to maintain healthy teeth.

Vitamin C
Vitamin C reduces gum inflammation and strengthens gums.

Vitamin D
Vitamin D assists with calcium absorption in the teeth.

Calcium
Calcium is necessary for strong teeth.

Phosphorus
Phosphorus is needed for strong teeth.

Fluoride
Fluoride is a trace element that strengthens tooth enamel and helps to protect against cavities.

Other Tips
- Calcium deficiency contributes to tooth loss.
- Use a mouth protector if you participate in activities that could result in injury to your mouth or teeth. These activities include contact sports, of course, but a fall from a bicycle could chip or crack teeth, so talk to your dentist about your particular needs.

What Can Go Wrong
Caries (Cavities)
The following factors increase your risk of tooth decay and cavities:

Blood types. Type O has a higher risk, types B and AB have a moderate risk, and type A has a low-to-moderate risk. Nonsecretors of all types have a higher risk.

Family history. Being born to a mother with a tendency to have cavities is a risk factor. Oral bacteria can be transferred from mother to baby, both before and after birth. Babies' mouths can be infected with cavity-causing bacteria before the teeth emerge.

Medications. Several medications, including antihistamines, antidepressants, mood-altering drugs such as Ritalin, and heart medications reduce the amount of saliva you produce, increasing your risk for cavities.

What you can do: Minimize the consumption of chewy, sticky foods, as they cling to the teeth and encourage the growth of cavity-causing bacteria. Talk to your dentist about tooth sealants. For more information, type DENTAL CAVITIES into an Internet search engine.

Tooth and Jaw Conditions That Tend to Run in Families

There are no known genetic links for this condition:
- Prognathism

Medical Conditions That Can Affect Dental Health

It is important to properly treat any medical condition with which you are diagnosed, because the condition may affect other parts of your body. The body's organs and systems are inextricably connected to one another, so what goes wrong in one part may create problems in another. Conditions that may affect dental health include:

- *Allergies*
- *Diabetes*—having type II diabetes increases the risk of developing periodontal disease.
- *Dry mouth*—saliva lubricates your mouth, helps to wash food away from teeth and gums, and works to counteract the acids produced by plaque. Certain medications, such as antihistamines, can contribute to dry mouth. Talk to your dentist about methods to help restore saliva flow.
- *Heart disease*
- *Osteoporosis*—bone loss and tooth loss are closely linked. Some studies suggest that tooth loss in the lower jaw is an early indicator of impending osteoporosis.
- *Pregnancy*
- *Stress*

Risky Behavior and Possible Consequences	
RISKY BEHAVIOR	POSSIBLE CONSEQUENCES
Too much sugar in the diet	Cavities
A diet low in calcium	Cavities
Vitamin deficiency	Gum infections
Using chewing tobacco	Cavities, especially at the root level
Diabetics who smoke	Increases the risk of tooth loss by twenty times

Visit www.healthwatchguide.com for updates on the teeth.

NOTES

The Testicles

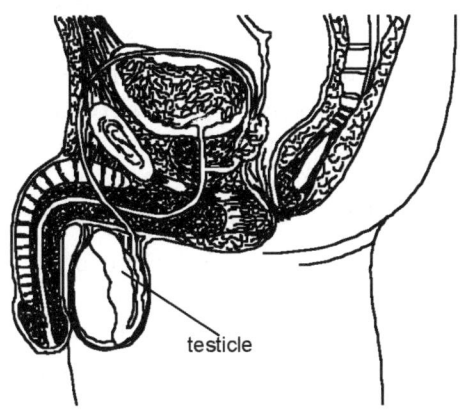
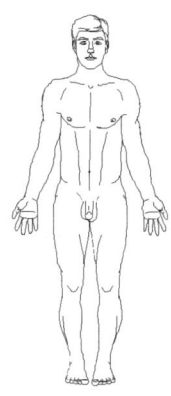

Function

The testicles are a pair of male sex glands located under the penis in a pouch called the scrotum. They produce and store sperm and are the body's primary source of male hormones, including testosterone and androgen. The testicles normally descend into the scrotum before birth.

Keeping the Testicles Healthy

- Protect against mumps-associated orchitis, an inflammation of the testicles that can lead to sterility, by being vaccinated against mumps.
- Use appropriate support and/or protection during athletic activities. Talk to your doctor or athletic trainer about the right kind of strap or cup to use.

Beneficial Foods and Nutrients

See Part Four, The Importance of Nutrients, for a list of foods containing the vitamins and trace elements mentioned in this section.

Vitamin A
Vitamin A is necessary for reproductive health.

Selenium
Selenium is necessary for healthy sperm cells and testosterone metabolism.

Zinc
Zinc supports sperm production.

Other Tips

A monthly testicular self-exam (TSE) is the best way to identify testicular cancer in its earliest stages.

How to perform a TSE: Right after a warm shower, when the skin of the scrotum is relaxed, gently roll the testicle between your thumb and fingers, feeling for a small, firm, painless lump or swelling. If you find one, call your doctor right away. Chances are that it is nothing more than a harmless cyst or enlarged blood vessel, but if it is cancer, early treatment is highly successful.

What Can Go Wrong

Testicular Cancer

Testicular cancer is the most common cancer in teenagers and young men. More than 7,000 cases are diagnosed annually. While the cancer cannot be prevented, early diagnosis and treatment can cure it in more than 95 percent of cases. The following factors increase your risk of developing testicular cancer.

Age. Most at risk are those aged fifteen to forty.

Ethnicity/ancestry. In descending order of risk: whites, Hispanics, Asians, Native Americans, and blacks.

Family history. Having relatives with testicular cancer increases your risk.

Personal history. Factors increasing risk include:
- Undescended testicle—risk remains even after surgery to place the testicle in the scrotum, and there is an increased risk of cancer in the other testicle, even if it descended properly
- Abnormal testicular development
- Cancer in one testicle increases the risk of developing cancer in the other
- Klinefelter's syndrome

What you can do: Know your personal risks. There are no standard medical screenings performed for testicular cancer, so make sure you perform a monthly self-exam. For more information, type TESTICULAR CANCER into an Internet search engine.

Hypogonadism

Hypogonadism is an inability of the testicles to produce testosterone and/or sperm. This condition affects two men per thousand. The following factors increase your risk of developing hypogonadism.

Age. This condition can occur during fetal development, in adolescence, or adulthood.

Personal history. The following factors increase risk:
- Having a mother who took diethylstilbestrol (DES) while pregnant with you
- Traumatic injury to the testes
- Treatment for cancer with chemotherapy or radiation
- Mumps that affect the testicles

Family history. A family history of hypogonadism may increase your risk.

Medical conditions. Conditions that increase risk include:
- Autoimmune disorders
- Disorders of the pituitary gland
- Hemochromatosis
- Hypothyroidism
- Kallman's syndrome
- Klinefelter's syndrome
- Sarcoidosis and other inflammatory diseases

What you can do: Minimize your controllable risks. Treat any medical conditions that are considered to be risk factors. For more information, type HYPOGONADISM into an Internet search engine.

Testicular Conditions That Tend to Run in Families

There are no known genetic links for this condition:
- Anorchism (missing one or both testicles)

Medical Conditions That Can Affect the Testicles

It is important to properly treat any medical condition with which you are diagnosed, because the condition may affect other parts of your body. The body's organs and systems are inextricably connected to one another, and what goes wrong in one part may create problems in another. Conditions that can affect the testicles include:

- *Mumps*—some 25 percent of boys or men who become infected with mumps will develop orchitis, an inflammation of the testicles that can lead to sterility in more than 50 percent of those affected. Immunization against mumps is the only way to prevent mumps-associated orchitis. The mumps vaccine is commonly given twice during childhood as part of the MMR (mumps, measles, rubella) series. See "Immunizations" in Part Two for more information.

Risky Behavior and Possible Consequences	
RISKY BEHAVIOR	**POSSIBLE CONSEQUENCES**
Unprotected sex resulting in an infection with chlamydia or gonorrhea	Orchitis
Multiple sexual partners	Orchitis
A sexual partner with a history of sexually transmitted diseases	Orchitis
Cigarette smoking	Decrease in sperm production
Alcohol abuse	Decrease in testosterone production
Excessive heat from saunas and hot tubs	Temporary decrease in sperm production (this is not a reliable form of birth control!)
Marijuana use	Hypogonadism

Visit www.healthwatchguide.com for updates on the testicles.

The Throat

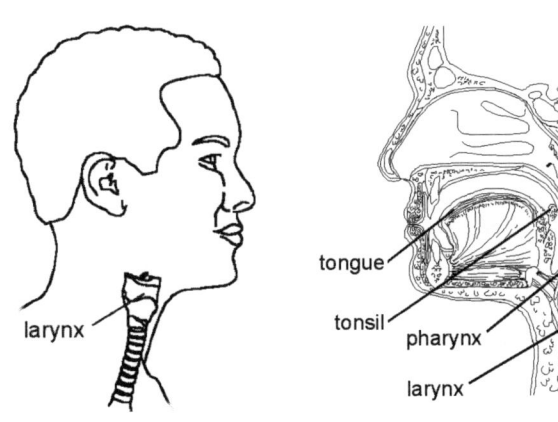

Function

The throat is the part of the digestive tract that connects the back of the mouth to the esophagus. It also is an important gateway in the immune system's barricades against infection. The tonsils are lymph nodes that trap germs trying to get into the body via the mouth and nose. Occasionally, the tonsils are dealing with so many germs that they become painfully swollen. The pain can be treated with analgesics, and possibly antibiotics, but removal is usually not recommended, because that would eliminate an important safeguard.

Keeping the Throat Healthy

- Avoid exposure to viruses, such as those that cause colds or influenza. These viruses are the most common causes of sore throats.
- Avoid exposure to bacterial infections, such as strep, as these can lead to rheumatic fever. Viral infections cannot be treated with antibiotics, but bacterial infections can, so if you suspect strep, seek treatment promptly.
- Keep your home, especially the bedrooms, well humidified during the dry winter months.

Beneficial Foods and Nutrients

See Part Four, The Importance of Nutrients, for a list of foods containing the vitamins and trace elements mentioned in this section.

Vitamin A
Vitamin A contributes to the health of the immune system.

Vitamin C
Vitamin C helps to ward off colds.

Zinc
Zinc strengthens the immune system.

Other Tips

People who smoke and drink heavily are putting themselves at a severe risk for cancer of the larynx.

What Can Go Wrong

Cancer of the Larynx and Hypolarynx

About 12,000 new cases are diagnosed each year in the United States. The following factors increase your risk of developing cancer of the larynx or hypolarynx.

Age. People aged fifty-five and over are most at risk.

Blood types. Types A and AB have a higher risk; types B and O have a moderate risk.

Ethnicity/ancestry. This cancer is more common in blacks than in whites.

Gender. This disease is ten times more common in men than in women.

Workplace. Exposure to asbestos is a risk factor.

What you can do: First of all, don't use tobacco. Smoking and/or excessive alcohol use are the two biggest risk factors for throat cancer. For more information, type THROAT CANCER into an Internet search engine.

Streptococcal Pharyngitis (Strep Throat)

Strep throat is most common in the winter months, especially in communities of people, such as businesses, schools, and day-care centers. Strep germs are spread through direct contact with nasal secretions or saliva. The following conditions increase your risk of developing streptococcal infections.

Age. People aged five to fifteen are most at risk.

Blood types. Type B has a higher risk; types A, AB, and O have a moderate risk.

What you can do: Strep infections can lead to rheumatic fever, which can have dangerous consequences. Avoid exposure to people with possible strep infections. Wash your hands thoroughly after touching any surface that may have been touched by someone else. Don't share silverware or cups. For more information, type STREPTOCOCCAL PHARYNGITIS into an Internet search engine.

Risky Behavior and Possible Consequences	
RISKY BEHAVIOR	POSSIBLE CONSEQUENCES
Smoking	Cancer of the larynx or throat
Excessive use of alcohol	Cancer of the larynx or throat

Visit www.healthwatchguide.com for updates on the throat.

NOTES

The Thyroid

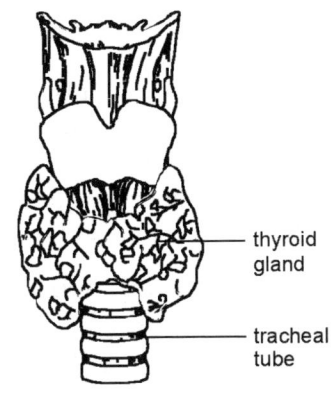
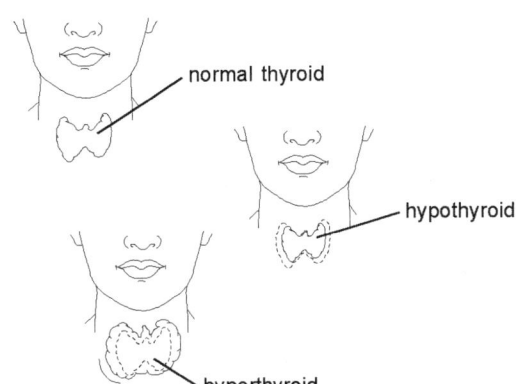

Function

The thyroid, a quarter-sized, butterfly-shaped gland, is located at the front of the neck, just beneath the larynx. It produces thyroid hormone, which affects heart rate, body temperature, energy level, and the oxidation rate of food products in the body's cells. The amount of hormone released is controlled by the pituitary gland.

Keeping the Thyroid Healthy

What You and Your Doctor Should Know

- Family history of thyroid cancer
- Personal history of radiation therapy

Beneficial Foods and Nutrients

See Part Four, The Importance of Nutrients, for a list of foods containing the trace elements mentioned in this section.

Iodine

Iodine is a key component in thyroid hormones. Lack of iodine can cause mental retardation and goiter.

Selenium

Selenium is used by the thyroid gland.

What Can Go Wrong

Thyroid Cancer

There are several forms of thyroid cancer. Each year in the United States some 15,000 cases are diagnosed in women, and 4,600 in men. The following factors increase the risk of developing thyroid cancer.

Age. This cancer is most common between ages twenty-five and sixty-five.

Blood types. Types A, B, and AB have a higher risk; type O has a moderate risk.

Note: Type A individuals with a history of thyroid tumors (benign or malignant) may have a very high risk of developing colon cancer.

Ethnicity/ancestry. In descending order of risk: Asians/Pacific Islanders, whites, Hispanics, blacks, and Native Americans/Alaska Natives.

Family history. The following factors increase risk:
- A history of familial medullary thyroid cancer, also called multiple endocrine neoplasia (MEN) syndrome
- A close relative with goiter

Gender. Women have two to three times the risk of men.

Genetic risks. Thyroid cancer can be caused by an altered gene (RET) that is passed from parent to child. Inheritance of this gene almost guarantees thyroid cancer.

Medical history. The following procedures increase risk:
- Radiation treatments for conditions in the head, neck, and throat
- X-ray analysis of tonsillitis conditions (common in the mid-to-late 1950s)

Personal history. Exposure to large doses of radiation, such as radioactive fallout, increases your risk. This fallout contains radioactive iodine, which collects in the thyroid.

What you can do: Know your family history! If thyroid cancer or goiter runs in your family, be sure to tell your doctor about it, as well as your personal history of radiation therapy. If appropriate, get genetic testing. Minimize your controllable risks. For more information, type THYROID CANCER into an Internet search engine.

Hyperthyroidism

Hyperthyroidism is caused by an overactive thyroid. The following conditions increase your risk of developing hyperthyroidism.

Blood types. Type O has a high risk; types A, AB, and B have a moderate risk. Nonsecretors of all types have a higher risk.

Medical conditions. These conditions are risk factors:
- Benign growths on the thyroid or pituitary glands
- Graves' disease (an autoimmune disorder that affects the thyroid, and the most common form of hyperthyroidism)
- Inflammation of the thyroid caused by infection
- Ingesting too much iodine
- Ingesting too much thyroid hormone
- Tumors on the testicles or ovaries

What you can do: There is no way to prevent hyperthyroidism, but treating conditions that can lead to hyperthyroidism is an important step. For more information, type HYPERTHYROIDISM into an Internet search engine.

Hypothyroidism

Hypothyroidism is caused by an underactive thyroid. The most common form is Hashimoto's thyroiditis, an immune system disorder. The following conditions increase your risk of developing hypothyroidism.

Age. Patients are usually over age fifty.

Blood types. For Hashimoto's thyroiditis: type O has a higher risk, type A has a moderate-to-high risk, and types B and AB have a moderate risk. For other forms of hypothyroidism: type A has a higher risk, and types B, AB, and O have a moderate risk.

Family history. This disease runs in families.

Gender. Women have eight times the risk of men.

Medical conditions. These conditions increase risk:
- Autoimmune disease—the body makes antibodies to the thyroid gland
- Congenital defect
- Disorder of the pituitary gland
- Inflammation of the thyroid caused by infection
- Radiation treatments of the throat and neck
- Removal of the thyroid gland

What you can do: This condition cannot be prevented, but it can be treated. Newborns can be screened for congenital hypothyroidism if there are symptoms present. For more information, type HYPOTHYROIDISM into an Internet search engine.

Thyroid Conditions That Tend to Run in Families

These conditions have no known genetic links:
- Chronic thyroiditis (Hashimoto's thyroiditis)
- Goiter
- Multiple endocrine neoplasia (MEN) II

Medical Conditions That Can Affect Thyroid Health

It is important to properly treat any medical condition with which you are diagnosed, because the condition may affect other parts of your body. The body's organs and systems are inextricably connected to one another, and what goes wrong in one part may create problems in another.

- *Depression* is associated with hypothyroidism. Lithium, which is used to treat depression, frequently causes hypothyroidism.
- *Stress* has been linked to thyroid disease.
- *Autoimmune diseases* often seen with thyroid disease:
  - *Addison's disease*
  - *Diabetes mellitus*
  - *Lupus*
  - *Pernicious anemia*
  - *Rheumatoid arthritis*
  - *Sjögren's syndrome*

Risky Behavior and Possible Consequences	
RISKY BEHAVIOR	**POSSIBLE CONSEQUENCES**
Extremely low-calorie diet	Thyroid disease
Lack of sufficient iodine in the diet	Goiter (a swollen thyroid) and hypothyroidism
Obesity	Hypothyroidism

Visit www.healthwatchguide.com for updates on the thyroid.

NOTES

The Urinary Tract

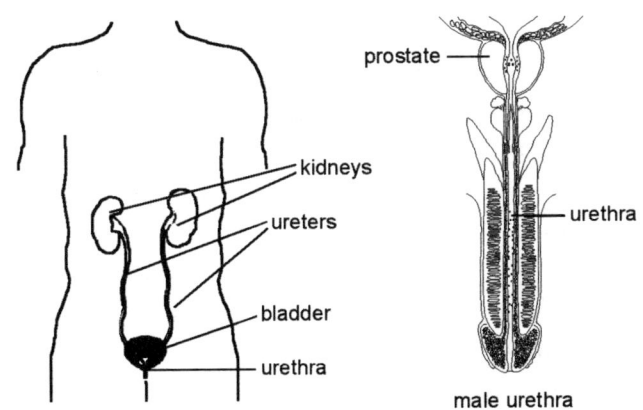

male urethra

Function

The urinary tract consists of the kidneys, the ureters (the tubes that run from the kidney to the bladder), the bladder, and the urethra (the tube that runs from the bladder to the outside of the body). Infections can occur at any point along this chain, so it is important to keep all of the components healthy. The urinary tract collects body wastes by filtering them out of the blood supply as it passes through the kidneys. The wastes are combined with water to form urine, which passes through the ureters to the bladder where the urine is stored until the bladder is emptied. The average adult passes about a quart and a half of urine daily.

Keeping the Urinary Tract Healthy

Urine is normally sterile—it contains no bacteria. Bacteria get into the urinary tract from the kidneys (this is more common in infants, whose filtration systems are immature, but is rare in adults) and from the outside world.

The body has a very good defense system to prevent external bacteria from getting to the urethra, the bladder, the ureters, and the kidneys. The urethral sphincter squeezes shut after urination, and the urethra is fairly long, making it difficult for bacteria to travel upward. The bladder is usually completely emptied at urination, flushing out bacteria with the flow of urine. In men, the prostate gland produces a substance that slows bacterial growth.

However, any activity that pushes bacteria into the urethral opening can put you at risk of a urinary tract infection. For instance, wiping from back to front rubs feces right over the urethral opening. For women, intercourse presses the external urethral tissue into the opening. Tight clothing, nylon crotches in underwear, and unchanged sanitary napkins all create a moist environment that encourages the growth of bacteria, and friction can result in raw patches on urethral tissue, which are susceptible to infection. Urinary tract infections can lead to more serious infections affecting the bladder, the ureters, and the kidneys.

- Wear cotton underwear, or underwear with cotton crotches.
- Don't wash underclothes with strong detergents or bleach.
- Drink six to eight glasses of water or other fluids daily. This keeps the whole urinary tract system adequately flushed and diluted.
- Urinate when you feel the urge. Holding back can be painful as the bladder fills, and it allows bacteria to breed to very unhealthy levels.

Women:

- Practice good personal hygiene. Blot or wipe gently from front to back after urination or a bowel movement. This helps to avoid spreading germs from your rectum to your vagina or urethra.
- Urinate and cleanse the genital area both before and after intercourse—but don't douche!
- Change sanitary napkins at least twice a day during your period.
- Use showers instead of tub baths.

Beneficial Foods and Nutrients

See Part Four, The Importance of Nutrients, for a list of foods containing the vitamins mentioned in this section.

Cranberry Juice

Cranberry juice contains acids that have been shown to fight the bacteria that cause urinary tract infections.

Vitamin A

Vitamin A contributes to the health of mucous membranes which fight off bacterial infection.

Vitamin C

Vitamin C contains ascorbic acid, which helps to kill germs.

Other Tips

- Wear protective clothing if your work environment exposes you to chemicals.

Women:

- If you wear pads during your period, change them at least twice a day. The warm, moist environment provides a perfect breeding ground for bacteria that cause bladder infections.

What Can Go Wrong

Urethral Cancer

This is a cancer affecting the urethra—the tube that carries urine from the bladder for excretion from the body. This is a rare cancer, affecting about 600 people annually. The following factors increase your risk of developing urethral cancer.

Age. Affects ages thirteen to ninety, with the most common diagnosis at around age seventy.

Ethnicity/ancestry. This disease is more common in whites than in blacks.

Gender. Women are more commonly affected than men.

Medical conditions. The following conditions increase risk:

- Bladder cancer
- Chronic inflammation or infection of the urethra

What you can do: Know your risk factors. Minimize your risks for urinary tract infections. For more information type URETHRAL CANCER into an Internet search engine.

Urinary Tract Infections (UTIs)

The following factors increase your risk of developing urinary tract infections:

Age. A person's risk of UTIs increases as he or she gets older.

Blood types. Types B and AB have a higher risk; types A and O have a moderate risk. All nonsecretors have a higher risk.

Gender. Women are much more at risk for UTIs than men largely because the urethra is so much shorter. Children also are at risk for UTIs; these often are undiagnosed because very young children are unable to describe how they feel. Males who were not circumcised as newborns are at risk.

Medical conditions. The following conditions increase risk:

- Anything requiring catheterization or extended bed rest
- Benign prostatic hyperplasia
- Diabetes
- Pregnancy

What you can do: Practice good hygiene and minimize your controllable risks. For more information, type URINARY TRACT INFECTIONS into an Internet search engine.

Urinary Tract Conditions That Tend to Run in Families

The following conditions have no known genetic links:

- Bladder
  - *Enuresis (bed-wetting)*
  - *Recurrent cystitis*
- Kidneys
  - *Berger's disease*
  - *Goodpasture's syndrome*
  - *Lupus nephritis*
  - *Nephrolithiasis (kidney stones)*
  - *Wilms' tumor*

Medical Conditions That Can Affect Urinary Tract Health

It is important to properly treat any medical condition with which you are diagnosed, because the condition may affect other parts of your body. The body's organs and systems are inextricably connected to one another, and what goes wrong in one part may create problems in another. Conditions that affect the urinary tract include:

- *Chronic bacterial prostatitis* increases the risk of UTIs for men.
- *Congenital abnormalities of the urinary tract* are the usual cause of UTIs in children.
- *Diabetes*—changes in the immune system cause a higher risk of UTIs.
- *Kidney stones* increase the risk of UTIs for men.
- *Pregnancy*—women who develop a UTI during pregnancy are at greater risk of kidney infections.
- *Urinary obstructions*
- *Vesicoureteral reflux*

Risky Behavior and Possible Consequences

RISKY BEHAVIOR	POSSIBLE CONSEQUENCES
Using colored toilet paper, bubble bath, perfumed soaps, douches, feminine hygiene deodorants, deodorant tampons and napkins	Urinary tract infection
Wearing tight clothing, such as bodysuits, tight pants, or nylon panty hose without cotton liners	Urinary tract infection
Routinely holding back when you need to urinate	Urinary tract infection
Unprotected sexual intercourse	Urinary tract infection, urethritis
Using a diaphragm	Urinary tract infection
Using condoms with spermicidal foam	Urinary tract infection
Using unlubricated condoms	Urinary tract infection
Contracting AIDS (men)	Reiter's syndrome (urethral arthritis)
Becoming infected with chlamydia (men)	Reiter's syndrome
Rectal intercourse	Urinary tract infection, urethritis
Infections from STDs	Urethral cancer
Infection with human papillomavirus (HPV)	Urethral cancer
Inadequate fluid intake	Urinary tract infection

Visit www.healthwatchguide.com for updates on the urinary tract.

The Uterus

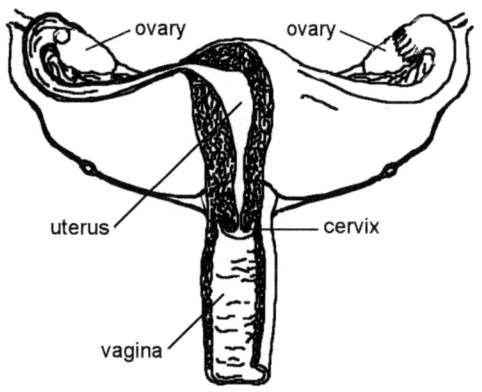

female reproductive tract (cross-section)

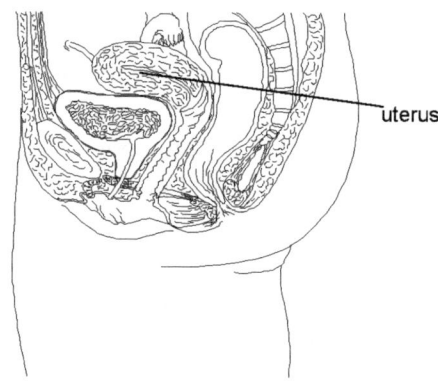

Function

The uterus, also known as the womb, is the reproductive organ in which the baby grows during pregnancy. It is located in the pelvic region, between the bladder and the rectum. Fallopian tubes run from the top of the uterus to each of the ovaries.

Keeping the Uterus Healthy

Excess estrogen is responsible for many cancers afflicting women. Estrogen is stored in the body's fat cells, so obesity is seen as a major risk factor for uterine cancer. Maintain a healthful weight.

What You and Your Doctor Should Know

Your personal history of:

- Childbirth
- Early menstruation
- Infertility
- Irregular periods
- Late menopause—over age fifty-five

Beneficial Foods and Nutrients

See Part Four, The Importance of Nutrients, for a list of foods containing vitamin A.

> **Definitions of Terms**
>
> **Fibroids**—benign tumors that very rarely develop into cancer. They are very common in women in their forties and usually need no treatment. They usually get smaller and sometimes disappear after menopause.
>
> **Endometriosis**—a benign, though sometimes painful, condition that occurs when bits of the endometrium (lining of the uterus) migrate to other parts of the body. As strange as it seems, this condition does not cause cancer.

Vitamin A

Vitamin A is necessary for healthy embryonic development.

What Can Go Wrong

Uterine or Endometrial Cancer

This is the most common gynecological cancer and the third most common cancer in women overall. Having increased levels of estrogen seems to be the biggest risk factor. The following factors also increase your risk of developing uterine cancer.

Age. This cancer is most commonly diagnosed in postmenopausal women between the ages of sixty and seventy, but it can occur earlier.

Blood types. Types A and AB have a higher risk; types B and O have a moderate risk. Nonsecretors of all types have the highest risk.

Ethnicity/ancestry. In descending order of risk: Hawaiians, whites, Japanese, blacks, Koreans, Vietnamese, and Native Americans.

Medical conditions. These conditions increase risk:
- Diabetes
- Endometrial hyperplasia
- Endometrial polyps
- Hereditary nonpolyposis colorectal cancer
- Hypertension (high blood pressure)
- Polycystic ovarian disease

Medications. Increased risk is associated with:
- Tamoxifen, used to treat breast cancer
- Drugs used to stimulate ovulation

Personal history. The following are risk factors:
- Early menstruation
- Infertility
- Irregular periods
- Late menopause—over age fifty-five
- Never having had children

What you can do: Know your risk factors. If you are on estrogen replacement therapy following menopause, be sure to follow your doctor's advice about checkups. Continue to have gynecological exams after menopause. The risks increase with age, so don't stop going to your ob/gyn or family doctor. Minimize your controllable risks. For more information, type ENDOMETRIAL CANCER into an Internet search engine.

Uterine Conditions That Tend to Run in Families

There are no known genetic links for this condition:
- Endometriosis

Risky Behavior and Possible Consequences	
RISKY BEHAVIOR	**POSSIBLE CONSEQUENCES**
Obesity	Uterine cancer
Using estrogen therapy with an intact uterus*	Uterine cancer
Hormone replacement therapy*	Uterine cancer

*Estrogen used in combination with progesterone does not increase the risk.

Visit www.healthwatchguide.com for updates on the uterus.

The Vagina

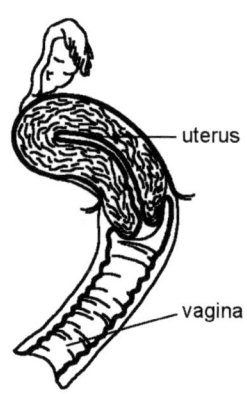
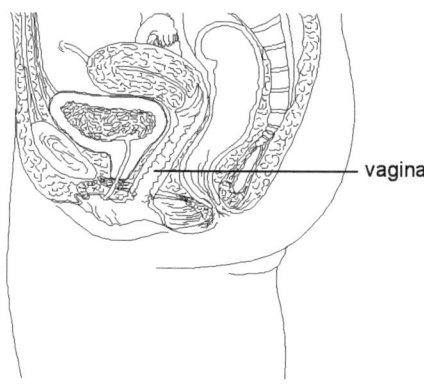

Function

The vagina is a muscular canal between the outside of the body and the cervix (the opening of the uteru). It is lined with mucous membranes that help to protect the body against bacteria.

Keeping the Vagina Healthy

- Avoid douching when possible. The vagina is designed to keep itself clean, and douching often kills beneficial bacteria, making it easier for infections to take hold.
- Practice good hygiene. Wipe from front to back after going to the bathroom to avoid pushing feces into the vagina.
- Replace tampons every couple of hours, and don't forget to remove the last one. Forgotten tampons are a common cause of vaginal infections.

What Can Go Wrong

Vaginal Cancer

Vaginal cancer—squamous cell vaginal carcinoma and clear cell vaginal adenocarcinoma—is a very rare primary cancer. Most vaginal cancers result from the spread of cervical or endometrial cancer.

Risk factors for squamous cell vaginal carcinoma include:

- Being over age fifty

- History of cervical cancer

Risk factors for clear cell vaginal adenocarcinoma include:
- Younger age at diagnosis, usually around nineteen
- Being born to a mother who took diethylstilbestrol (DES) during the first trimester

What you can do: Early detection can make a difference. Be sure to have annual Pap smears and pelvic exams. For more information, type VAGINAL CANCER into an Internet search engine.

Medical Conditions that Can Affect Vaginal Health

It is important to properly treat any medical condition with which you are diagnosed, because the condition may affect other parts of your body. The body's organs and systems are inextricably connected to one another, so what goes wrong in one part may create problems in another. The following conditions are risk factors for vaginal yeast infections:

- *Diabetes*
- *Pregnancy*
- *Sustained use of antibiotics*, especially tetracycline

Risky Behavior and Possible Consequences

RISKY BEHAVIOR	POSSIBLE CONSEQUENCES
Using oral contraceptives containing estrogen	Vaginal yeast infections
Infection with AIDS	Vaginal yeast infections
Wearing tight underwear or underwear with non-cotton crotches	Vaginal yeast infections
Abrasions of the vagina	Vaginal yeast infections
Intercourse with an infected partner	Trichomoniasis (a vaginal infection)
Becoming infected with an STD	Vaginitis

Visit www.healthwatchguide.com for updates on the vagina.

NOTES

ADDITIONAL NOTES

References

Blood Type Information

D'Adamo, Peter J., with Catherine Whitney. *The Eat Right for Your Type Complete Blood Type Encyclopedia.* New York; Riverhead Books, 2002.

Vitamin, Minerals, Trace Elements, and Food Information

The Food and Nutrition Board, The National Academies Institute of Medicine. http://www.iom.edu/iomhome/nsf/pages/Food+And+Nutrition+Board?OpenDocument.

Hendler, Sheldon S., and David Rorvik. *PDR for Nutritional Supplements.* Montvale, NJ: Medical Economics, Thompson Healthcare, 2001.

Higdon, J. V. (2001) *Vitamins, Minerals.* Oregon State University, Linus Pauling Institute Micronutrient Information Center. http://lpi.oregonstate.edu/infocenter/index.html.

Office of Dietary Supplements, National Institutes of Health. http://dietary-supplements.info.nih.gov/

Diseases and Medical Conditions

Centers for Disease Control and Prevention. http://www.cdc.gov.

MedLine Plus: Medical Encyclopedia, U.S. National Library of Medicine and the National Institutes of Health. http://www.nlm.nih.gov/medlineplus/encyclopedia.html

National Cancer Institute, National Institutes of Health. http://cancer.gov.

National Institute of Diabetes and Digestive and Kidney Disorders (NIDDK), National Institutes of Health. http://www.niddk.nih.gov.

Osteoporosis and Related Bone Diseases—National Resource Center, National Institutes of Health. http://www.osteo.org.

Index

Entries that appear in **bold** indicate forms.

A

Abetalipoproteinemia, 159
Acetaminophen, 253, 254, 258
Achalasia, 221
Acid rain, 215
Acne, 147
Acquired immunity, 238
Acrodermatitis enteropathica, 183
Acromegaly, 233
Acrylonitrile, 203
Acute otitis media (inner ear), 218
Addison's disease, 170, 304
Adenoids, 263
Adequate intake (AI), 145
Adrenal glands, 235, 236
Adrenaline, 234
Adrenocorticotropic hormone (ACTH), 235
Adult Immunizations, 68–75
Advanced Practice Nurse (A.P.N.), 141
African-Americans, 232, 257
AIDS (acquired immune deficiency syndrome), 211, 227, 239–240, 242, 261, 264, 265, 281, 307, 311
AIDS-related lymphoma, 265
Air-contrast barium enema, 42, 243
Air pressure, 217
Alcohol, 9, 145, 147, 149, 152, 156, 164, 168, 184, 189, 196, 198, 201, 202, 205, 208, 209, 211, 213, 219, 221, 230, 232, 234, 237, 243, 247, 250, 254, 257, 262, 266, 271, 273, 277, 279, 283, 284, 292, 295, 300, 302
Alcoholic neuropathy, 271
Aldosterone, 236
Alimentary canal, 243
Allergies, 218, 242, 261, 262, 272, 273, 289, 298
   drug, 289
   food, 238, 289
Allergies, 20

Aluminum hydroxide, 169
Alzheimer's disease, 158, 205
AMACR, 100
Amblyopia (lazy eye), 224, 227
Amebiasis, 247
Amphetamines, 234
Amyotrophic lateral sclerosis (ALS), 205, 268, 270
Androgens, 236, 299
Anemia, 41, 164, 189, 193, 216. *See also* Folate deficiency anemia; Iron deficiency anemia; Megaloblastic macrocytic anemia; Pernicious anemia; Sickle-cell anemia; Sideroblastic anemia; Vitamin B_{12} deficiency anemia.
Anesthesiologist, 141
Aneurysm, 213–214
Ankylosing spondylitis (AS), 262, 291, 292
Anorchism, 300
Anorexia nervosa, 201
Antacids, 144, 169, 175, 253
Antibacterial ointments, 288
Antibiotics, 8, 311
Antibodies, 190
Antigens, 190, 238
Antioxidants, 150, 155, 158, 202, 232
Anus, 284
Aortic insufficiency, 234
Apolipoproteins A, 231, 232
Apolipoproteins B, 231, 232
Arrhythmias, 234
Arsenic, 187, 188, 256, 258
Arteries, 212
Arthritis, 249, 250
   psoriatic (PA), 249, 250
   rheumatoid, 226, 230, 241, 248, 249, 250, 262, 304
   See also Osteoarthritis.
Artichokes, 255
Ascorbic acid. *See* Vitamin C (ascorbic acid).
Aspirin, 204, 205, 206, 218, 244, 258, 279, 284, 295

Asthma, 200, 239, 259–260, 263
Astigmatism, 223
Atheroembolic renal disease, 251–252, 253
Atherosclerosis, 214, 216, 233
Athletes, 179
Atrial myxoma, 233
Attention deficit disorder, 205, 206
Autism, 62, 205
Autoimmune diseases, 240–241, 304

B

Bacteria, 244, 259, 294, 295
Balance, 217
Barrett's esophagus, 221
Basal cell carcinoma, 288–289
Bed rest, 200
Bed-wetting. See Enuresis.
Beer, 277
Bell's palsy, 226
Benign hypermobility joint syndrome (BHJS), 248, 250
Benign prostatic hyperplasia (BPH), 283
Benzene, 196
Berger's disease, 253, 307
Beriberi, 149
Beta-carotene, 146, 147, 148, 178
Betel nuts, 266
Bicycles, 280
Bile, 228
Biotin, 161, 165
Biotin deficiency facies, 161
Bipolar affective disorder, 205
Birth control pills. See Oral contraceptives.
Bladder, 187–189, 305
    stones, 189
Bladder infection. See Cystitis.
Bleach, 244, 294
Bleeding disorders, 159
Blinking, 223
Blockages, 170
Blood, 190–196, 231, 242, 244, 251, 256
    coagulation, 159, 160
    clots. See Thrombosis.
    plasma, 190
    platelets, 190
    red cells, 190
    white cells, 190, 238, 241
Blood-clotting disorders, 159, 196. See also Thrombosis.
Blood pressure, 41, 42, 167, 172, 205
    high. See Hypertension.
    reading, 43, 212
Blood types, 5, 190, 191
    type A, 154, 190, 191, 241
    type AB, 190, 191
    type B, 190, 191, 192, 242
    type O, 159, 190, 191, 192, 242, 244
    See also Rh factor; Secretors and nonsecretors.
Body mass index (BMI), 6, 41
Bone Density Screenings, 77–78
Bone mineral density (BMD), 42, 77, 198
Bones, 158, 166, 175, 197–201
Bottle feeding, 218
Bowel movements. See Defecation.
Brain, 202–206
    damage, 176
    tumors. See Cancer, brain.
Breast Exams, 106–108
Breastfeeding, 9, 144, 158, 163, 169, 178, 184, 200, 207, 208, 217, 218, 242, 244, 275, 288
Breasts, 106, 207–209
    cysts, 207
    exams, 42, 106, 208
    self-exams, 106, 208
Breathing, 239
Bronchial tubes, 259
Bronchitis, chronic, 233, 260, 262
Burkitt's lymphoma, 264

C

Caffeine, 9, 144, 145, 149, 198, 213, 218, 219, 221, 234, 284, 295
Calciferol. See Vitamin D (calciferol).
Calcium, 144, 156, 166–167, 168, 169, 171, 175, 178, 179, 184, 192, 197, 198, 200, 201, 232, 236, 237, 239, 251, 252, 253, 267, 270, 284, 297, 298
Calories, 213, 231
Cancer, 43, 156
    adrenal cortex, 200
    anal, 286
    bile duct, 257
    bladder, 187–188, 189
    bone, 200
    brain, 203
    breast, 207, 208, 209
    bronchial, 262
    cervical, 210–211, 280
    colon, 42, 83, 243, 244, 245, 284, 303
    colorectal, 246, 247, 284, 285, 286, 286
    endometrial. See Cancer, uterine.

esophageal, 221
gallbladder, 228
gastric. *See* Cancer, stomach.
hypolarynx, 302
kidney, 252, 253
larynx, 302
liver, 256, 257, 258
lung, 260–261, 262
male breast, 209
nasal cavity. *See* Cancer, nasopharyneal.
nasopharyneal, 273
oral, 266
oropharynx, 266
ovarian, 275–276
pancreatic, 277, 279
penile, 280–281
prostate, 42, 43, 100, 282, 282–283
sinus. *See* Cancer, nasopharyneal.
skin, 5, 156, 281, 288, 289
stomach, 171, 221, 293, 294, 295
testicular, 3, 299–300
thyroid, 176, 303–304
urethral, 306, 307
uterine, 309
vaginal, 310–311
See also Basal cell carcinoma; Hodgkin's lymphoma; Leukemia; Melanoma of the eye; Multiple myeloma; Myeloma; Non-Hodgkin's lymphoma; Osteosarcoma; Squamous cell carcinoma.
Carbon dioxide, 190, 212
Cardiologist, 141
Cardiomyopathy, 234. *See also* Peripartum cardiomyopathy.
Caries, 297–298
Carpal tunnel syndrome, 229, 270
Cataracts
   adult, 224, 226, 227
   congenital, 224, 227
Cavities. *See* Caries.
Celiac disease, 200, 243, 244–245, 246
Certified Registered Midwife (C.N.M.), 141
Certified Registered Nurse Anesthetist (C.R.N.A.), 141
Cervical erosion, 211
Cervicitis, 211
Cervix, 210
Checkups, 7. *See also* Dental checkups.
Chemicals, 254
Chemotherapy, 200

Chicken pox, 63, 65, 206, 258
Childhood Immunizations, 66–67
Children, 202. *See also* Infants.
Chiropractor, 141
Chlamydia, 43, 189, 211, 227, 281, 283, 300, 307
Chlamydiae pneumoniae, 233
Cholangiocarcinoma. *See* Cancer, bile duct.
Cholera, 244, 247, 295
Cholesteatoma, 218
Cholesterol, 42, 79–80, 205, 212–213, 216, 229, 231, 232, 234, 253
   ratio, 79–80
Cholesterol Screenings, 80–82
Cholethiasis. *See* Gallstones (cholethiasis).
Choline, 162, 202, 213, 228, 232, 251, 255, 270
Choroiditis, 226
Chromium, 173, 255, 277
Chronic fatigue syndrome, 239
Chronic obstructive pulmonary disease (COPD). *See* Bronchitis, chronic.
Churg-Strauss vasculitis, 253
Cilia, 259, 272
Cinnamon, 244, 293
Circulatory system, 212–216
Circumcision, 280, 281
Cirrhosis. *See* Liver, disease.
Clear cell vaginal adenocarcinoma. *See* Cancer, vaginal.
Cleft lip, 266
Cleft palate, 266
Clinical Nurse Specialist (C.N.S.), 141
Clothing, 287, 305, 306, 307, 311
Cobalamin. *See* Vitamin B_{12} (cobalamin).
Cocaine, 206, 234
Coenzyme A, 165
Coffee. *See* Caffeine.
Colitis, 200
   ulcerative, 243, 246, 286
Colon Cancer Screenings, 83–85
Colonoscopy, 42, 83, 86, 243, 245
Colonoscopy, 86
Color vision deficiency, 226
Complete blood count (CBC), 191
Condoms, 189, 307
Cones, 222
Congenital hypothyroidism, 177
Congestion, nasal, 272–273
Conjunctivitis, 227
Constipation, 247
Contraceptive History, 23–24

Cooking, 244, 293, 294
Cookware, 175
Copper, 174, 183, 198, 223, 232, 239, 255, 270, 288
Corn, 144, 151
Cornea, 222
Cortisol, 235, 235, 236, 241
Coyotes, 254, 255
C-reactive protein, 212, 231
Cretinism. *See* Congential hypothyroidism.
Crohn's disease, 168, 200, 243, 246
Crutches, 269
Cushing's syndrome, 236
Cutting boards, 244, 294
Cyclophosphamide, 188
Cystic fibrosis, 159
Cystitis, 189, 190, 307
Cystoscopy, 188

D

Dairy products, 239. *See also* Milk.
De Quervain's disease, 230
Decongestants, 273
DEET, 288
Defecation, 243, 284, 286
Defects, genetic, 25–28
    autosomal dominant, 25, 27
    autosomal recessive, 25, 26
    chromosomal, 28
    congenital, 25
    X-linked, 25, 28
    X-linked dominant, 25, 28
    X-linked recessive, 25, 27
Dehydration, 170
Dementia, 205
Dental checkups, 10, 41, 42, 43, 87–88, 266, 296, 297
Dental Examinations and Treatments, 90–95
Dental Records—Baby Teeth, 87
Dental Records—Permanent Teeth, 88–89
Dental surgery, 232
Dentist, 141
Dentists—Dentists, Orthodontists, Endodontists, and Periodontists, 129–132
Dentures, 266
Depression, 205, 304
Dermatitis, 289
Dermatologist, 141
Diabetes, 42, 96, 168, 170, 173, 204, 206, 226, 219, 229, 230, 233, 253, 271, 275, 276, 277–279, 298, 304, 307, 311
    insipidus, 278–279
    type I (juvenile), 277–278
    type II (adult-onset), 278, 279
Diabetes mellitus. *See* Diabetes, type II (adult-onset).
Diabetes Screenings, 96–97
Diabetic retinopathy, 226
Diaphragm, 189, 307
Diarrhea, 168, 170, 244, 247
Diastolic number, 43, 212
Diet. *See* Nutrition.
Diethylstilbestrol (DES), 210, 211
Dieting, 152, 304
Digestive tract, 243, 250, 293, 301
Diphtheria, 62, 63, 64, 259, 262, 295
Disks, 290, 292
Diverticulosis, 247
Douches, 211, 306, 310
Down syndrome, 205
Drinks, soft, 253
Drugs, illicit, 205, 234, 242, 255, 257. *See also* Amphetamines; Cocaine; Marijuana.
Drugs, over-the-counter, 10
Drugs, prescription, 7–8, 9–10, 148, 149, 150, 151, 153, 154, 156, 158, 159, 160, 161, 162, 164, 165, 167, 169, 170, 175, 179, 180, 182
DTaP: Diphteria, Tetanus, Pertussis (whooping cough) vaccine, 62–63
Duodenum, 246
Dupuytren's contracture, 230

E

E. coli, 244, 253, 293
Ear infections, 218
Earlobes, 218
Ears, 217–219
Eczema, 288, 289
Eggs, 208
Ejaculations, 282
Emphysema, 262
Encephalitis, 202, 205
Endocarditis, 232
Endocrinologist, 141
Endometriosis, 309
Enteritis, 168
Enuresis, 188, 271, 307
Epilepsy, 205
Epstein-Barr infection, 264
Erectile dysfunction, 280
Erythroplakia, 266

Esophagus, 220–221
Essential tremors, 271
Estrogen, 77, 158, 166, 167, 197, 199, 207, 208, 235, 244, 274, 275, 308, 309, 311
Exercise, 3, 5, 10, 197, 201, 202, 208, 212, 231, 238, 243, 248, 251, 267, 277, 278, 284, 293
Exstrophy, 188
Eye Medical Records, 98
Eye Prescriptions, 99
Eye-Care Specialists—Ophthalmologists, Optometrists, and Opticians, 132–134
Eyes, 41, 42, 98, 222–227
   dry, 226, 227
   color, 223
   exams, 223
   See also Hyperopia; Myopia; Presbyopia; Vision, peripheral.
Eyestrain, 223

F

Fallopian tubes, 274, 308
Familial Mediterranean fever, 262
Family Medical History, 34–39
Family Practitioner, 141
Farsightedness. *See* Hyperopia.
Fascia, 230
Fat, 213, 216, 231, 247, 250, 253, 277, 279, 283, 286
Fatty acids, 231
   Omega-3, 213, 223, 232
Febrile seizures, 205, 271
Fecal occult blood test, 42, 83, 243
Feces, 226, 247, 255, 257, 284, 305, 310
Feet, 216
Fertility, 235
Fertilization, 274–275
Fetus, 231
Fiber, 213, 243, 247, 253, 277, 279, 284, 286
Fibroadenomas, 207
Fibroids, 309
Fibromyalgia, 240, 268
Fish, 244
   Cantonese salted, 273
   oil, 148
Flavonoids, 232
Flossing, 296, 297
Flu shots, 63, 64, 64, 259
Fluids, 9, 187, 189, 259, 284, 306, 307
Fluoride, 144, 175, 198, 297
Folate. *See* Folic acid (folate).
Folate deficiency anemia, 194–195, 196
Folic acid (folate), 9, 144, 153, 154, 192, 194–195, 202, 208, 213, 232, 244, 284–285, 291, 292
Follicle stimulating hormone, 235
Food, 143, 145, 297
   allium, 282
   diuretic, 251
   preparation, 243, 244, 247, 293, 294, 295
   See also Nutrition.
Footwear, 7
Foreskin, 280
Formaldehyde, 203
Foxes, 254, 255
Fractures, 201
Free radicals, 158, 174, 232, 242
Fruits, 5, 147, 220, 244, 255, 294, 297
   citrus, 248

G

G-6-PD deficiency, 156
Gallbladder, 228–229
   disease, 279
Gallstones (cholethiasis), 228
Garlic, 243–244, 293
Gastritis, 293, 294–295
Gastroenterologist, 141
Gastroesophageal reflux disease. *See* GERD (gastroesophageal reflux disease).
General Guidelines for Pregnant Women, 9–10
Generalist, 141
Genetics, 25–26
   screenings, 42
   testing, 9, 26
Genital herpes, 206, 281
Genital warts, 210, 280
Genitalia, ambiguous, 281
GERD (Gastroesophageal reflux disease), 220, 221, 243, 293
German measles. *See* Rubella (German measles).
Giant cell arteritis (GCA), 214, 216
Gilbert's syndrome, 289
Glaucoma, 223, 224–225, 226
Glucagon, 277
Glucose, 96, 173, 277
Gluten intolerance, 168
Goiters, 176, 177, 303, 304
Goitrogens, 176
Gonorrhea, 189, 281, 283, 300
Goodpasture's syndrome, 253, 307
Gout, 230, 249, 250
Graves' disease, 226, 241

Graves' opthalmopathy, 226
Growth hormone, 235
Gum, 297
Gynecologist, 141
Gynecomastia, 209

H

H. pylori, 233
Haemophilus influenza B, 63
Hamburger, 243–244, 293
Hands, 216, 229–230
    washing, 5, 9, 224, 247, 302
Hashimoto's thyroiditis, 241, 304
HCS-B27 antigen, 291
HDL (high-density lipoprotein), 79, 184, 213
Head, 41
Headaches, 202. *See also* Migraines.
Health
    managing, 7–8
    personal, 7, 10
Healthcare providers, 125–142
    definitions, 141–142
Hearing, 41, 42
    loss of, 219
Heart, 212, 231–234
    attack, 232, 233, 234
    disease, 170, 216, 231, 298
Heartburn. *See* GERD (gastroesophageal reflux disease).
Height, 41, 42
Hematocrit (HCT), 41, 191
Hemoccult test. *See* Fecal occult blood test.
Hemochromatosis, 156, 173, 179, 195–196, 205, 233, 257
    Sub-Saharan African, 257
Hemoglobin (HGB), 41, 177, 190, 191
Hemophilia, 159, 196
Hemorroids, 286
Hepatitis A, 255, 257
    vaccine, 63
Hepatitis B, 63, 64, 253, 256, 257, 258
    vaccine, 63, 64–65, 254, 255, 256
Hepatitis C, 255, 256, 257, 258
Hepatitis D, 255, 257
Hepatitis E, 257
Hepatocellular carcinoma. *See* Cancer, liver.
Hereditary conditions, 25–27
Hernia, 247
Herpes simplex, 226
Herpes zoster, 226

HIB: H. Influenza Type B vaccine, 63, 202
HIV (human immunodeficiency virus), 211, 240, 273
Hives, 289
Hodgkin's lymphoma, 263
Home safety, 10
Homeopath, 141
Homocysteine, 153, 154, 231, 232
Hookworms, 247
Hormone replacement therapy (HRT), 209, 276, 309
Hormones, 235–237
Hot tubs, 300
Human papillomavirus (HPV), 210, 211, 280, 281, 286, 307
Humidity, 239, 301
Hydrochloric acid, 293
Hydrogen peroxide, 288
Hyperactivity, 203
Hypercalcemia, 157, 167
Hyperglycemia, 173
Hypernatremia, 171
Hyperopia, 223
Hyperparathyroidism, primary, 200, 236–237
Hypertension, 206, 214–215, 216, 226, 231, 253, 278
Hyperthyroidism, 177, 304
Hypoglycemia, 173
Hypogonadism, 275, 300
Hypokalemia, 170
Hypospadias, 281
Hypothyroidism, 289, 304

I

Ichthyosis vulgaris, 289
Iguanas, 293
Immune system, 238–242
Immunizations, 7, 62–76
Immunologist, 141
Indoles, 282
Infants, 7, 158, 160, 174, 177, 178, 184, 218, 244, 288
    premature, 156, 169
Infections and/or Illnesses Requiring Medical Treatment, 14
Inflammation, 238
Influenza vaccine. *See* Flu shots.
Insect repellents, 288
Insulin, 96, 277
Insurance Companies, 138–139
Intern, 141

Internist, 141
Interstitial lung disease, 261, 262
Intestines, 243–247, 293
Intrinsic factor, 293
Iodine, 176–177, 182, 288, 303, 304
   allergy to, 177
IPV or OPV (polio) vaccine, 63
Iris, 222
Iron, 9, 144, 147, 155, 156, 166, 174, 177–179, 180, 183, 192, 194, 195, 196, 232, 239, 257, 259
   types, 178
Iron deficiency anemia, 178, 184, 194
Irritable bowel syndrome, 247
Isoflavones, 213
IV patients, 161, 174, 182

J

Joints, 248–250
Juices, 144
   apple, 244, 293
   cranberry, 187, 251, 306

K

Keshan disease, 182
Kidneys, 168, 251–253, 305
   disease, 170, 205, 233, 250, 253
   stones, 156, 166, 167, 237, 252, 253, 307

L

Lactose intolerance, 200, 246
Lamellar ichthyosis, 289
Laxatives 247
Lazy eye. *See* Amblyopia (Lazy eye)
LDL (low-density lipoprotein), 79, 213
Lead, 42, 206
Leber's disease, 154
Legionnaire's disease, 259
Lens, 222
Leukemia, 192–193, 196
Leukoplakia, 266
Licensed Practical Nurse (L.P.N.), 141
Licorice, 170
Lifestyle, 3, 5–8, 185, 201, 231, 234, 239, 247, 253, 271
Lifting, 290, 292
Ligaments, 248
Lipoprotein (a), 231
Lithium, 304
Liver, 254–258
   disease, 205, 229, 257, 258

Lou Gehrig's disease. *See* Amyotrophic lateral sclerosis (ALS).
Lungs, 259–262
   disease, 233
Lupus. *See* Systemic lupus erythematosus.
Lupus nephritis, 253, 307
Luteinizing hormone (LH), 235
Lycopene, 282
Lyme disease, 65
   vaccine, 65
Lymph nodes, 262
Lymphatic system, 238, 263–264
Lymphocytes, 263
Lymphoma, 244

M

Macula, 222
Macular degeneration, 225, 226, 227
Magnesium, 167–168, 180, 198, 213, 232, 268, 270
Malabsorption syndrome, 145
Mammograms, 42, 106, 207
Manganese, 180, 198, 255, 277, 288
Manic depression disorder, 205
Maple suger urine disorder, 205
Marfan's syndrome, 233
Marijuana, 205, 209, 300
Marrow, 197
Mastoiditis, 218
Mayonnaise, 244, 294
Measles, 62
Meat, 244, 293, 294
   raw, 244, 294
   See also Hamburger.
Medical conditions, 7–8
   fat-absorption, 157
   predisposition for, 29–33
Medical Conditions That Tend to Run in Families, 29–33
Medical Doctor (M.D.), 141
Medical history, 5, 11–40
   family, 5, 25–40, 185
   personal, 12–24, 185
Medical tests, 41–124
   children, 41–42
   adults, 42–43
   men, 100–102
   women, 103–123
Medicare/Medicaid Information, 140
Medications. *See* Drugs, prescription; Drugs, over-the-counter.

Megaloblastic macrocytic anemia, 153, 163
Melanin, 223
Melanocytes, 288
Melanoma. *See* Cancer, skin.
Melanoma of the eye, 225
Melatonin, 235, 244, 287
Membranous nephropathy, 252–253
Men's health, 188, 277
Ménière's disease, 218–219
Meningitis, 203, 205, 206
    vaccine, 64
Menkes' disease, 174
Menopause, 3, 77, 123, 274
Menstrual Record, 109–123
Menstruation, 109, 201, 275, 306
Mercurochrome, 288
Merthiolate, 288
Metals, heavy, 206, 271
Micropenis, 281
Migraines, 205
Milk, 179, 218, 288
    fortified, 157, 178
Mineral oil, 159
Minerals, 143–144, 166–172, 295
Mitral stenosis, 233
Mitral valve prolapse, 233
MMR: Measles, Mumps, Rubella (German Measles) vaccine, 62, 65, 300
Moles, 287
Molybdenum, 181
Mononucleosis, 264
Mouth, 265–266
Mouthwashes, 266
Movies, 203
Mucus, 218, 238, 239, 259, 272–273, 293
Multiple endocrine neoplasia (MEN), 279, 304
Multiple myeloma, 193
Multiple sclerosis (MS), 240, 270, 271
Mumps, 62, 299, 300
Muscles, 267–268
Muscular dystrophy, 268
Myasthenia gravis, 168, 240–241, 268
Myeloma, 199
Myocardial infarction. *See* Heart, attacks.
Myoglobin, 177
Myopia, 223

N

Naturopath, 141
Nearsightedness. *See* Myopia.

Nephrolithiasis. *See* Kidneys, stones.
Nephrologist, 141
Nervous system, 269–271
Neuralgia, 271
Neurofibromatosis type 2, 219
Neurogenic bladder, 189
Neurologist, 142
Neurosarcoidosis, 271
Neurosyphilis, 271
Nevi. *See* Moles.
Niacin. *See* Vitamin B_3 (niacin).
Night blindness, 223, 225
Noise, 217, 219, 271
Non-Hodgkin's lymphoma (NHL), 263–264
Nose, 272–273
NSAIDs (nonsteroidal anti-inflammatory drugs), 295
Nurse Practitioner (N.P.), 142
Nutrition, 3, 5, 9, 143–144, 172, 216, 231, 238, 242, 243, 253, 279, 286, 287, 293, 294, 297. *See also* Vegetarians.

O

Obesity, 3, 6, 189, 209, 211, 216, 229, 231, 234, 248, 250, 253, 257, 276, 278, 283, 286, 292, 295, 304, 308, 309
Obstetrician, 142
Olfactory cells, 272
Olivopontocerebellar atrophy, 205
Oncologist, 142
Ophthalmologist, 142
Optic nerve, 222
Oral contraceptives, 145, 165, 208, 209, 211, 216, 234, 275, 311
Orchitis, 299, 300
Orthodontist, 142
Orthopedist, 142
Osteitis fibrosa, 200
Osteoarthritis, 200, 249, 250
Osteomalacia, 157, 200, 201
Osteopath (D.O.), 142
Osteoporosis, 3, 77, 166, 167, 171, 197, 198–199, 201, 298
Osteosarcoma, 198, 200, 226
Other Practitioners—Chiropractors, Physical Therapists, and Other Practitioners, 135–137
Otitis externa, 219
Otorhinolaryngologist, 142
Otosclerosis, 219
Ova, 274

Ovaries, 274–276
Over-the-Counter Medication, Herbs, and Other Products, 19
Ovulation, 275
Oxalates, 198, 253

P

Pancreas, 96, 277–279
Pancreatitis, 279
Pantothenic acid, 165, 213, 232, 235, 239, 255, 270
Pap smears, 43, 103, 210, 211, 311
Pap Smears, 103–105
Parasites, 244, 247, 294
Parathyroid glands, 236
Parathyroid hormone (PTH), 236, 237
Parkinson's disease, 203–204, 205
Pediatrician, 142
Pellagra, 151
Pelvic exams, 42, 311
Penis, 280–281
Peppermint, 243, 293
Pepsin, 293
Periodontal disease, 198, 233, 239, 266, 279
Periodontist, 142
Peripartum cardiomyopathy, 233, 234
Peripheral artery disease, 215
Peripheral neuropathy, 159
Pernicious anemia, 195, 241, 285, 304
Personal Medical History, 12–13
Pertussis (whooping cough), 62, 63
Peyronie's disease, 280, 281
Phosphorus, 156, 157, 169, 197, 198, 200, 232, 236, 251, 268, 270, 297
Photoreceptors, 222
Physical Therapist, 142
Physician Assistant (P.A.), 142
Physicians—Family Practice, Obstetrics and Gynecology, and Specialists, 125–128
Phytates, 178, 184
Pick's disease, 205
Piercings, 257
Pituary gland, 235, 303
Plummer-Vinson syndrome, 221
Pneumococcal conjugate vaccine (Prevnar), 63, 202, 218
Pneumococcal polysaccharide vaccine, 64
Pneumonia, 64, 259, 261, 262
Polio vaccine. *See* IPV or OPV (polio) vaccine.
Polio. *See* Poliomyelitis.
Poliomyelitis, 62

Pollutants and toxins, 9, 223, 242
Polycystic ovary disease, 275, 276, 279
Polyphenols, 178, 208, 243, 277, 282
Polyps, 210, 243
    colon, 245–246, 247, 284
    colorectal, 285–286
Posture, 290, 292
Potassium, 168, 170, 171, 213, 268, 270
Poultry, 244, 294
Preeclampsia. *See* Toxemia (preeclampsia).
Pregnancy and Childbirth History, 21–22
Pregnancy, 9–10, 148, 154, 161, 163, 164, 167, 177, 178, 184, 191, 200, 204, 205, 207, 215–216, 234, 238, 242, 253, 255, 257, 266, 275, 298, 307, 311
Prenatal care, 9
Presbyopia, 223
Prescription Record, 15–18
Prevnar. *See* Pneumococcal conjugate vaccine (Prevnar).
Primary biliary cirrhosis, 257
Proctitis, 286
Progesterone, 274, 275
Prognathism, 298
Prolactin, 235
Prolactinoma, 235–236
Prostate, 282–283, 305
    exams, 42, 43, 100, 282, 283
Prostate Exams, 101–102, 282
Prostate-specific antigen (PSA), 43
    blood test, 100, 282
Prostatitis, 283, 307
Protein, animal, 198. *See also* Meat; Poultry.
Prunes, 213, 244, 293
Psoriasis, 249, 289
Psychiatrist, 142
Psychologist, 142
Pulmonary stenosis, 233
Pupil, 222
Pus, 238
Pyridoxine. *See* Vitamin B_6 (pyridoxine).

R

Raccoons, 202–203
Radiation, 189, 196, 200, 227, 295, 303, 304
Radiologist, 142
Radishes, 255
Recommended Adult Tests and Examinations for Men, 54–61, 282
Recommended Adult Tests and Examinations for Women, 46–53

Recommended dietary allowance (RDA), 144
Recommended Tests for Children, 44–45
Rectal exam, digital, 42, 100, 282, 283
Rectum, 284–286
Reflux, 220
Registered Nurse (R.N.), 142
Rehabilitative Therapist, 142
Reiter's syndrome, 226, 227, 281, 307
Relaxation, 202
Renal cell carcinoma. *See* Cancer, kidney.
Renal insufficiency, 156
Repetitive movements, 205, 229, 248, 270
Reproduction, 274–275
Retina, 222
Retinal detachment, 226
Retinitis pigmentosa, 159
Retinoblastoma, 226
Retinoic acid, 234
Retinol, 146
Reye's syndrome, 206, 258
Rh factor, 188, 191
Rheumatic fever, 232, 234, 301, 302
Rheumatologist, 142
Riboflavin. *See* Vitamin B_2 (riboflavin).
Rickets, 157, 169, 200, 201
Ringing in the ears. *See* Tinnitus.
Risk factors, 3, 185
Rodents, 255
Rods, 222
Rubella (German measles), 7, 206, 227, 234, 257
    vaccine, 62, 64, 202
Russell-Silver syndrome, 200

S

Saffron flower, 232
Saliva, 293, 297, 298
Salivary glands, 265
Salmonella, 244, 247, 293, 295
Salt. *See* Sodium.
Sanitary napkins, 305, 306
Sarcoidosis, 167, 225–226, 241, 256, 261, 262, 264, 289
Saunas, 10, 300
Scarlet fever, 232
Schizophrenia, 204, 205
Sclera, 222
Scleroderma, 253, 262
Sclerosing cholangitis, 256–257
Scoliosis, 291, 292
Scrotum, 299

Scurvy, 155
Seasonal affective disorder (SAD), 202
Secretors and nonsecretors, 188, 191, 242
Seizures, 205
Selective mutism, 205
Selenium, 158, 182, 239, 282, 284, 299, 303
Semen, 281
Seminal fluid, 282
Senility, 205
Sexual intercourse, 3, 6, 189, 211, 227, 242, 247, 255, 257, 280, 281, 283, 286, 300, 307, 311
    safe, 3, 6, 210, 242, 256, 280
Sexually transmitted diseases (STDs), 6, 42, 43, 211, 281, 300, 307, 311
    screening, 42
    See also Gonorrhea; Syphilis.
Shigella, 247, 295
Sickle-cell anemia, 156, 195, 226, 253
Sideroblastic anemia, 156
Sinusitis, 273
Sjögren's syndrome, 241, 304
Skeleton, 197
Skin, 238, 287–289
Sleep, 10, 231, 234, 238, 271
Sleepwalking, 205
Smallpox, 62
Smoking, 3, 5, 9, 148, 156, 189, 196, 201, 205, 211, 213, 216, 219, 221, 223, 231, 234, 242, 247, 253, 258, 259, 260, 261, 262, 266, 273, 279, 281, 286, 294, 298, 300, 302
Sneezing, 273
Snow shoveling, 234
Sodium, 170, 171–172, 175, 198, 213, 219, 232, 268, 270
Soy, 213
Speculum, 103
Sperm, 299, 300
Spermicides, 189, 307
SPF (sun protection factor), 287
Spina bifida, 291–292
Spinal cord, 290
Spine, 290–292
Spleen, 238, 263, 264
Squamous cell carcinoma, 288–289
Squamous cell vaginal carcinoma. *See* Cancer, vaginal.
STDs. *See* Sexually transmitted diseases (STDs).
Stein-Leventhal syndrome. *See* Polycystic ovary disease.
Sterilization, 288

Steroids, 158, 201, 256, 258
Stomach, 243, 293–295
    acid, 238
Stool guaiac test. *See* Fecal occult blood test.
Strabismus, 223
Strep throat, 232, 301, 302
Streptococcal pharyngitis. *See* Strep throat.
Streptococcus pneumoniae, 63, 64
Stress, 206, 211, 213, 216, 219, 231, 234, 236, 242, 247, 262, 271, 289, 295, 298, 304
Strokes, 200, 204, 205, 206, 234
Stuttering, 271
Sugars, 216, 223
Sunburns, 289
Sunglasses, 224, 226, 227
Sunlight, 5, 156, 197, 200, 201, 202, 223, 234, 238, 266, 287
Sunscreen, 287, 288
Surgeon, 142
Swabs, 217
Swimmer's ear. *See* Otitis externa.
Swimming, 217, 219, 226
Syndrome X, 234
Syphilis, 206, 211, 219, 253, 271
Systemic lupus erythematosus, 233, 240, 241, 262, 304
Systolic number, 43, 212

T

T scores, 77
Tampons, 211, 310
Tapeworms, 254–255, 294
Taste buds, 265
Tattoos, 257
Tea, 144, 149, 178, 297
    black, 198, 297
    green, 187, 198, 208, 213, 221, 232, 239, 243, 277, 282, 284, 293, 297
Tears, 238
Teeth, 10, 41, 42, 43, 87–88, 157, 166, 175, 198, 296–298. *See also* Dental checkups; Dental surgery; Periodontal disease.
Television, 203
Temperature, 43
Tendons, 248
Tennis elbow, 248
Testicles, 299–300
    protection of, 280, 299
Testicular self-exam (TSE), 41, 43, 100, 299
Testosterone, 201, 235, 236, 237, 299, 300

Tetanus, 63, 64
Tetanus-diphtheria booster, 64
Tetracycline, 311
Thalassemia, 156
Thiamine. *See* Vitamin B_1 (thiamine).
Throat, 301–302
    sore, 301
Thrombosis, 234, 251
Thymus gland, 238, 239, 263, 268
Thyroid, 176, 182, 234, 235, 250, 303–304
    hormone, 303
    screening, 43
Thyrotropic-stimulating hormone (TSH), 235
Tinnitus, 219
Tobacco, chewing, 221, 266, 298
Tocopherol. *See* Vitamin E (tocopherol).
Tongue, 265
Tonsils, 263, 301
Toothbrushes, 296–297
Toothpaste, 175, 296
Toxemia (preeclampsia), 215–216, 253
Toxins. *See* Pollutants and toxins.
Toxoplasmosis, 10, 226
Trace elements, 144
Trachoma, 227
Trachomatous, 227
Transfusions, 190, 239
Transient ischemic attack (TIA), 204–205
Trichomoniasis, 311
Tricuspid regurgitation, 233
Triglycerides, 79, 213, 232
Tuberculosis (TB), 42, 261
Typhoid fever, 247, 262, 295
Tyramine, 205

U

Ulcers, 170, 243, 244, 295
    duodenal, 246
    gastric, 295
    peptic, 295
Underwear, 306, 311
Ureters, 305
Urethra, 281, 305
Urethritis, 211, 307
Uric acid, 249
Urinalysis, 41, 42, 43
Urinary incontinence, 189
Urinary tract, 305–307
    infections (UTIs), 187, 188, 189, 305, 306–307
Urination, 10, 168, 187, 251, 280, 305, 306, 307

Urine, 187, 251, 252, 305
Urologist, 142
Uterus, 308–309

V

Vaccinations. *See* Immunizations.
Vagina, 310–311
Vaginitis, 311
Varicose veins, 216
Vegans. *See* Vegetarians.
Vegetables, 5, 147, 201, 220–221, 244, 255, 294, 297
    cruciferous, 282
Vegetarians, 145, 148, 154, 169, 178, 183
Veins, 212
Vertebrae, 290, 295
Vesicoureteral reflux, 188, 307
Video games, 203
Vinyl chloride, 203
Vision, peripheral, 222
Vitamin A, 146–148, 160, 187, 192, 198, 223, 239, 244, 259, 266, 287, 293, 297, 299, 301, 306, 309
Vitamin B_1 (thiamine), 144, 149, 232, 244, 267, 270, 293
Vitamin B_{12} (cobalamin), 144, 164, 164, 192, 193–194, 202, 213, 232, 270, 293
Vitamin B_{12} deficiency anemia, 193–194, 196
Vitamin B_2 (riboflavin), 150, 192, 223, 239, 255, 287
Vitamin B_3 (niacin), 144, 213, 232, 244, 266, 270, 287, 294
Vitamin B_5. *See* Pantothenic acid.
Vitamin B_6 (pyridoxine), 152–153, 192, 208, 213, 232, 239, 263, 270, 277, 287, 297
Vitamin B_9. *See* Folic acid (folate).
Vitamin C (ascorbic acid), 144, 173, 178, 179, 187, 192, 232, 239, 255, 259, 266, 270, 273, 287, 297, 301, 306
Vitamin D (calciferol), 156–158, 166, 197, 198, 200, 201, 239, 251, 267, 277, 287
Vitamin E (tocopherol), 144, 155, 160, 192, 239, 255, 259, 280, 282, 287
Vitamin H. *See* Biotin.
Vitamin K, 159, 160, 192, 198
Vitamins, 143, 144, 146–165, 196, 291
    deficiency, 145, 295, 298
    definitions, 145
    overdosing, 145
Vitiligo, 289
Vomiting, 221, 295
VZV: Varicella (chicken pox) vaccine, 63, 65

W

Water, 9, 187, 243, 251, 284, 306
    contaminated, 247, 256, 258
    treated with fluoride, 175
Wax, ear, 218
Weight, 5–6, 10, 41, 42, 201, 213, 231, 248, 270, 277, 278, 290, 295, 308. *See also* Obesity.
Whooping cough. *See* Pertussis (whooping cough).
Wilms' tumor, 253, 307
Wilson's disease, 174
Wine, 277
Women
    health, 148, 158, 164, 178, 179, 188
    postmenopausal, 158, 166, 167, 197, 198, 199, 279
Wood, pressure-treated, 187, 188
Workplace, 185, 244
Wrists, 229

X

Xerophthalmia, 147
X-rays, 10, 242

Y

Yeast infections, 311
Yogurt, 238

Z

Z scores, 77
Zinc, 147, 178, 183, 239, 244, 248, 266, 273, 277, 288, 294, 299, 301

About the Author

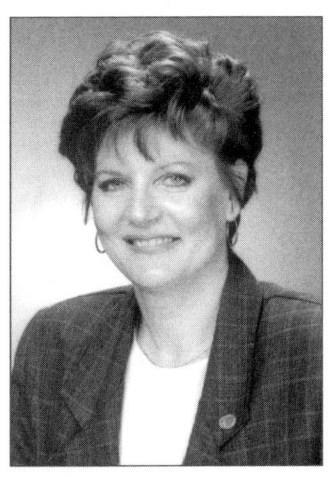

Kim Hendrickson Leffler was born and educated in Michigan. Throughout her career, she has held positions as a reporter for *The Detroit News*, public relations account supervisor for the J. Walter Thompson advertising agency, radio-television writer-producer for J. Walter Thompson and BBDO, Marketing Communications Coordinator for a division of 3M Company, Marketing and International Specialist for Data General Corporation, Consumer Products Marketing Manager for Aladan Corporation, Vice President of Marketing for the Greater Richmond Partnership, and Deputy Director of the Hanover County, Virginia, Department of Economic Development.

In her spare time, Kim is active in a number of community organizations. She lives with her family in Hanover County, Virginia.